FIRST AID FOR THE

PEDIATRICS clerkship

THE STUDENT TO STUDENT GUIDE

SERIES EDITORS:

LATHA G. STEAD, MD
Assistant Professor of Emergency Medicine
Mayo Clinic College of Medicine
Rochester, Minnesota

S. MATTHEW STEAD, MD, PhD
Fellow in Pediatric Neurology
Mayo Graduate School of Medicine
Rochester, Minnesota

MATTHEW S. KAUFMAN, MD
Resident in Internal Medicine
Long Island Jewish Medical Center
New Hyde Park, New York

TITLE EDITORS:

ELIZABETH N. JACOBSON
Class of 2004
Mayo Clinic College of Medicine
Rochester, Minnesota

MARYAM Y. NAIM, MD
Resident in Pediatrics
Mayo Graduate School of Medicine
Rochester, Minnesota

McGraw-Hill
Medical Publishing Division

New York   Chicago   San Francisco   Lisbon   London   Madrid
Mexico City   Milan   New Delhi   San Juan   Seoul
Singapore   Sydney   Toronto

First Aid for the Pediatrics Clerkship

1 2 3 4 5 6 7 8 9 0   QPD/QPD   0 9 8 7 6 5 4

ISBN 0-07-136424-2

Notice

Medicine is an ever-changing science. As new research and clinical experience broaden our knowledge, changes in treatment and drug therapy are required. The authors and the publisher of this work have checked with sources believed to be reliable in their efforts to provide information that is complete and generally in accord with the standards accepted at the time of publication. However, in view of the possibility of human error or changes in medical sciences, neither the authors nor the publisher nor any other party who has been involved in the preparation or publication of this work warrants that the information contained herein is in every respect accurate or complete, and they disclaim all responsibility for any errors or omissions or for the results obtained from use of the information contained in this work. Readers are encouraged to confirm the information contained herein with other sources. For example and in particular, readers are advised to check the product information sheet included in the package of each drug they plan to administer to be certain that the information contained in this work is accurate and that changes have not been made in the recommended dose or in the contraindications for administration. This recommendation is of particular importance in connection with new or infrequently used drugs.

This book was set in Goudy by Rainbow Graphics.
The editor was Catherine A. Johnson.
The production supervisor was Catherine H. Saggese.
Project management was provided by Rainbow Graphics.
The index was prepared by Angie Wiley Indexing Services.
Quebecor Dubuque was the printer and binder.
This book is printed on acid-free paper.

Cataloging-in-Publication Data is on file for this title at the Library of Congress.

Contributing Authors

NISHANT ANAND
Class of 2004, Mayo Clinic College of Medicine
Rochester, MN
Immunologic Disease

RACHEL ANDERSON, MD
Resident in Pediatrics
Houston, TX
Growth & Development

SANDHYA R. BEHERA, MBBS
Research Student
Dept. of Emergency Medicine, Mayo Clinic
Rochester, MN
Respiratory Tract Disease; Gastrointestinal Disease

JOHN BREINHOLT III, MD
Fellow in Pediatric Cardiology
Baylor College of Medicine
Houston, TX
Cardiovascular Disease

ALEX GONZALES, MD
Resident in Pediatrics
Houston, TX
Prevention, Health Supervision, & Child Abuse

FRANK ILLUZZI, MD
Attending Physician, Emergency Medicine
St. Vincent's Hospital
Bridgeport, CT
Pediatric Life Support

SERGEY KUNKOV, MD
Attending Physician, Pediatric Emergency Medicine
Jacobi Medical Center
Bronx, NY
*Gestation & Birth; Issues Unique to Newborns & Prematurity;
    Prevention, Health Supervision, & Child Abuse*

RON LIEBERMAN, MD
Attending Physician, Emergency Medicine
Encino, CA
Renal & Genitourinary Disease

MATTHEW JAMES LOE
Class of 2005, Mayo Clinic College of Medicine
Rochester, MN
Neurologic Disease

LYNDA MARTINS, DO
Resident in Emergency Medicine
Jacobi-Montefiore EM Residency
Bronx, NY
Special Organs: Eye, Ear, Nose

JAMES MELTZER, MD
Resident in Pediatrics
Montefiore Medical Center
Bronx, NY
Nutrition

BRIAN NOBIE, MD
Attending Physician, Emergency Medicine
Orlando, FL
Gastrointestinal Disease

TANIA PARSA, MD
Fellow in Pediatric Emergency Medicine
New Canaan, CT
Metabolic Disease; Psychiatric Disease

BENJAMIN PEAKE
Class of 2005, Mayo Clinic College of Medicine
Rochester, MN
Infectious Disease

JENNIFER SATO
Class of 2004, Mayo Clinic College of Medicine
Rochester, MN
Renal & Genitourinary Disease

MIA SVENSSON, MD
Resident in Pediatrics
Weill Medical College, Cornell University
New York, NY
Respiratory Tract Disease

CHITRA J. VARADACHARI, MD
Resident in Internal Medicine
Mayo Graduate School of Medicine
Rochester, MN
Cardiovascular Disease

MUHAMMAD WASEEM, MD
Asst. Professor of Pediatrics & Emergency Medicine
Weill Medical College, Cornell University
New York, NY
*Immunologic Disease; Hematologic Disease; Endocrine
    Disease; Musculoskeletal Disease/Orthopedics*

Faculty Reviewers

MARK S. MANNENBACH, MD
Division Head of Pediatric Emergency Medicine
Assistant Professor of Pediatric & Adolescent Medicine
Mayo Clinic
Rochester, MN

BRIAN R. MOORE, MD, FAAP
Pediatric Medical Director, Mayo Medical Transport
Senior Associate Consultant, Division of Pediatric
    Emergency Medicine
Instructor of Pediatric & Adolescent Medicine
Mayo Clinic
Rochester, MN

JULIA A. ROSEKRANS, MD, FAAP
Former Pediatrics Residency Director
Assistant Professor of Pediatrics & Adolescent
    Medicine
Mayo Clinic
Rochester, MN

GREGORY J. SCHEARS, MD
Assistant Professor of Anesthesiology and Pediatrics &
    Adolescent Medicine
Mayo Clinic
Rochester, MN

Contents

How to Succeed in the Pediatrics Clerkship

INTRODUCTION

This clinical study aid was designed in the tradition of the First Aid series of books. You will find that rather than simply preparing you for success on the clerkship exam, this resource will also help guide you in the clinical diagnosis and treatment of many of the problems seen by pediatricians. The content of the book is based on the objectives for medical students laid out by the Council on Medical Student Education in Pediatrics (COMSEP). Each of the chapters contains the major topics central to the practice of pediatrics and has been specifically designed for the third-year medical student learning level.

The content of the text is organized in the format similar to other texts in the First Aid series. Topics are listed by bold headings, and the "meat" of the topic provides essential information. The outside margins contain mnemonics, diagrams, summary or warning statements, and tips. Tips are categorized into typical scenarios **Typical Scenario**, exam tips 📝 , and ward tips 🩺 .

The pediatric clerkship is unique among all the medical school rotations. Even if you are sure you do not want to be a pediatrician, it can be a very fun and rewarding experience. There are three key components to the rotation: (1) what to do on the wards, (2) what to do on outpatient, and (3) how to study for the exam.

ON THE WARDS . . .

Be on time. Most ward teams begin rounding around 8 A.M. If you are expected to "pre-round," you should give yourself at least 15 minutes per patient that you are following to see the patient, look up any tests, and learn about the events that occurred overnight. Like all working professionals, you will face occasional obstacles to punctuality, but make sure this is occasional. When you first start a rotation, try to show up at least an extra 15 minutes early until you get the routine figured out. There will often be "table rounds" followed by walking rounds.

Find a way to keep your patient information organized and handy. By this rotation, you may have figured out the best way for you to track your patients, a miniature physical, medications, labs, test results, and daily progress. If not, ask around—other medical students or your interns can show you what works for them and may even make a copy for you of the template they use. We suggest index cards, a notebook, or a page-long template for each patient kept on a clipboard.

Dress in a professional manner. Even if the resident wears scrubs and the attending wears stiletto heels, you must dress in a professional, conservative manner. It would be appropriate to ask your resident what would be suitable for you to wear (it may not need to be a full suit and tie or the female equivalent). Wear a short white coat over your clothes unless discouraged.

> **Men** should wear long pants, with cuffs covering the ankle, a long-sleeved, collared shirt, and a tie—no jeans, no sneakers, no short-sleeved shirts.
> **Women** should wear long pants or a knee-length skirt and blouse or dressy sweater—no jeans, sneakers, heels greater than 1½ inches, or open-toed shoes.
> **Both men and women** may wear scrubs during overnight call. Do not make this your uniform.

Act in a pleasant manner. Inpatient rotations can be difficult, stressful, and tiring. Smooth out your experience by being nice to be around. Smile a lot and learn everyone's name. If you do not understand or disagree with a treatment plan or diagnosis, do not "challenge." Instead, say "I'm sorry, I don't quite understand, could you please explain . . ." Be empathetic toward patients.

Be aware of the hierarchy. The way in which this will affect you will vary from hospital to hospital and team to team, but it is always present to some degree. In general, address your questions regarding ward functioning to interns or residents. Address your medical questions to residents, your senior, or the attending. Make an effort to be somewhat informed on your subject prior to asking attendings medical questions.

Address patients and staff in a respectful way. Address your pediatric patients by first name. Address their parents as Sir, Ma'am, or Mr., Mrs., or Miss. Do not address parents as "honey," "sweetie," and the like. Although you may feel these names are friendly, parents will think you have forgotten their name, that you are being inappropriately familiar, or both. Address all physicians as "doctor" unless told otherwise. Nurses, technicians, and other staff are indispensable and can teach you a lot. Please treat them respectfully.

Take responsibility for your patients. Know everything there is to know about your patients—their history, test results, details about their medical problem, and prognosis. Keep your intern or resident informed of new developments that he or she might not be aware of, and ask for any updates of which you might not be aware. Assist the team in developing a plan, and speak to radiology, consultants, and family. Never give bad news to patients or family members without the assistance of your supervising resident or attending.

Respect patients' rights.
- All patients have the right to have their personal medical information kept private. This means do not discuss the patient's information with family members without that patient's consent, and do not discuss any patient in hallways, elevators, or cafeterias.
- All patients have the right to refuse treatment. This means they can refuse treatment by a specific individual (e.g., you, the medical student) or of a specific type (e.g., no nasogastric tube). Patients can even refuse lifesaving treatment. The only exceptions to this rule are patients who are deemed to not have the capacity to make decisions or understand situations, in which case a health care proxy should be sought, and patients who are suicidal or homicidal.
- All patients should be informed of the right to seek advanced directives on admission (particularly DNR/DNI orders). Often, this is done in a booklet by the admissions staff. If your patient is chronically ill or has a life-threatening illness, address the subject of advanced directives. The most effective way to handle this is to address this issue with every patient. This will help to avoid awkward conversations, even with less ill patients, because you can honestly tell them that you ask these questions of all your patients. These issues are particularly imminent with critically ill patients; however, the unexpected can happen with any patient.

Volunteer. Be self-propelled, self-motivated. Volunteer to help with a procedure or a difficult task. Volunteer to give a 20-minute talk on a topic of your choice. Volunteer to take additional patients. Volunteer to stay late. Bring in relevant articles regarding patients and their issues—this shows your enthusiasm, your curiosity, your outside reading, and your interest in evidence-based medicine.

Be a team player. Help other medical students with their tasks; teach them information you have learned. Support your supervising intern or resident whenever possible. Never steal the spotlight, steal a procedure, or make a fellow medical student or resident look bad.

Be prepared. Always have medical tools (stethoscope, reflex hammer, penlight, measuring tape), medical tape, pocket references, patient information, a small toy for distraction/gaze tracking, and stickers for rewards readily available. That way you will have what you need when you need it, and possibly more importantly, you will have what someone else needs when they are looking for it! The key is to have the necessary items with you without looking like you can barely haul around your heavy white coat.

Be honest. If you don't understand, don't know, or didn't do it, make sure you always say that. Never say or document information that is false (a common example: "bowel sounds normal" when you did not listen).

Present patient information in an organized manner. The presentation of a new patient will be much more thorough than the update given at rounds every morning. Vital information that should be included in a presentation differs by age group. Always begin with a succinct chief complaint—always a symptom, not a diagnosis (e.g., "wheezing," not "asthma")—and its duration. The next line should include identifiers (age, sex) and important diagnoses carried (e.g., this is where you could state "known asthmatic" or other important information in a wheezer).

Here is a template for the "bullet" presentation for inpatients the days subsequent to admission:

> This is a [age] year old [gender] with a history of [major/pertinent history such as asthma, prematurity, etc. or otherwise healthy] who presented on [date] with [major symptoms, such as cough, fever, and chills], and was found to have [working diagnosis]. [Tests done] showed [results]. Yesterday/overnight the patient [state important changes, new plan, new tests, new medications]. This morning the patient feels [state the patient's words], and the physical exam is significant for [state major findings]. Plan is [state plan].

Some patients have extensive histories. The whole history should be present in the admission note, but in a ward presentation it is often too much to absorb. In these cases it will be very much appreciated by your team if you can generate a good summary that maintains an accurate picture of the patient. This usually takes some thought, but it is worth it.

How to Present a Chest Radiograph (CXR)

Always take time to look at each of your patients' radiographs; don't just rely on the report. It is good clinical practice and your attending will likely ask you if you did. Plus, it will help you look like a star on rounds if you have seen the film before.

- First, confirm that the CXR belongs to your patient and is the most recent one.
- If possible, compare to a previous film.

Then, present in a systematic manner:
1. *Technique*
   Rotation, anteroposterior (AP) or posteroanterior (PA), penetration, inspiratory effort (number of ribs visible in lungfields).

(continued)

2. *Bony structures*
   Look for rib, clavicle, scapula, and sternum fractures.

3. *Airway*
   Look at the glottal area (steeple sign, thumbprint, foreign body, etc.), as well as for tracheal deviation, pneumothorax, pneumomediastinum.

4. *Pleural space*
   Look for fluid collections, which can represent hemothorax, chylothorax, pleural effusion.

5. *Lung parenchyma*
   Look for infiltrates and consolidations. These can represent pneumonia, pulmonary contusions, hematoma, or aspiration. The location of an infiltrate can provide a clue to the location of a pneumonia:

   - Obscured right (R) costophrenic angle = right lower lobe
   - Obscured left (L) costophrenic angle = left lower lobe
   - Obscured R heart border = right middle lobe
   - Obscured L heart border = left upper lobe

6. *Mediastinum*
   - Look at size of mediastinum—a widened one (> 8 cm) suggests aortic rupture.
   - Look for enlarged cardiac silhouette (> ½ thoracic width at base of heart), which may represent congestive heart failure (CHF), cardiomyopathy, hemopericardium, or pneumopericardium.

7. *Diaphragm*
   - Look for free air under the diaphragm (suggests perforation).
   - Look for stomach, bowel, or NG tube above diaphragm (suggests diaphragmatic rupture).

8. *Tubes and lines*
   - Identify all tubes and lines.
   - An endotracheal tube should be 2 cm above the carina. A common mistake is right mainstem bronchus intubation.
   - A chest tube (including the most proximal hole) should be in the pleural space (not in the lung parenchyma).
   - An NGT should be in the stomach and uncoiled.
   - The tip of a central venous catheter (central line) should be in the superior vena cava (not in the right atrium).
   - The tip of a Swan–Ganz catheter should be in the pulmonary artery.
   - The tip of a transvenous pacemaker should be in the right atrium.

A sample CXR presentation may sound like:

This is the CXR of [child's name]. The film is an AP view with good inspiratory effort. There is an isolated fracture of the 8th rib on the right. There is no tracheal deviation or mediastinal shift. There is no pneumo- or hemothorax. The cardiac silhouette appears to be of normal size. The diaphragm and heart borders on both sides are clear, no infiltrates are noted. There is a central venous catheter present, the tip of which is in the superior vena cava. This shows improvement over the CXR from [number of days ago] as the right lower lobe infiltrate is no longer present.

How to Present an Electrocardiogram (ECG)

See chapter on cardiovascular disease for specific rhythms.

- First, confirm that the ECG belongs to your patient and is most recent one.
- If possible, compare to a previous tracing. *(continued)*

Then, present in a systematic manner:

1. Rate (see Figure 1-1)
   "The rate is [number of] beats per minute."
   - The ECG paper is scored so that one big box is .20 seconds. These big boxes consist of five little boxes, each of which are 0.04 seconds.
   - A quick way to calculate rate when the rhythm is regular is the mantra: 300, 150, 100, 75, 60, 50 (= 300 / # large boxes), which is measured as the number of large boxes between two QRS complexes. Therefore, a distance of one large box between two adjacent QRS complexes would be a rate of 300, while a distance of five large boxes between two adjacent QRS complexes would be a rate of 60.
   - For irregular rhythms, count the number of complexes that occur in a 6-second interval (30 large boxes) and multiply by 10 to get a rate in bpm.

2. Rhythm
   "The rhythm is [sinus]/[atrial fibrillation]/[atrial flutter]"
   - If p waves are present in all leads, and upright in leads I & AVF, then the rhythm is sinus. Lack of p waves usually suggests an atrial rhythm. A ventricular rhythm (V Fib or V Tach) is an unstable one (could spell imminent death)—and you should be getting ready for advanced cardiac life support (ACLS).

3. Axis (see Figure 1-2 on page 8)
   "The axis is [normal]/[deviated to the right]/[deviated to the left]."
   - If I and aVF are both upright or positive, then the axis is normal.
   - If I is upright and aVF is upside down, then there is left axis deviation (LAD).
   - If I is upside down and aVF is upright, then there is right axis deviation (RAD).
   - If I and aVF are both upside down or negative, then there is extreme RAD.

4. Intervals (see Figure 1-3 on page 8)
   "The [PR]/[QRS] intervals are [normal]/[shortened]/[widened]."
   - Normal PR interval = .12–.20 seconds.
   - Short PR is associated with Wolff–Parkinson–White syndrome (WPW).
   - Long PR interval is associated with heart block of which there are three types:
     - First-degree block: PR interval > .20 seconds (one big box).
     - Second-degree (Wenckebach) block: PR interval lengthens progressively until a QRS is dropped.
     - Second-degree (Mobitz) block: PR interval is constant, but one QRS is dropped at a fixed interval.
     - Third-degree block: Complete AV dissociation, prolonged presence is incompatible with life.
   - Normal QRS interval ≤ .12 seconds.
   - Prolonged QRS is seen when the beat is initiated in the ventricle rather than the sinoatrial node, when there is a bundle branch block, and when the heart is artificially paced with longer QRS intervals. Prolonged QRS is also noted in tricyclic overdose and WPW.

5. Wave morphology (see Figure 1-4 on page 8)
   a. Ventricular hypertrophy
      - "There [is/is no] [left/right] [ventricular/atrial] hypertrophy."
   b. Atrial hypertrophy
      - Clue is presence of tall p waves.
   c. Ischemic changes
      - "There [are/are no] S-T wave [depressions/elevations] or [flattened/inverted] T waves." Presence of Q wave indicates an old infarct.
   d. Bundle branch block (BBB)
      - "There [is/is no] [left/right] bundle branch block."
      - Clues:
      - Presence of RSR' wave in leads V1–V3 with ST depression and T wave inversion goes with RBBB.
      - Presence of notched R wave in leads I, aVL, and V4–V6 goes with LBBB.

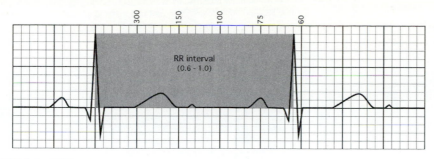

FIGURE 1-1. ECG rate.

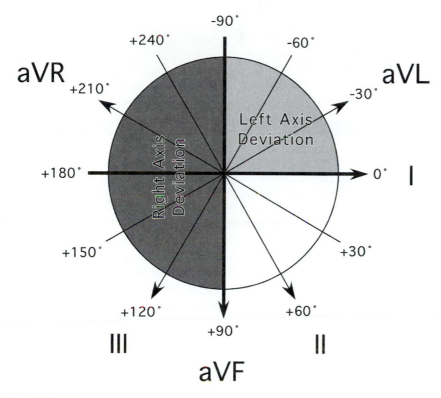

FIGURE 1-2. ECG axes.

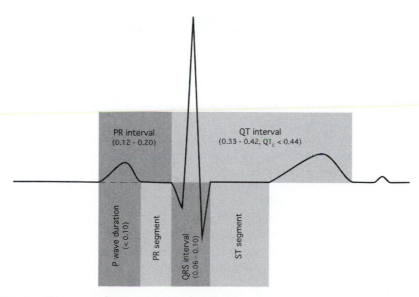

FIGURE 1-3. ECG segments.

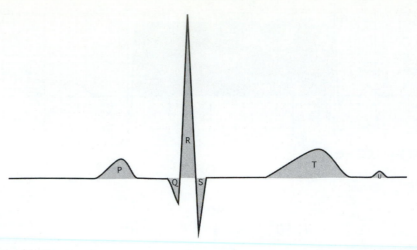

FIGURE 1-4. ECG waves.

ON OUTPATIENT

The ambulatory part of the pediatrics rotation consists of mainly two parts—focused histories and physicals for acute problems and well-child visits. In the general pediatrics clinic, you will see the common ailments of children, but don't overlook the possibilty of less common ones. Usually, you will see the patient first, to take the history and do the physical exam. It is important to strike a balance between obtaining a thorough exam and not upsetting the child so much that the attending won't be able to recheck any pertinent parts of it. For acute cases, present the patient distinctly, including an appropriate differential diagnosis and plan. In this section, be sure to include possible etiologies, such as specific bacteria, as well as a specific treatment (e.g., a particular antibiotic, dose, and course of treatment). For presentation of well-child visits, cover all the bases, but focus on the patients' concerns and your findings. There are specific issues to discuss depending on the age of the child. Past history and development is important, but so is anticipatory guidance–prevention and expectations for what is to come. The goal is to be both efficient and thorough.

YOUR ROTATION GRADE

Usually, the clerkship grade is broken down into three or four components:
- *Inpatient evaluation:* This includes evaluation of your ward time by residents and attendings and is based on your performance on the ward. Usually, this makes up about half your grade, and can be largely subjective.
- *Ambulatory evaluation:* This includes your performance in clinic, including clinic notes and any procedures performed in the outpatient setting.
- *National Board of Medical Examiners (NBME) examination:* This portion of the grade is anywhere from 20% to 50%, so performance on this multiple-choice test is vital to achieving honors in the clerkship.
- *Objective Structured Clinical Examination (OSCE):* Some schools now include an OCSE as part of their clerkship evaluation. This is basically an exam that involves standardized patients and allows assessment of a student's bedside manner and physical examination skills. This may com-

Pediatric History and Physical Exam

HISTORY
ID/CC: Age, sex, symptom, duration

HPI:
Symptoms—location, quality, quantity, aggravating and alleviating factors
Time course—onset, duration, frequency, change over time
Rx/Intervention—medications, medical help sought, other actions taken
Exposures, ill contacts, travel

Current Health:
Nutrition—breast milk/formula/food, quantity, frequency, supplements, problems (poor suck/swallow, reflux)
Sleep—quantity, quality, disturbances (snoring, apnea, bedwetting, restlessness), intervention, wakes up refreshed
Elimination—bowel movement frequency/quality, urination frequency, problems, toilet training
Behavior—toward family, friends, discipline
Development—gross motor, fine motor, language, cognition, social/emotional

PMH:
Pregnancy (be sensitive to adoption issues)—gravida/para status, maternal age, duration, exposures (medications, alcohol, tobacco, drugs, infections, radiation); complications (bleeding, gestational diabetes, hypertension, etc.), occurred on contraception?, planned?, emotions regarding pregnancy, problems with past pregnancies
Labor and delivery—length of labor, rupture of membranes, fetal movement, medications, presentation/delivery, mode of delivery, assistance (forceps, vacuum), complications, Apgars, immediate breathe/cry, oxygen requirement/intubation and duration
Neonatal—birth height/weight, abnormalities/injuries, length of hospital stay, complications (respiratory distress, cyanosis, anemia, jaundice, seizures, anomalies, infections), behavior, maternal concerns
Infancy—temperament, feeding, family reactions to infant
Illnesses/hospitalizations/surgeries/accidents/injuries—dates, medications/interventions, impact on child/family—don't forget circumcision
Medications—past (antibiotics, especially), present, reactions
Allergies—include reaction
Immunizations—up to date, reactions
Family history—relatives, ages, health problems, deaths (age/cause), miscarriages/stillbirths/deaths of infants or children
Social history—parents' education and occupation, living arrangements, pets, water (city or well), lead exposure (old house, paint), smoke exposure, religion, finances, family dynamics, risk-taking behaviors, school/daycare, other caregivers

ROS:
General—fever, activity, growth
Head—trauma, size, shape
Eyes—erythema, drainage, acuity, tearing, trauma
Ears—infection, drainage, hearing
Nose—drainage, congestion, sneezing, bleeding, frequent colds
Mouth—eruption/condition of teeth, lesions, infection, odor
Throat—sore, tonsils, recurrent strep pharyngitis
Neck—stiff, lumps, tenderness
Respiratory—cough, wheeze, chest pain, pneumonia, retractions, apnea, stridor
Cardiovascular—murmur, exercise intolerance, diaphoresis, syncope
Gastrointestinal—appetite, constipation, diarrhea, poor suck, swallow, abdominal pain, jaundice, vomiting, change in bowel movements, blood, food intolerances
GU—urine output, stream, urgency, frequency, discharge, blood, fussy during menstruation, sexually active
Endocrine—polyuria/polydipsia/polyphagia, puberty, thyroid, growth/stature
Musculoskeletal—pain, swelling, redness, warmth, movement, trauma
Neurologic—headache, dizziness, convulsions, visual changes, loss of consciousness, gait, coordination, handedness
Skin—bruises, rash, itching, hair loss, color (cyanosis)
Lymph—swelling, redness, tender glands

(continued)

PHYSICAL EXAM

General—smiling, playful, cooperative, irritable, lethargic, tired, hydration status
Vitals—temperature, heart rate, respiratory rate, blood pressure
Growth—weight, height, head circumference and percentiles, BMI if applicable
Skin—inspect, palpate, birthmarks, rash, jaundice, cyanosis
Hair—whorl, lanugo, Tanner stage
Head—anterior fontanelle, sutures
Eyes—redness, swelling, discharge, red reflex, strabismus, scleral icterus
Ears—tympanic membranes (DO LAST!)
Nose—patent nares, flaring nostrils
Mouth—teeth, palate, thrush
Throat—oropharynx (red, moist, injection, exudate)
Neck—range of motion, meningeal signs
Lymph—cervical, axillary, inguinal
Cardiovascular—heart rate, murmur, rub, pulses (central/peripheral; bilateral upper and lower extremities including femoral), perfusion/color
Respiratory—rate, retractions, grunting, crackles, wheezes
Abdomen—bowel sounds, distention, tenderness, hepatosplenomegaly, masses, umbilicus, rectal
Back—scoliosis, dimples
Musculoskeletal—joints—erythema, warmth, swelling tenderness, range of motion
Neurologic—gait, symmetric extremity movement, strength/tone/bulk, reflexes (age-appropriate and deep tendon reflexes), mentation, coordination
Genitalia—circumcision, testes, labia, hymen, Tanner staging

prise up to one fourth of a student's grade. It is a tool that will probably become increasingly popular over the next few years. It is not a frequent part of the pediatrics rotation at this point in time, though some assessment of clinical thinking or skills is likely to occur.

HOW TO STUDY

Make a list of core material to learn. This list should reflect common symptoms, illnesses, and areas in which you have particular interest or in which you feel particularly weak. Do not try to learn every possible topic.

Symptoms
- Fever
- Failure to thrive
- Sore throat
- Wheezing
- Vomiting
- Diarrhea
- Abdominal pain
- Jaundice
- Fluid and electrolyte imbalance
- Seizures

The knowledge you need on the wards is the day-to-day management know-how (though just about anything is game for pimping!). The knowledge you want by the end-of-rotation examination is the epidemiology, risk factors, pathophysiology, diagnosis, and treatment of major diseases seen in pediatrics.

As you see patients, note their major symptoms and diagnosis for review. Your reading on the symptom-based topics above should be done with a specific patient in mind. For example, if a patient comes in with diarrhea, read about common infectious causes of gastroenteritis and the differences between and complications of them, noninfectious causes, and dehydration in the review book that night.

Select your study material. We recommend:

- This review book, *First Aid for Pediatrics*
- A major pediatric textbook—*Nelson's Textbook of Pediatrics* (also available on MD Consult) and its very good counterpart, *Nelson's Essentials*
- *The Harriet Lane Handbook*—the bible of pediatrics: medicine, medications, and lab values as they apply to children
- A full-text online journal database, such as *www.mdconsult.com* (subscription is $99/year for students)

Prepare a talk on a topic. You may be asked to give a small talk once or twice during your rotation. If not, you should volunteer! Feel free to choose a topic that is on your list; however, realize that the people who hear the lecture may consider this dull. The ideal topic is slightly uncommon but not rare, for example, Kawasaki disease. To prepare a talk on a topic, read about it in a major textbook and a review article not more than 2 years old. Then search online or in the library for recent developments or changes in treatment.

Procedures. You may have the opportunity to perform a couple of procedures on your pediatrics rotation. Be sure to volunteer to do them whenever you can, and at least actively observe if participation is not allowed. These may include:

- Lumbar puncture
- Intravenous line placement
- Nasogastric tube placement
- Venipuncture (blood draw)
- Pulling central (and other) lines
- Foley (urinary) catheter placement
- Ankle–brachial index (ABI) measurement
- Transillumination of scrotum

HOW TO PREPARE FOR THE CLINICAL CLERKSHIP EXAMINATION

If you have read about your core illnesses and core symptoms, you will know a great deal about pediatrics. It is difficult but vital to balance reading about your specific patients and covering all of the core topics of pediatrics. To study for the clerkship exam, we recommend:

2–3 weeks before exam: Read this entire review book, taking notes.
10 days before exam: Read the notes you took during the rotation on your core content list, and the corresponding review book sections.
5 days before exam: Read the entire review book, concentrating on lists and mnemonics.
2 days before exam: Exercise, eat well, skim the book, and go to bed early.
1 day before exam: Exercise, eat well, review your notes and the mnemonics, and go to bed on time. Do not have any caffeine after 2 P.M.

Other helpful studying strategies include:

Study with friends. Group studying can be very helpful. Other people may point out areas that you have not studied enough and may help you focus on the goal. If you tend to get distracted by other people in the room, limit this to less than half of your study time.

Study in a bright room. Find the room in your house or in your library that has the best, brightest light. This will help prevent you from falling asleep. If you don't have a bright light, get a halogen desk lamp or a light that simulates sunlight (not a tanning lamp).

Eat light, balanced meals. Make sure your meals are balanced, with lean protein, fruits and vegetables, and fiber. A high-sugar, high-carbohydrate meal will give you an initial burst of energy for 1 to 2 hours, but then you'll drop.

Take practice exams. The point of practice exams is not so much the content that is contained in the questions, but the training of sitting still for 3 hours and trying to pick the best answer for each and every question.

Tips for answering questions. All questions are intended to have one best answer. When answering questions, follow these guidelines:

> **Read the answers first.** For all questions longer than two sentences, reading the answers first can help you sift through the question for the key information.
> **Look for the words "EXCEPT, MOST, LEAST, NOT, BEST, WORST, TRUE, FALSE, CORRECT, INCORRECT, ALWAYS and NEVER."** If you find one of these words, circle or underline it for later comparison with the answer.

Finally, remember—children are not just small adults. They present with a whole new set of medical and social issues. More than ever, you are treating families, not just individual patients.

High-Yield Facts

Gestation and Birth

EMBRYOLOGY

Gestational/Embryologic Landmarks
See Table 2-1.

Germ Layers
See Table 2-2.

Heart
- Week 3:
  - Paired heart tubes begin to work.
- Week 4:
  - Primordial atrium is divided into left and right by septa primum and secundum.

The main source of energy for a growing fetus is carbohydrates.

VSD is the most common congenital heart defect.

TABLE 2-1. Gestational/embryologic landmarks.	
Week 1	Fertilization, usually in fallopian tube ampulla Implantation begins
Week 2	Implantation complete Endoderm and ectoderm form (bilaminar embryo)
Week 3	Mesoderm formed (trilaminar embryo)
Week 5	Subdivisions of forebrain, midbrain, and hindbrain are formed
Week 7	Heart formed
Week 8	Primary organogenesis complete Placentation occurs
Week 9	Permanent kidneys begin functioning
Week 10	Midgut returns from umbilical cord, where it was developing, to abdominal cavity, while undergoing counterclockwise rotation
Week 24	Primitive alveoli are formed and surfactant production begins
Week 26	Testicles descend

TABLE 2-2. Summary of germ layer derivatives.

Ectoderm	Neural Crest Cells (Ectoderm)	Mesoderm	Endoderm
▪ CNS, peripheral nervous system (PNS) ▪ Sensory epithelia of eye, ear, nose ▪ Epidermis, hair, nails ▪ Mammary glands, pituitary gland, subcutaneous glands ▪ Tooth enamel	▪ Spinal nerves; cranial nerves V, VII, IX, X; sensory neurons ▪ Autonomic ganglia ▪ Adrenal medulla ▪ Meninges ▪ Pigment cells, glial cells of peripheral nerves	▪ Connective tissue, cartilage, bone ▪ Striated and smooth muscle ▪ Blood and lymphatic systems ▪ Ovaries, testes, genital ducts ▪ Serous membranes lining body cavities ▪ Spleen, adrenal cortex	▪ Epithelial lining of gastrointestinal tract, respiratory tract, and middle ear, including eustachian tube ▪ Tonsil parenchyma ▪ Thymus ▪ Parathyroid and thyroid glands ▪ Liver, pancreas

- Septum primum forms the valve of the foramen ovale, which closes about 3 months after birth.
- Failure of the foramen ovale to close results in an **atrial septal defect (ASD).**
  - Week 7:
    - The single ventricle is divided into left and right; prior to that the interventricular foramen communicates between left and right sides.
    - Failure of the interventricular foramen to close results in a **ventricular septal defect (VSD).**

Circulation

- See Figure 2-1.
- Well-oxygenated blood returns from placenta through umbilical vein, where half of it enters the inferior vena cava through the ductus venosus (continuation of the umbilical vein beyond the branching of the left and right portal veins), and the rest enters the hepatic circulation (preferentially through the left portal vein).
- Despite the fact that the umbilical venous blood joins the inferior vena cava prior to entering the right atrium, the streams do not mix substantially. Blood from the umbilical artery is preferentially shunted through the foramen ovale to the left atrium, while blood from the lower inferior vena cava, right hepatic circulation, and superior vena cava enters the right ventricle.
- The major portion of blood exiting the right ventricle is then shunted to the aorta through the ductus arteriosus because the lungs are collapsed and pulmonary artery pressures are high.
- Sixty-five percent of blood in the descending aorta returns to the umbilical arteries for reoxygenation at the placenta; the remainder supplies the inferior part of the body.
- After birth, pulmonary artery pressure drops because the lungs expand, reducing flow across the ductus arteriosus and stimulating its closure (usually within first few days of life).
- Pressure in the left atrium becomes higher than that in the right atrium after birth due to the increased pulmonary return, which stimulates closure of the foramen ovale (usually complete by third month of life). (See Figure 2-2.)

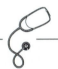

Upper portion of fetal body is perfused much better than lower because of the way fetal circulation functions.

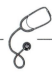

Closure of the ductus arteriosus can be aborted by prostaglandin E$_1$ and facilitated by indomethacin (via inhibition of prostaglandin synthesis).

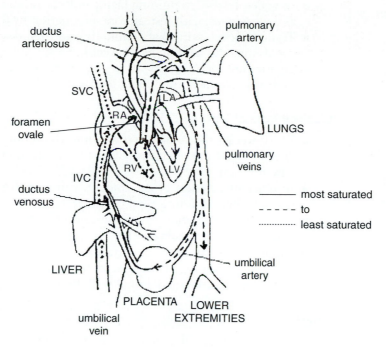

TO BRAIN, HEART
UPPER EXTREMITIES

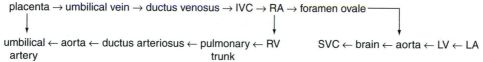

placenta → umbilical vein → ductus venosus → IVC → RA → foramen ovale

umbilical ← aorta ← ductus arteriosus ← pulmonary ← RV   SVC ← brain ← aorta ← LV ← LA
artery   trunk

FIGURE 2-1. Fetal circulation. (Artwork by Elizabeth N. Jacobson.)

Hemoglobin

Fetal erythropoiesis occurs in the yolk sac (3–8 weeks), liver (6–8 weeks), spleen (9–28 weeks), and then bone marrow (28 weeks onward).

Genitourinary Tract

- Metanephri (permanent kidneys) start functioning at 9 weeks; urine is excreted into amniotic cavity.
- Initially, kidneys lie in the pelvis; by 8 weeks they migrate into their adult position.

Failure of kidneys to develop can lead to **oligohydramnios** (decreased fluid in the amniotic cavity).

Failure of kidneys to migrate can lead to ectopic kidneys.

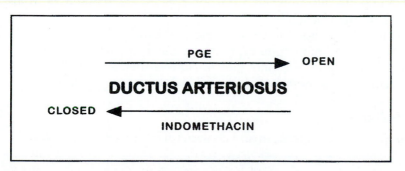

FIGURE 2-2. Mechanism of ductus arteriosus patency/closure.

A horseshoe kidney gets caught on the inferior mesenteric artery (IMA) during ascent.

Failure of testicle(s) to descend, cryptorchidism, may need to be corrected surgically to prevent progressive dysplasia and may affect fertility.

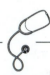

Infants born prior to 30 weeks are given exogenous surfactant to prevent respiratory distress syndrome (RDS). Mom is given steroids.

Lecithin to sphingomyelin ratio in the amniotic fluid greater than 3 indicates fetal lung maturity.

Folic acid supplements during pregnancy reduce incidence of neural tube defects.

- Morphologic sexual characteristics do not develop until 7 weeks' gestation.
- In males, testis-determining factor induces primary sex cords to develop as male gonads, with testosterone production by 8 weeks.
- Testicles develop intra-abdominally and then descend through inguinal canals into the scrotum by 26 weeks.
- Ovaries are identified by 10 weeks; primary sex cords develop into female gonads with primordial follicles developing prenatally.

Gastrointestinal Tract

- By 10 weeks, the midgut returns from the umbilical cord, where it was developing, to the abdominal cavity, while undergoing counterclockwise rotation.
- Insufficient rotation of the midgut, called **malrotation,** can present in neonatal period as intestinal obstruction.
- Incomplete separation of foregut and primitive airway can lead to **tracheoesophageal fistula (TEF).**
- Failure of the intestine to return to the abdominal cavity with intestinal contents remaining at the base of the umbilical cord causes **gastroschisis,** a full-thickness abdominal wall defect with extruded intestine.

Lungs

By 24 weeks, primitive alveoli are formed and surfactant production is begun.

Central Nervous System (CNS)

- During week 3, the neural tube is formed on the ectodermal surface.
- Neural tube openings (rostral and caudal) are closed by 25 to 27 days.
- By week 5, subdivisions of forebrain, midbrain, and hindbrain are formed.
- Failure of neural tube to close completely can result in **spina bifida** (unfused vertebral arch with or without unfused dura mater and spinal cord), commonly seen in the lumbar area.

PLACENTA

Development

- Fetal portion of placenta is formed from chorionic sac.
- Maternal portion is derived from endometrium.

Transport

- Nutrients, electrolytes, water, and gases are diffused or transported across the placenta.
- Most drugs pass through placenta and can be detected in fetal plasma (e.g., warfarin, morphine, propylthiouracil, and drugs of abuse).
- A few substances cannot pass because of their size or charge (e.g., heparin); protein hormones (e.g., insulin) do not cross placenta.

Metabolism

Placenta synthesizes glycogen and cholesterol.

Endocrine Function

Placenta produces β-human chorionic gonadotropin (β-hCG), human chorionic adrenocorticotropic hormone (ACTH), human placental lactogen, and human chorionic somatomammotropin.

PRENATAL DISTURBANCES

Infections

Infants who have experienced an intrauterine infection have a higher-than-average incidence of being small for gestational age, hepatosplenomegaly, congenital defects, microcephaly, and intracranial calcifications.

TOXOPLASMOSIS

- Maternal infection is due to ingestion of oocysts from feces of infected cats and is asymptomatic.
- Clinical features in infants include microcephaly, hydrocephalus, intracranial calcifications, choreoretinitis, and seizures.

RUBELLA

- Congenital rubella syndrome is rare due to the effectiveness of the rubella vaccine.
- Maternal infection early in pregnancy can result in congenital rubella syndrome, which includes meningoencephalitis, microcephaly, cataracts, sensorineural hearing loss, and congenital heart disease (patent ductus arteriosus and pulmonary artery stenosis).

CYTOMEGALOVIRUS (CMV)

- Common—occurs in 1% of newborns.
- Newborn disease is associated with primary maternal infection with a 50% chance of infection.
- In those affected, only 5% have neurologic deficits.
- Infection occurs in 1% of pregnancies with recurrent or reactivated infection.
- CMV transmitted intrapartum, through infected blood or through breast milk, is not associated with neurologic deficits.
- Clinical features include intrauterine growth retardation (IUGR), low birth weight, petechiae and purpura, jaundice and hepatosplenomegaly, microcephaly, chorioretinitis, and intracranial calcifications.
- Late manifestations like learning and hearing deficits can occur in 10% of clinically inapparent infections.

Toxins and Teratogens

ALCOHOL

- Most common teratogen.
- The amount of alcohol consumed correlates with the severity of spectrum of effects in the neonate, ranging from mild reduction in cerebral function to classic fetal alcohol syndrome (see Figure 2-3).
- Clinical manifestations include microcephaly and mental retardation, IUGR, facial dysmorphism (midfacial hypoplasia, micrognathia, shortened nasal philtrum, short palpebral fissures, and a thin vermillion border), renal and cardiac defects, and hypospadias.

Maternal α-fetoprotein (AFP) is *high* in:
- Multiple gestations (most common)
- Fetal neural tube defects
- Gastroschisis

Maternal AFP is *low* in trisomies 21 (Down's) and 18.

Incorrect dates is the most common cause for abnormal AFP.

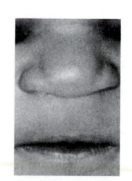

FIGURE 2-3. Fetal Alcohol Syndrome. Notice the depressed nasal bridge, flat philtrum, long upper lip, and thin vermillion border. (Reproduced, with permission, from Stoler JM, Holmes LB. Underrecognition of prenatal alcohol effects in infants of known alcohol abusing women. *The Journal of Pediatrics* 135(4): 430–436, 1999.)

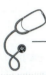

Testing urine for β-hCG allows early detection of pregnancy.

Prenatal infections that most commonly cause birth defects:

TORCH

Toxoplasmosis
Other (hepatitis B, syphilis, varicella-zoster virus)
Rubella
Cytomegalovirus
Herpes simplex virus/human immunodeficiency virus (HSV/HIV)
See Figure 2-4.

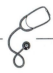

Among women infected with toxoplasmosis, only 50% will give birth to an infected neonate.

COCAINE

- Causes maternal hypertension and constriction of placental circulation leading to decreased uterine blood flow and fetal hypoxia.
- Associated with a higher risk of spontaneous abortion, placental abruption, fetal distress, meconium staining, preterm birth, IUGR, and low Apgar scores at birth.
- Associated with intracranial hemorrhage and necrotizing enterocolitis; cardiac, skull, and genitourinary malformations; and increased incidence of sudden infant death syndrome (SIDS).
- Cocaine withdrawal in an infant causes irritability, increased tremulousness, and poor feeding, as well as increased incidence of learning difficulties and attention and concentration deficits later on.

NARCOTICS

Heroin and methadone are associated with IUGR, SIDS, and infant narcotic withdrawal syndrome.

TOBACCO

Smoking is associated with decreased birth weight.

PHENYTOIN

Phenytoin is associated with fetal hydantoin syndrome, which includes IUGR, mental retardation, dysmorphic facies, and hypoplasia of nails and distal phalanges.

TETRACYCLINE

Tetracycline causes tooth discoloration and inhibits bone formation.

ISOTRETINOIN (ACCUTANE)

Accutane is associated with hydrocephalus, microtia, micrognathia, and aortic arch abnormalities.

WARFARIN

Warfarin causes abnormal cartilage development, mental retardation, deafness, and blindness.

MATERNAL CONDITIONS

Diabetes

- Associated with macrosomia (weight > 4 kg), which can lead to birth-related injury.
- Fetal complications are related to degree of control of maternal diabetes.
- Other fetal/neonatal complications include metabolic disorders (hypoglycemia, hypocalcemia, and hypomagnesemia), perinatal asphyxia, respiratory distress syndrome, hyperbilirubinemia, polycythemia and hyperviscosity, and congenital malformations including cardiac, renal, gastrointestinal, neurologic, and skeletal defects.

Others

- Hypertension and renal and cardiac disease are associated with small-for-gestational-age babies and prematurity.
- Maternal lupus is related to first-degree atrioventricular (AV) block in affected infants.

Delivery Room Care

- Once the head is delivered, the nose and mouth are suctioned.
- Once the whole body is delivered, the newborn is held at the level of the table and the umbilical cord is clamped.
- Newborn is then placed under radiant warmer and is dried with warm towels.
- Mouth and nose are gently suctioned.
- Gentle rubbing of the back or flicking of the soles of the feet, if needed to stimulate breathing.

Apgar Scoring

- Practical method of assessing newborn infants immediately after birth to help identify those requiring resuscitation on a scale of 0 to 10.
- Assessment at 1 and 5 minutes; further assessments at 10 and 15 minutes may indicate success of resuscitation (see Table 2-3).
- Does not predict neonatal mortality or subsequent cerebral palsy.

Prophylaxis

- Gonococcal and chlamydial eye infection prophylaxis is with 1% silver nitrate drops and erythromycin or tetracycline ointment.
- Vitamin K is given intramuscularly (IM) to prevent hemorrhagic disease of the newborn.

Cord Blood/Stem Cells

- Can be used to test for infants' blood type
- Rich in stem cells, which are pleuripotential cells that have potential use in malignancies and gene therapy

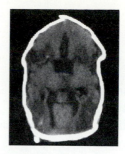

FIGURE 2-4. Head CT consistent with TORCH infection—marked ventricular dilation, extensive encephalomalacia involving both cerebral hemispheres, absent corpus callosum, periventricular calcifications, skull deformity with overriding sutures.

Pregnant women should not change a cat's litter box, due to risk of toxoplasmosis.

HIGH-YIELD FACTS

Gestation and Birth

General Appearance

Plethora (high hematocrit secondary to chronic fetal hypoxia), jaundice, sepsis and TORCH infections, cyanosis (with congenital heart and lung disease), pallor (anemia, shock, patent ductus arteriosus).

TABLE 2-3. Apgar scoring.

	Activity (Muscle Tone)	Pulse	Grimace (Reflex Irritability)	Appearance (Skin Color)	Respiration
0	Absent	Absent	No response	Blue-gray, pale all over	Absent
1	Arms and legs flexed	Below 100 bpm	Grimace	Normal, except for extremities	Slow, irregular
2	Active movement	Above 100 bpm	Sneeze, cough, pull away	Normal all over	Good crying

Total out of 10: 7–10 normal newborn; 4–7 may require some resuscitative measures; ≤ 3 require immediate resuscitation.

Incidence of fetal alcohol syndrome is higher in the Native American population because of the higher incidence of alcoholism.

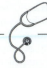

Cocaine use is associated with placental abruption.

Typical Scenario

Term, 5-lb., 2-day-old infant has irritability, nasal stuffiness, and coarse tremors. He feeds poorly and has diarrhea. *Think:* Cocaine or heroin withdrawal.

Infants of narcotic-abusing mothers should never be given naloxone in the delivery room because it may precipitate seizures.

Elevation of maternal glucose causes elevated fetal glucose leading to fetal hyperinsulinism, this can lead to hypoglycemia in the newborn.

Skin

- Erythema toxicum is a pustular rash distributed over the trunk, face, and extremities, which resolves over a week.
- Mongolian spots are bluish spots present over the buttocks and back that are seen in infants of African, Asian, and Native American descent that tend to fade over a year.
- Capillary hemangiomas ("stork bites") are pink spots over the eyelids, forehead, and back of the neck that tend to fade with time.
- See chapter on dermatology.

Head

- Anterior fontanelle closes at 9 to 12 months.
- Large fontanelle is seen in hypothyroidism, osteogenesis imperfecta, and some chromosomal abnormalities.

Face

- Mouth—look for cleft lip/palate and macroglossia (large tongue is seen with hypothyroidism, Down's, and Beckwith–Wiedemann syndrome).
- Look for dysmorphic features, including micrognathia, bossing of the forehead, hypertelorism (widely spaced eyes), and low-set ears (Down's) (see chapter on congenital malformations and chromosomal abnormalities).

Eyes

- Check for red reflex with ophthalmoscope.
- Look for cataracts, Brushfield spots (salt-and-pepper speckling of the iris seen in Down's syndrome), leukocoria (white pupil) with retinoblastoma (rare), and subconjunctival hemorrhage, which can occur after a traumatic delivery.
- See chapter on special organs.

Neck

Inspect for thyroid enlargement and palpate along the sternocleidomastoid for hematoma.

Chest

- Symmetry/equality of breath sounds.
- Retractions and grunting may signify respiratory distress (nasal flaring, intercostal retractions, use of accessory muscles).
- Breasts may be enlarged from the effects of maternal estrogens.

Cardiovascular

- Heart rate rhythm, quality of heart sounds, and the presence of a murmur.
- Check pulses.

Abdomen

- Palpate for masses.
- Examine umbilicus for omphalocele and gastroschesis.
- Inspect the umbilical cord for single umbilical artery (normally two); if present, may indicate congenital anomalies.

Extremities

- Ensure that clavicles are intact.
- Primitive reflexes (see chapter on growth and development).

Back

Look for dimples or tufts of hair that may indicate spina bifida.

Genitalia

- Girls may have vaginal bleeding and swollen labia secondary to withdrawal of maternal estrogens.
- In boys, palpate for the presence of testicles in scrotum and look for hypo- or epispadias (urethral opening proximal to normal position either on the dorsal or ventral surface).

SMALL OR LARGE FOR GESTATIONAL AGE

Small for Gestational Age (SGA)

- Birth weight less than the tenth percentile for gestational age.
- There are two broad categories, early and late onset.
- Early onset:
  - Insult that begins before 28 weeks' gestational age.
  - Head circumference and height are proportionally small-sized (symmetric).
  - Seen in infants born to mothers with severe vascular disease with hypertension, renal diseases, congenital anomalies, infections, and chromosomal abnormalities.
- Late onset or asymmetric IUGR.
  - Occurs with an insult after 28 weeks' gestational age.
  - Sparing of the head circumference.
  - Can occur with multiple gestation and preeclampsia.

LARGE FOR GESTATIONAL AGE (LGA)

- Birth weight greater than the 90th percentile for gestational age.
- Those at risk are infants of diabetic mothers, postmature infants, and those with Beckwith–Wiedemann syndrome.
- Most LGA infants have large parents and are constitutionally large.
- Macrosomic infants are those with a birth weight > 4 kg.

BIRTH TRAUMA

Clavicular Fracture

- Most common bone fracture during delivery.
- Complete fracture symptoms involve decreased or absent movement, gross deformity of clavicle, tenderness on palpation, and localized crepitus.
- Greenstick (partial) fractures have no symptoms and the diagnosis is made at 7 to 10 days because of callus formation.

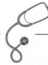

Acrocyanosis (blue hands and feet only) can be normal in a newborn.

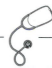

A bulging fontanelle is seen with increased intracranial pressure, hydrocephalus, and meningitis.

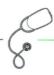

Papilledema does not occur in infants with open cranial sutures.

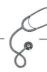

Absent breath sounds may signify a tension pneumothorax or atelectasis; bowel sounds in the thorax may indicate congenital diaphragmatic hernia.

Diminished femoral pulses are seen in coarctation of the aorta.

HIGH-YIELD FACTS

Gestation and Birth

The most common cause of an abdominal mass in a newborn is an enlarged kidney.

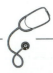

Circumcision should be avoided in boys with hypo- or epispadias as foreskin can be used to repair these defects later on.

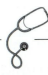

All macrosomic infants should be examined for signs of birth trauma and checked for hypoglycemia.

Complete clavicular fractures will lead to absence of Moro's reflex.

Caput Succedaneum

- Area of edema over the presenting portion of the scalp during a vertex delivery.
- Associated with bruising and petechiae.

Cephalohematoma

- Caused by bleeding that occurs below the periosteum of the overlying bone (usually the parietal).
- Associated with skull fractures in 5–10%, most often linear.

Skull Fracture/Epidural Hematoma

- Skull fractures are uncommon; most are linear and associated with cephalohematoma. Depressed fractures are often visible and may require surgery.
- Epidural hematomas are rare and may require prompt surgical evacuation.

Molding

- Temporary asymmetry of the skull from the overlapping of bones that occurs following prolonged labor and vaginal deliveries.
- Normal head shape is regained within a week.

Klumpke's Palsy

- Involves the lower arm and affects the seventh and eighth cervical and first thoracic nerve roots. The hand is paralyzed and has an absent grasp reflex, causing a "claw hand" deformity.
- It is rare to have an isolated Klumpke's palsy.
- Is often accompanied by Horner's syndrome.

Erb's Palsy

- Erb–Duchenne involves the upper arm and is the most common type.
- Involves the fifth and sixth cervical roots, and the arm is adducted and internally rotated, but the grasp reflex is intact (see Figure 2-5).

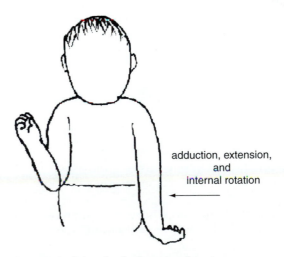

adduction, extension, and internal rotation

FIGURE 2-5. Erb's palsy. (Artwork by Elizabeth N. Jacobson)

Risk Factors

- Rupture of amniotic membranes for 18 hours or more
- Choreoamnionitis
- Intrapartum maternal fever
- Maternal group B streptococcus colonization
- Prematurity

Group B Streptococcus (GBS)

- Major cause of severe systemic infection in neonates.
- Vertical transmission most important route of transmission.
- Two patterns of disease:
  - Early-onset disease:
    - Presents shortly after birth with a sepsis-like clinical picture (respiratory distress, apnea, cyanosis, and hypotension).
  - Late-onset disease:
    - Occurs after the first week of life and manifests as meningitis in the majority of patients with bulging fontanelle, lethargy, irritability, vomiting, and seizures.
- Diagnosis is confirmed by GBS isolation from sterile body fluid (blood, cerebrospinal fluid).
- Treatment is with penicillin G.

Escherichia coli

- Principal cause of gram-negative sepsis and meningitis in newborn.
- Commonly colonize genitourinary (GU) and gastrointestinal (GI) tracts.
- Risk factors include maternal urinary tract infection (UTI) during last month of pregnancy in addition to previously mentioned risk factors.
- Clinical manifestations include sepsis, meningitis, UTI, pneumonia.
- Diagnosis is confirmed by *E. coli* isolation from normally sterile body fluids.
- Treatment should be based on antibiotic sensitivity data.

Listeria monocytogenes

- Important cause of neonatal sepsis.
- Colonizes GU tract.
- Clinical manifestations include sepsis and meningitis.
- Diagnosis is confirmed by *L. monocytogenes* isolation from sterile body fluid.
- Treatment is with penicillin or ampicillin.

Herpes Simplex

- Prevalence rate for adults with genital herpes is about 20%.
- Risk of neonatal disease is much higher with primary maternal infection (44%), and only 3% for a recurrent one.
- Ninety percent of neonatal infection is acquired through infected secretions during birth.
- There are three distinct patterns of disease:
  - Cutaneous disease:
    - Involves skin, mouth, and eyes.
    - Vesicular eruptions appear around 7 to 10 days of life, usually on presenting part.
    - If not recognized promptly, can progress to disseminated disease.
  - Encephalitic disease:
    - Occurs at second to third week of life.

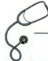

Caput succedaneum is external to the periosteum and crosses the midline of the skull and suture lines versus a cephalohematoma, which is below the periosteum and does not cross suture lines.

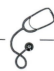

Brachial plexus injuries can occur during birth when traction is used with shoulder dystocia.

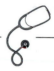

Degree of functional return in birth brachial plexus injuries depends on the severity of the nerve injury (stretch, rupture, avulsion).

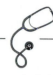

Twenty percent of pregnant women are colonized with GBS. It is recommended that all pregnant women be screened (vaginal, rectal swabs) at 35 to 37 weeks of gestation, and be given intrapartum penicillin if positive.

HIGH-YIELD FACTS

Gestation and Birth

- Clinical signs include lethargy, irritability, poor suck, seizures.
- Cutaneous lesions may be absent.
  - Disseminated disease:
    - Sepsis-like clinical picture (apnea, irritability, hypotonia, hypotension).
    - Cutaneous lesions may be absent.

DIAGNOSIS

- HSV can be isolated in cell culture from skin lesions or nasopharyngeal swabs.
- Polymerase chain reaction (PCR) is a sensitive tool for HSV detection.

TREATMENT

- Acyclovir is very effective in treatment of HSV infection.
- Course of treatment is often prolonged (21 days) for encephalitic and disseminated forms.

Chlamydia

- Acquired during passage through the birth canal of an infected mother.
- Causes conjunctivitis (few days to several days) and pneumonia (between 3 and 19 weeks).

DIAGNOSIS

Culture.

TREATMENT

Erythromycin orally for 14 days.

Syphilis

- Results from transplacental transfer of *Treponema pallidum*.
- Common features include intermittent fever, osteitis and osteochondritis, hepatosplenomegaly, lymphadenopathy, persistent rhinitis ("snuffles"), and a maculopapular rash involving the palms and the soles.
- Late manifestations include a saddle nose deformity, saber shins, frontal bossing, Hutchison teeth and mulberry molars, sensorineural, and Clutton's joints (painless joint effusions).

DIAGNOSIS

- Rapid plasma reagin (RPR) titers and the flourescent treponemal antibody-absorption test (FTA-ABS).
- Treponemes can also be seen on darkfield microscopy of nasal discharge.

TREATMENT

Penicillin G.

HIV

- Eighty percent of pediatric acquired immune deficiency syndrome (AIDS) results from maternal–fetal vertical transmission.
- Transmission from infected breast milk can occur.
- Clinical features in the infant include persistent thrush, lymphadenopathy and hepatosplenomegaly, severe diarrhea, failure to thrive, and recurrent infections.

Cesarean section is performed for women with primary genital herpes and vaginal lesions in late gestation.

Typical Scenario

Three-week-old infant presents with paroxysmal cough and tachypnea, but no fever; bilateral diffuse crackles, hyperinflation, and patchy infiltrates on x-ray; had conjunctivitis at 10 days of age. *Think: Chlamydia trachomatis.*

Maternal treatment with zidovudine (AZT) in the second trimester reduces the rate of transmission by > 60%.

Diagnosis

- Detection of p24 antigen in peripheral blood, PCR to detect viral nucleic acid in peripheral blood, and enzyme-linked immunosorbent assay (ELISA) for the detection of antibodies.

Treatment

- Nutritional support, *Pneumocystis carinii* prophylaxis, antiviral therapy, and anti-infective agents for specific infections.

SELECTED PROBLEMS IN FULL-TERM INFANTS

Developmental Dysplasia of the Hip (DDH)

- Occurs in ~1 in 800 births.
- More common in white females, with breech presentation, and is more likely to be unilateral and involve the left hip.
- Signs include asymmetry of the skin folds in the groin and shortening of the affected leg.
- Evaluation maneuvers:
  - Ortolani—abduction of the hips by using gentle inward and upward pressure over the greater trochanter.
  - Barlow—adduct the hips by using the thumb to apply outward and backward pressure; clicks of reduction and dislocation are elicited in patients with hip dislocation.
- Diagnosis is confirmed by ultrasound.
- Can be treated with a special brace (Pavlik harness) or sometimes casting. See chapter on musculoskeletal disease.

Meconium Ileus/Aspiration

- Meconium is the first intestinal discharge of a newborn infant and is composed of epithelial calls, fetal hair, mucus, and bile.
- Intrauterine stress may cause passage of meconium into the amniotic fluid, which can cause airway obstruction and a severe inflammatory response, leading to severe respiratory distress known as meconium aspiration syndrome.
- Meconium ileus occurs when meconium becomes obstructed in the terminal ileum; presentation is with failure to pass stool, abdominal distention, and vomiting.

Hypoxic/Ischemic Encephalopathy

- Hypoxic ischemic encephalopathy is an important cause of permanent damage to the cells of the CNS that occurs secondary to hypoxia (decreased oxygen delivery) and ischemia (decreased blood flow).
- Can be caused by maternal conditions (hypertension), placental insufficiency, severe neonatal blood loss, and overwhelming infection.
- Neurologic manifestations include hypotonia, coma, and seizures.
- It can result in death, cerebral palsy (CP), and mental retardation.

Diaphragmatic Hernia

- Associated with chromosomal abnormalities, low birth weight, and IUGR.
- Signs and symptoms include respiratory distress immediately on delivery, tachypnea, poor breath sounds over affected side of chest, and scaphoid abdomen.

Delivery room management of a meconium-stained infant consists of nasopharyngeal suctioning before the delivery of the thorax. Infants with respiratory depression require intubation and tracheal suctioning.

Typical Scenario

Postmature, 41-week gestational age newborn on first day of life has grunting respirations, signs of air trapping, and RR 100/min. *Think:* Meconium aspiration.

Meconium ileus is the most common presentation of cystic fibrosis in the neonatal period.

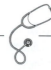

Ninety percent of full-term infants pass their first stool within the first 24 hours of life.

High indirect serum bilirubin levels in the first 24 hours of life are never physiologic.

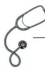

In neonates there is a cephalopedal progression of jaundice; approximate levels for involvement:

- Head and neck: 4 to 8 mg/dL
- Upper trunk: 5 to 12 mg/dL
- Lower trunk and thighs: 8 to 16 mg/dL
- Arms and lower legs: 11 to 18 mg/dL
- Palms and soles: > 15 mg/dL

Early diagnosis of hypothyroidism and treatment with thyroid hormone prior to 3 months of age can greatly improve intellectual outcome.

Jaundice

- Common causes of hyperbilirubinemia include ABO incompatibility, breast milk jaundice (see chapter on nutrition), Rh iso-immunization, and infection.
- **Conjugated hyperbilirubinemia (direct):**
  - When an infant's direct (conjugated) bilirubin is > 3 mg/dL.
  - Most common causes are idiopathic neonatal hepatitis (diagnosis of exclusion) and biliary atresia.
- **Unconjugated hyperbilirubinemia (indirect):**
  - When an infant's indirect (unconjugated) serum bilirubin level is > 10 mg/dL.
  - Most common cause of neonatal jaundice, seen in up to 50% of neonates.
  - Secondary to increased bilirubin load, defective uptake and conjugation, and impaired excretion into bile.
  - Physiologic hyperbilirubinemia is seen after the first 24 hours of life, peaks at 3 days, and resolves over 2 weeks.
- **Kernicterus:**
  - Bilirubin neurotoxicity secondary to persistently elevated bilirubin levels, which exceed albumin-binding capacity of the blood resulting in deposition of bilirubin in the basal ganglia.
  - This can result in subtle neurologic deficits, hearing loss, profound encephalopathy, and death.
- Treatment is initiated to prevent kernicterus:
  - Phototherapy with blue-green light converts bilirubin in skin to non-toxic isomers that are excreted without conjugation.
  - Elevated bilirubin levels (12–20 mg/dL) are usually treated with phototherapy.
  - Exchange transfusion should be considered at higher levels (20–25 mg/dL).

NEWBORN SCREENING

Neonatal Screening

- Available for various genetic, metabolic, hematologic, and endocrine disorders.
- All states have screening programs, although specific tests required vary.
- Tests performed on heel puncture include those for hypothyroidism, galactosemia, adrenal hyperplasia, cystic fibrosis, phenylketonuria, and other organic acid- and aminoacidopathies.

Auditory Screening

- Hearing impairment can affect speech and language development and occurs in 5 in 1,000 births.
- All infants should be screened with otoacoustic emission hearing testing.

Prematurity

PREMATURITY

DEFINITIONS

- Premature infant—live-born newborn delivered prior to 37 weeks from the first day of last menstrual period
- Low-birth-weight infant—weight less than 2,500 g
- Very-low-birth-weight infant—weight less than 1,500 g

ETIOLOGY

- Most premature births have no identifiable causes.
- Identifiable contributors include maternal, fetal, and obstetric:
  - Maternal:
    - Low socioeconomic status
    - Preeclampsia
    - Infections (urinary tract infections, group B streptococcus, etc.)
    - Chronic medical illness (hypertension, renal disease, diabetes, cyanotic heart disease, etc.)
    - Drug use
  - Obstetric:
    - Incompetent cervix
    - Polyhydramnios
    - Chorioamnionitis
    - Premature rupture of membranes
    - Placenta previa and abruptio placenta
  - Fetal:
    - Multiple gestation
    - Fetal distress (from hypoxia, etc.)
    - Congenital anomalies

Placing a healthy premature neonate in a neutral thermal environment reduces calories burned.

COMMON PROBLEMS IN PREMATURE NEWBORNS

Respiratory Distress Syndrome (RDS) (Hyaline Membrane Disease of the Newborn)

ETIOLOGY/PATHOPHYSIOLOGY

- Occurs secondary to insufficiency of lung surfactant due to immaturity of surfactant producing type 2 alveolar cells.
- Alveoli are small, inflate with difficulty, and do not remain gas-filled between inspirations.

- Ribcage is weak and compliant.
- High surface tension and propensity for alveolar collapse.
- Alveolar collapse results in progressive atelectasis, intrapulmonary shunting, hypoxemia, and cyanosis.

EPIDEMIOLOGY

Usually seen in infants < 32 weeks' gestational age.

SIGNS AND SYMPTOMS

- Seen within the first 3 hours of birth
- Tachypnea
- Grunting
- Cyanosis

DIAGNOSIS

Chest x-ray with fine, diffuse reticulogranular or "ground glass" pattern and air bronchograms (see Figure 3-1).

TREATMENT

- Aggressive respiratory support, including oxygen, continuous positive airway pressure (CPAP), intubation, and mechanical ventilation.
- To decrease barotrauma, novel methods of ventilation are sometimes used—high-frequency oscillation, jet ventilation, and liquid ventilation.
- Exogenous surfactant replacement (instillation via endotracheal tube) has dramatically reduced mortality in infants with RDS.

Bronchopulmonary Dysplasia (BPD) (Wilson–Mikity Syndrome)

DEFINITION

- Need for supplemental oxygen beyond 28 days of life.
- Characterized by squamous metaplasia and hypertrophy of small airways.

Production of surfactant can be accelerated by maternal steroid (betamethasone) administration; best if given 24 to 48 hours prior to delivery.

Most of these neonates also receive antibiotics because clinically and radiographically RDS and congenital pneumonia are indistinguishable.

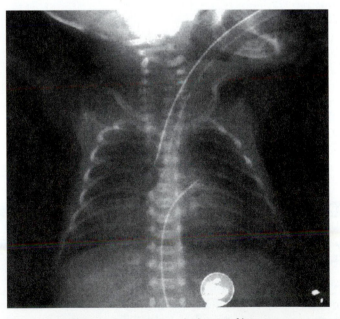

FIGURE 3-1. Chest x-ray demonstrating "ground glass" infiltrates consistent with respiratory distress syndrome (with a more focal area of infiltrate or atelectasis in the medial right lung base).

ETIOLOGY

- Multifactorial
  - Lung immaturity
  - Prolonged mechanical ventilation
  - Barotrauma (from mechanical ventilation)
  - Oxygen toxicity to the lungs

DIAGNOSIS

Chest x-ray with hyperaeration and atelectasis.

TREATMENT

- Supplemental oxygen as needed
- Oral steroids
- Bronchodilators

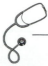

Necrotizing Enterocolitis (NEC)

ETIOLOGY

- Seen primarily in premature infants, although described in full-term neonates as well.
- Caused by bowel ischemia and bacterial invasion of intestinal wall.

SIGNS AND SYMPTOMS

- Intolerance of oral feeding (vomiting, bilious aspirates, and large volume residue in stomach)
- Abdominal distention
- Temperature instability
- Respiratory distress
- Acidosis, sepsis, shock

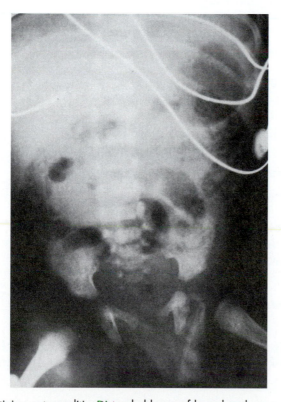

FIGURE 3-2. Necrotizing enterocolitis. Distended loops of bowel and pneumatosis intestinalis.

Serious sequelae of NEC include intestinal strictures, malabsorption, fistulae, and short bowel syndrome (in case of surgery).

Typical Scenario

Six-day-old, 2 lb. neonate develops episodes of apnea, abdominal distention, and bloody diarrhea. *Think:* Necrotizing enterocolitis.

Currently, severe retinopathy of prematurity is rare due to judicious use of oxygen.

DIAGNOSIS

- Distended loops of bowel
- Abdominal x-ray with "pneumatosis intestinalis"—air bubbles within the bowel wall (see Figure 3-2)
- Air in portal vein
- Free air under diaphragm (in case of perforation)
- Occult blood in stool

TREATMENT

- Discontinue feeds
- Place nasogastric tube
- Intravenous fluids
- Antibiotics
- Surgery in severe cases

Retinopathy of Prematurity (ROP)

ETIOLOGY

- Caused by proliferation of immature retinal vessels due to excessive use of oxygen.
- Can lead to retinal detachment and blindness in severe cases.

DIAGNOSIS

All very-low-birth-weight infants should be screened for ROP with an ophthalmoscopic exam.

TREATMENT

Laser surgery may be needed in severe cases.

Intraventricular Hemorrhage (IVH)

DEFINITION

Rupture of germinal matrix blood vessels due to hypoxic or hypotensive injury.

PREDISPOSING FACTORS

- Prematurity
- RDS
- Hypo- or hypervolemia
- Shock

SIGNS AND SYMPTOMS

- Most asymptomatic
- Lethargy
- Poor suck
- High-pitched cry
- Bulging fontanelle

DIAGNOSIS

Cranial ultrasound (through anterior fontanelle).

TREATMENT

- Directed toward correction of underlying conditions (RDS, shock, etc.).
- In cases of associated hydrocephalus, placement of ventriculoperitoneal shunt may be required.

Rickets of Prematurity

ETIOLOGY

- Transfer of calcium and phosphorous occurs most rapidly during third trimester (which is most likely to be "missed" by preemies).
- Vitamin D deficiency.

SIGNS AND SYMPTOMS

- Hypotonia
- Pathologic fractures
- Craniotabes (occipital flattening)
- Harrison's groove (indentation of the ribs at the diaphragmatic level)
- "Rachitic rosary"(swelling of costochondral junctions)

DIAGNOSIS

- Based on x-ray findings
  - Cupping, fraying of metaphyses
  - Subperiosteal new bone formation
  - Osteopenia

TREATMENT

- Vitamin D administration
- Calcium supplements

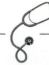

All premature, very-low-birth-weight infants should have a cranial ultrasound in the first week of life to look for intraventricular hemorrhage.

Serum calcium and phosphorus are not good indicators of presence of rickets; serum alkaline phosphatase level is elevated in this condition.

SURVIVAL OF PREMATURE NEONATES

- Birth weight (BW) is a very strong predictor of survival.
- Only 20% of neonates with BW of 500 to 600 g survive.
- Survival of infant with BW of 1,250 to 1,500 g is about 90%.
- There is no worldwide, universal gestational age that defines viability.
- In the United States, chance of normal survival is 50% after 24 weeks.

SPECIAL NEEDS OF EX-PREEMIES

- Due to their bronchopulmonary dysplasia, ex-preemies can experience recurrent wheezing episodes and severe course of respiratory infections, especially respiratory syncytial virus (RSV).
- Due to increased work of breathing and "catch-up" growth, ex-preemies should receive high-calorie diet to allow for this additional caloric expenditure.
- Routine vaccination should be given based on postnatal (not gestational) age.
- Early identification and intervention is needed for infants with developmental problems.

Ex-preemies can receive RSV prophylaxis with RSV monoclonal antibodies during RSV season (IM injections once a month).

Growth and Development

GROWTH

- Understanding normal growth patterns of childhood is important because it is an indication of the overall health of a child.
- Growth is influenced by both genetics and environment.

Growth Charts

- Height, weight, and head circumference are plotted on growth curves to compare the patient to the population.
- Serial plotting of patient's growth allows the clinician to observe patterns of growth over time.
- Potential limitations of particular growth charts include possible development from small population sizes, ethnic differences, and whether they represent growth potential versus proper care and feeding.
- Specialized charts exist for children who are premature (Babson), have Down's syndrome, myelomeningocele, Prader–Willi syndrome, cerebral palsy, or Williams syndrome.

Having only one point on a growth chart is like having no point; the trend over time is what is important.

Early Growth Trends

- A term infant regains to birth weight by 2 weeks.
- During the first 3 months, a child is expected to gain 1 kg per month.
- A child should be three times birth weight by his or her first birthday.

Intrauterine Factors

- Insulin-like growth factor (IGF) is important for fetal growth.
- Growth hormone and IGF are both important for postnatal growth.
- Thyroid hormone is important for central nervous system (CNS) development, but not important for fetal growth.
- Fetal weight gain is greatest during the third trimester.
- Teratogens and chromosomal abnormalities (trisomy 21, Turner's syndrome) can impair fetal growth.

In the normal child, the greatest growth occurs in the first year of life.

Teeth

- By age 2½, children should have all of their primary teeth including their second molars.
- Central incisors are first to erupt, between 5 and 8 months.
- Second molars are last to erupt, between 20 and 30 months.

- Secondary (permanent) teeth begin to erupt by age 6 to 7 years.
- Early or late tooth eruption may be within normal limits, though it can be an indicator of a nutritional, genetic, or metabolic problem.

SPECIFIC GROWTH PROBLEMS

Microcephaly

DEFINITION

Head circumference > 3 standard deviations below the mean.

ETIOLOGY

- Genetic diseases (familial, trisomy 21, trisomy 18, cri-du-chat, Prader–Willi syndrome)
- Prenatal insults (maternal drug use, TORCH infections, maternal phenylketonuria [PKU], decreased placental blood flow)
- Structural malformation (e.g., lissencephaly)

IMPACT

A small brain predisposes to cognitive/motor delay and seizures.

Macrocephaly

DEFINITION

Head circumference > 3 standard deviations above the mean.

ETIOLOGY

- Familial in 50% of cases
- Hydrocephalus
- Other causes: Large brain (megalencephaly), cranioskeletal dysplasia, Sotos syndrome

Failure to Thrive (FTT)

DEFINITION

FTT is defined as a weight below the third percentile or a fall off the growth chart by two percentiles.

ETIOLOGY

- Organic causes include disease of any organ system.
- Nonorganic causes include abuse, neglect, and improper feeding. (See Table 4-1.)

SIGNS AND SYMPTOMS

- Expected age norms for height and weight not met
- Hair loss
- Loss of muscle mass
- Subcutaneous fat loss
- Dermatitis
- Lethargy
- Recurrent infection
- Kwashiorkor—protein malnutrition
- Marasmus—inadequate nutrition

Measure parents' and siblings' head circumference to check for familial cause of macrocephaly.

Weight is affected first in FTT, followed by height and head circumference.

Psychosocial reasons account for most cases of FTT in the United States.

Signs of FTT:
SMALL KID
Subcutaneous fat loss
Muscle atrophy
Alopecia
Lagging behind norms
Lethargy
Kwashiorkor/marasmus
Infection
Dermatitis

TABLE 4-1. Etiology of FTT.

Gastrointestinal

Nutritional
- Kwashiorkor
- Marasmus
- Zinc/iron deficiency

Feeding Disorder
- Oral–motor apraxia
- Cleft palate
- Dentition disorder

Vomiting
- Gastrointestinal reflux
- Structural anomalies
- Pyloric stenosis
- CNS lesions
- Hirschsprung's disease

Diarrhea
- Chronic toddler diarrhea
- Milk protein allergy/intolerance
- Infectious
  - Bacterial
  - Parasitic
- Malabsorption
  - Cystic fibrosis
  - Celiac disease
  - Inflammatory bowel disease

Hepatic
- Chronic hepatitis
- Glycogen storage disease

Infectious
- Tuberculosis
- HIV

Cardiac
- Congenital heart malformations

Pulmonary
- Tonsillar hypertrophy
- Cystic fibrosis
- Bronchopulmonary dysplasia
- Asthma
- Structural abnormalities
- Obstructive sleep apnea

Renal
- Chronic pyelonephritis
- Renal tubular acidosis
- Fanconi's syndrome
- Chronic renal insufficiency
- Urinary tract infection
- Diabetes insipidus

Endocrine
- Hypothyroidism
- Rickets
- Vitamin D deficiency
- Vitamin D resistance
- Hypophosphatemia
- Growth hormone resistance/deficiency
- Adrenal insufficiency/excess
- Parathyroid disorders
- Diabetes mellitus

CNS
- Pituitary insufficiency
- Diencephalic syndrome
- Cerebral palsy
- Cerebral hemorrhages
- Degenerative disorders

Congenital
- Inborn errors of metabolism
- Trisomy 13, 18, 21
- Russell–Silver syndrome
- Prader–Willi syndrome
- Cornelia de Lange's syndrome
- Perinatal infection
- Fetal alcohol syndrome

Other
- Prematurity
- Oncologic disease/treatment
- Immunodeficiency
- Collagen vascular disease
- Lead poisoning

DIAGNOSIS

- Detailed history—gestation, labor and delivery, neonatal problems (feeding or otherwise), breast-feeding mother's diet and medications; types and amounts of food, who prepares, who feeds; vomiting, diarrhea, infection; sick parents or siblings; major family life events/chronic stressors; travel outside the United States; any injuries to child.
- Observation of parent–child interactions, especially at feedings, is critical for diagnosis. Lack of weight gain after adequate caloric feedings is characteristic of nonorganic failure to thrive.

- Screening tests for common causes include complete blood count (CBC), electrolytes, blood urea nitrogen (BUN), creatinine, and albumin.

TREATMENT

- If a nonorganic cause is suspected or the child is severely malnourished, hospitalization may be required.
- If organic, treat the cause.

PROGNOSIS

FTT during the first year of life has a poor outcome due to the rapid growth of the brain during the first 6 months.

DEVELOPMENT

- Attainment of developmental milestones is an indicator of a child's overall neurologic function.
- Maturation of intellectual, social, and motor function should occur in a predictable manner.
- It is essential that the physician recognize normal patterns in order to identify deviations.

Developmental Milestones

- Each new motor, language, and social skill should be acquired during an expected age range in a child's life.
- Each new skill is built on an earlier skill, and skills are rarely skipped. (See Table 4-2.)

Neurologic Development

- Myelination of the nervous system begins midgestation and continues until 2 years of age.
- Myelination occurs in an orderly fashion, from head to toe (cephalo-caudal).
- Primitive reflexes are present after birth and diminish by 6 months (see Table 4-3).

Age Adjustment for Preterm Infants

- Preterm infants may differ from full-term infants with regard to development.
- Age correction should be done until the child is 18 to 24 months old for children born more than 2 weeks early.
- Use the corrected age when assessing developmental progress and growth.

DEVELOPMENT DELAY

DEFINITION

Performance significantly below average in a given skill area.

ETIOLOGY

- Cerebral palsy
- Mental retardation
- Learning disabilities

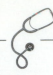

Organic versus nonorganic FTT is best distinguished by a detailed history and physical exam.

Typical Scenario

A child smiles spontaneously, babbles, sits without support, reaches, feeds herself a cookie but has no pincer grasp. What is her approximate age? *Think:* 8 to 9 months (pincer grasp at 10 months).

Unilateral loss of Moro's reflex is associated with clavicle or humerus fracture and brachial plexus palsy.

For age adjustment between birth and two years, subtract the number of days of prematurity from the chronological age.

TABLE 4-2. Developmental milestones.

Age	Motor	Language	Social	Other
1 month	■ Reacts to pain	■ Responds to noise	■ Regards human face ■ Establishes eye contact	
2 months	■ Eyes follow object to midline ■ **Head up prone**	■ Vocalizes	■ Social **smile** ■ Recognizes parent	
4 months	■ Eyes follow object past midline ■ **Rolls over**	■ **Laughs and squeals**	■ **Regards hand**	
6 months	■ **Sits well unsupported** ■ Transfers objects hand to hand (switches hands) ■ **Rolls prone to supine**	■ **Babbles**	■ Recognizes strangers	■ 6abbles (babbles) ■ *Six* strangers switch sitting at *six months*
9 months	■ **Pincer grasp (10 months)** ■ **Crawls** ■ Cruises (walks holding furniture)	■ Mama/dada ■ Bye-bye	■ Starts to explore	■ Can crawl, therefore can explore ■ It takes 9 months to be a "mama" ■ Pinches furniture to walk
12 months	■ **Walks** ■ Throws object	■ **1–3 words** ■ **Follows 1-step commands**	■ Stranger and separation anxiety	■ Walking away from mom causes anxiety ■ Knows 1 word at 1 year
2 years	■ **Walks up and down stairs** ■ Copies a line ■ **Runs** ■ **Kicks ball**	■ **2–3-word phrases** ■ One half of speech is understood by strangers ■ Refers to self by name ■ **Pronouns**	■ Parallel play	■ Puts 2 words together at 2 ■ At age 2, ¼ (½) of speech understood by strangers
3 years	■ **Copies a circle** ■ **Pedals a tricycle** ■ Can build a bridge of 3 cubes ■ Repeats 3 numbers	■ Speaks in sentences ■ Three fourths of speech is understood by strangers ■ Recognizes 3 colors	■ Group play ■ **Plays simple games** ■ Knows gender ■ Knows first and last name	■ *Tricycle*, 3 cubes, 3 numbers, 3 colors, 3 kids make a group ■ At age 3, ¾ of speech understood by strangers
4 years	■ Identifies body parts ■ Copies a cross ■ Copies a square (4.5 years) ■ **Hops on one foot** ■ **Throws overhand**	■ Speech is completely understood by strangers ■ Uses past tense ■ **Tells a story**	■ Plays with kids, social interaction	■ Song "head, shoulder, knees, and toes," 4 parts reminds you that at age 4 can identify body parts ■ At age 4, ¾ of speech is understood by strangers ■ When using past tense, speaks of things that happened be*fore* ■ If a 2 year old can copy one line, a 4 year old can copy two lines to draw a cross and a square, which has 4 sides

(continues)

TABLE 4-2. Developmental milestones (continued).

Age	Motor	Language	Social	Other
5 years	■ Copies a triangle ■ Catches a ball ■ Partially dresses self	■ Writes name ■ Counts 10 objects		
6 years	■ Draws a person with 6 parts ■ Ties shoes ■ Skips with alternating feet	■ Identifies left and right		■ At 6 years: *skips, shoes, person with 6 parts*

Typical Scenario

An 18-month-old infant brought in for temper tantrums has normal gross and fine motor skills but lacks language development and is cooperative and alert on exam. *Think:* Hearing loss.

■ Hearing and vision deficits
■ Autism
■ Neglect
■ Attention deficit hyperactivity disorder (ADHD)

DIAGNOSIS

■ The Denver Development Assessment Test (Denver II) is a screening tool intended to be performed at well-child visits to identify children with developmental delay.
■ Evaluates personal–social, fine motor, gross motor, and language skills.
■ Clinical Adaptive Test (CAT)/Clinical Linguistic Auditory and Milestone Scale (CLAMS) rates problem solving, visual motor ability, and language development from birth to 36 months of age.

TABLE 4-3. Primitive reflexes.

Reflex	Timing	Elicit	Response
Moro	Birth to 3–6 months	While supine, allow head to suddenly fall back approximately 3 cm	Symmetric extension and adduction, then flexion, of limbs
Startle	From when Moro disappears to 1 year	Startle	Arms and legs flex immediately
Galant	Birth to 2–6 months	While prone, stroke the paravertebral region of the back	Pelvis will move in the direction of the stimulated side
Sucking	Becomes voluntary at 3 months	Stimulate lips	Sucks
Babinski	Birth to 4 months	Stroke from toes to heel	Fanning of toes
Tonic neck	Birth to 4–6 months	While supine, rotate head laterally	Extension of limbs on chin side, and flexion of limbs on opposite side (fencing posture)
Rooting	Birth to 4–6 months	Stroke finger from mouth to earlobe	Head turns toward stimulus and mouth opens
Palmar/plantar grasp	Birth to 4–9 months	Stimulation of palm or plantar surface of foot	Palmar grasp/plantar flexion
Parachute	Appears at 9 months	Horizontal suspension and quick thrusting movement toward surface	Extension of extremities

LEARNING DISABILITIES

- Present in 5–10% of children.
- Include difficulties with reading, arithmetic, and writing.
- Dyslexia.
  - One of the most common learning disabilities.
  - Failure to acquire reading skills in the usual time course.
  - These children have excellent spoken language.
  - Dyslexia presents with different degrees of severity.

SLEEP PATTERNS

- Infants sleep 18 hours per day, with 50% rapid eye movement (REM) sleep, compared to an adult with 20% REM sleep.
- By age 4 months, nighttime sleep becomes consolidated.
- Two sleep stages are REM (irregular pulse and time when dreaming occurs) and non-REM (deep sleep).
- Parasomnias (sleep disorders) begin near age 3 years.
- Nightmares occur during REM sleep—the child awakens in distress about a dream.
- Night terrors occur in non-REM sleep—the child appears awake and frightened but is not responsive, and then is amnestic about the event the next morning.
- Somnambulism (sleepwalking) occurs in non-REM sleep; most common in ages 4 to 8 years.
- Somniloquy (talking) is very common throughout life, sometimes accompanying night terrors and sleepwalking.

At age 1 year, a child uses one word, and follows a one-step command.

At age 2 years, a child uses two- to three-word phrases and follows two-step commands, and others can understand half of the child's language.

At age 3 years, a child uses three-word sentences, and others can understand three fourths of the child's language.

At age 4 years, a child should be 40 lbs. and 40 inches tall and be able to draw a four-sided figure.

Growth and Development

Nutrition

NEWBORN NUTRITION

Newborn Feeding Tips

- Newborns require 110 to 115 kcal/kg/day and grow at a rate of about 30 g/day.
- Newborns usually begin feeding within the first 6 hours of life.
- Newborns should be breast or formula fed every 3 to 4 hours thereafter.
- *Supply = demand*—the more often the baby breast-feeds, the more milk will be produced.
- If the child has stopped losing weight by 5 to 7 days and begins to gain weight by 12 to 14 days, then feeding is adequate.
- Hunger is not the only reason infants cry. They don't need to be fed every time they cry.

Colostrum

- The milk secreted from the breasts toward the end of pregnancy and for 2 to 4 days after delivery.
- Usually a deep lemon color.
- High in protein, minerals, and immunologic factors; low in carbohydrates.

Benefits of Breast-Feeding

- Infant:
  - Decreases incidence of infection (i.e., otitis media, pneumonia, meningitis, bacteremia, diarrhea, urinary tract infection [UTI], botulism, necrotizing enterocolitis).
    - *Higher levels of immunologic factors*—immunoglobulins, complement, interferon, lactoferrin, lysozyme
    - *Decreased exposure to enteropathogens*
  - Other postulated benefits include higher IQ, better vision, decreased risk of sudden infant death syndrome (SIDS), less fussy eaters.
  - Decreased incidence of chronic disease (Type 1 diabetes, lymphoma, Crohn's/ulcerative colitis [UC], allergies).
- Maternal (increased maternal oxytocin levels):
  - Decreased postpartum bleeding
  - More rapid involution of uterus
  - Less menstrual blood loss

Term infants, due to loss of extracellular water and suboptimal caloric intake, lose 5% of birth weight in the first few days of life but regain their birth weight by the end of the second week.

Don't put baby to sleep with a bottle; it can lead to dental caries.

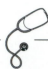

Immunoglobulin A (IgA) accounts for 80% of the protein in colostrum.

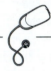

Whole cow's milk is not recommended before 1 year of age, because an infant's gastrointestinal (GI) tract is not developed enough to digest, predisposing to allergy, leading to GI blood loss and iron deficiency.

Tell the breast-feeding mother: If the baby doesn't let go, break the suction by inserting finger into corner of mouth; don't pull.

- Delayed ovulation
- Improved bone mineralization
- Decreased risk of ovarian and breast cancer
- Psychological benefits:
  - Increased maternal–child bonding
- Other:
  - Save money for family and society, no risk of mixing errors, correct temperature, convenient, no preparation

Common Problems with Breast-Feeding

- Soreness of nipples
  - Not due to prolonged feeding—due to improper positioning and poor removal
  - Engorgement
  - Unpleasant/painful swelling of the breasts when feeding cycle is decreased suddenly (relieved by increasing feeding on affected breast)
- Maternal fatigue, stress, and anxiety
  - Affects hormones needed for lactation
- Fear of inadequate milk production leading to formula milk supplementation
  - As the infants begins to feed less often, less milk is naturally produced. This often causes mother to misconceive that she is not producing enough milk to nourish the baby. Because of this, mother will frequently begin supplementing her milk with bottle milk, beginning a cycle of longer intervals between feeding, which causes less and less milk to actually be produced.
- Jaundice (see Table 5-1 and chapter on gestation and birth)
- Possible vitamin deficiencies—A, D, K, B_{12}, thiamine, riboflavin
- Infants who are exclusively breast-fed should receive vitamin drops after age 4 months.

Contraindications to Breast-Feeding

- Breast cancer
- Cancer chemotherapy
- Some medications (most are okay; check the label)
- Street drugs
- Herpetic breast lesions
- Untreated, active tuberculosis
- Cytomegalovirus (CMV) infection
- Human immunodeficiency virus (HIV) infection
  - In developing countries where food is scarce and HIV is endemic, the World Health Organization recommends breast-feeding by HIV-infected moms because the benefits outweigh the risks.
- Infant galactosemia

Signs of Insufficient Feeding of Infant

- Fewer than six wet diapers per day after age 1 week (before that, count one wet diaper per day for first week of life)
- Continual hunger, crying
- Continually sleepy, lethargic baby
- Fewer than seven feeds per day
- Long intervals between feedings
- Sleeping through the night without feeding
- Loss of > 10% of weight
- Increasing jaundice

TABLE 5-1. Breast-feeding versus breast milk jaundice.

Breast-Feeding Jaundice	Breast Milk Jaundice
Also called "not enough milk jaundice"—usually due to decreased or poor milk intake	Syndrome of prolonged unconjugated hyperbilirubinemia that is thought to be due to an inhibitor to bilirubin conjugation in the breast milk of some mothers
Occurs *during* first week of life	Begins *after* first week of life—peaks usually after second to third week
Reduced enteral intake leading to infrequent and scanty bowel movements and increased enterohepatic circulation of bilirubin	Transient; unless severe unconjugated hyperbilirubinemia No treatment necessary

Breast **F**eeding jaundice occurs in the **F**irst week. Breast **M**ilk jaundice occurs **M**any weeks later.

Not every woman will feel "milk letdown" despite proper breast-feeding.

Reasons for Failure to Grow and Gain Weight

- Improper formula preparation
- Use of skim and 2% milk before age 2
- Prolonged used of diluted formula
- Prolonged used of BRAT (bananas, rice, applesauce, toast) diet after illness
- Excessive juice or water
- Inconsistent care
- Inappropriate feeding schedule

Formula

- Types (see Table 5-2)
- Inappropriate formulas (see Table 5-3)

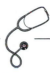

The common cold and flu are not contraindications to breast-feeding.

Solid Foods

- Solid food should be introduced between 4 and 6 months; introducing solids before this time does not contribute to a healthier child nor does it help the infant to sleep better.
- New foods should be introduced individually and about a week apart; this is done to identify any allergies and intolerance the child may have. There are many suggested orders in which to introduce new food. A common one is vegetables first, green to orange, then fruits, to introduce foods from most bland to sweetest.

Mastitis—tender erythematous swelling of portion of breast usually associated with fever. Most common organism is *Staphylococcus*, transmitted from oropharynx of asymptomatic infant. Infant should continue to feed on affected breast.

Readiness for Solid Foods

- Hand-to-mouth coordination
- Decreased tongue protrusion reflex
- Sits with support
- Improved head control
- Drooling
- Opens mouth to spoon

Caloric Requirements

Estimated average requirement = basal metabolic rate × physical activity level (see Table 5-4).

Undernutrition has the greatest effect on brain development from 1 to 3 months of age.

Feed at earliest sign of hunger; stop at earliest sign of satiety.

Do not give an infant under 6 months of age water or juice (water fills them up; juice contains empty calories, and excess sugar can cause diarrhea).

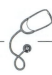

Do not use 2% milk before 2 years of age or skim milk before 5 years.

Typical formulas contain 20 kcal per ounce.

Avoid foods that are choking risks, including small fruits, raw vegetables, nuts, candy, and gum.

TABLE 5-2. Formulas.

Formula	Indications	Formulations
Cow's milk based	Premature Transitional	Lactose-free Low electrolyte Low iron Whey hydrosylate
Soy protein based	Galactosemia Lactose intolerance	Carbohydrate free Fiber-containing Sucrose free
Protein hydrosylate	Malabsorption Food allergies	
Amino acid based	Food allergies Short gut	
High medium-chain triglyceride oil	Chylous ascites Chylothorax	
Metabolic		Lofenelac Phenex-1—PKU Propimex-1—propionic acidemia

FLUID MANAGEMENT

Physiologic Compartments

TOTAL BODY WATER (TBW)

TBW makes up 50–75% of the total body mass depending on age, sex, and fat content.

DISTRIBUTION

- Intracellular fluid accounts for two thirds of TBW and 50% of total body mass.
- Extracellular fluid accounts for one third of TBW and 25% of total body mass.

TABLE 5-3. Inappropriate formulas.

Cow's milk	Decreased iron, essential fatty acids, vitamin E Increased sodium, potassium, chloride, and protein
Goat's milk	Allergen potential Very high potential renal solute load Low in folate and iron Questionable pasteurization
Rice milk	Very low in protein and fat Low in electrolytes and almost all vitamins and minerals
Commercial soy milk (not soy formula)	Soy induces L-thyroxine depletion through fecal waste, creating an increased requirement for iodine, potentially leading to goiter

46

TABLE 5-4. Daily caloric requirements.

Age	Males (kcal)	Females (kcal)
0–3 months	545	515
4–6 months	690	645
7–9 months	825	765
10–12 months	920	865
1–3 years	1,230	1,165
4–6 years	1,715	1,545
7–10 years	1,970	1,740
11–14 years	2,220	1,845
15–18 years	2,755	2,110

EXTRACELLULAR FLUID (ECF)

ECF is composed of plasma (intravascular volume) and interstitial fluid (ISF).

DEHYDRATION

- Definition: Body fluid depletion (see Table 5-5)
- Causes can be divided into two categories:
  - Poor intake
  - Excessive loss (e.g., vomiting, diarrhea)
- Leads to hypovolemia, gradually affecting each organ system

Fluid Therapy

GOALS

Rapidly expand the ECF volume and restore tissue perfusion, replenish fluid and electrolyte deficits, meet the patient's nutritional needs, and replace ongoing losses.

Neonates have a greater percentage of TBW per weight than do adults (about 70–75%).

You know a patient is dehydrated when he or she is **PARCHED**:
Pee, **P**ressure (blood)
Anterior fontanelle
Refill, capillary
Crying
Heart rate
Elasticity of skin
Dryness of mucous membranes

Percentage of dehydration can be estimated using (pre-illness weight − illness weight/pre-illness weight) × 100%.

TABLE 5-5. Signs and symptoms of dehydration.

	Mild	Moderate	Severe
% Body weight loss	3–5%	6–9%	> 10%
General	Consolable	Irritable	Lethargic/obtunded
Heart rate	Regular	Increased	More increased
Blood pressure	Normal	Normal/low	Low
Tears	Normal	Reduced	None
Urine	Normal	Reduced	Oliguric/anuric
Skin turgor	Normal	Tenting	None
Anterior fontanelle	Flat	Soft	Sunken
Capillary refill	< 2 sec	2–3 sec	> 3 sec
Mucous membranes	Moist	Dry	Parched/cracked

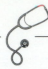
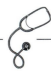

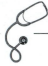
METHODS

- Fluid requirements can be determined from caloric expenditure.
- For each 100 kcal metabolized in 24 hours, the average patient will require 100 mL of water, 2 to 4 mEq Na^+, and 2 to 3 mEq K^+.
- This method overestimates fluid requirements in neonates under 3 kg.
- For a child over 20 kg, give 1,500 mL + 20 mL/kg for each kilogram over 20 kg.

MAINTENANCE

- Replacement of *normal* body fluid loss
- Causes of normal fluid loss include:
  - Insensible fluid loss (i.e., lungs and skin)
  - Urinary loss

DEFICIT

- Replacement of *abnormal* fluid and electrolyte loss (i.e., from vomiting, diarrhea, etc.).

- Example
- For a 25-kg patient:
  100 (for first 10 kg) × 10 +
  50 (for second 10 kg) × 10 +
  20 (for remainder) × 10 = 1,600 mL/day or
  65 mL/hr when divided by 24 hours

Deficit Therapy

HYPONATREMIA

In hypotonic (hyponatremic) dehydration, serum Na^+ < 130 mEq/L.

Epidemiology

- Most common electrolyte abnormality
- More common in infants fed on tap water

Etiology

- Hypervolemic hyponatremia—fluid retention:
  - Congestive heart failure (CHF)
  - Cirrhosis
  - Nephrotic syndrome
  - Acute or chronic renal failure
- Hypovolemic hyponatremia—increased sodium loss:
  - Due to renal loss
    - Diuretic excess, osmotic diuresis, salt-wasting diuresis
    - Adrenal insufficiency, pseudohypoaldosteronism

TABLE 5-6. Calculating maintenance fluids per day.		
Body Weight (kg)	**Milliliters per Day**	**Milliliters per Hour**
0–10	100/kg	4/kg
11–20	1,000 + 50/kg over 10	40 + 2/kg over 10
> 20	1,500 + 20/kg over 20	60+ 1/kg over 20

HIGH-YIELD FACTS

Nutrition

- Proximal renal tubular acidosis
- Metabolic alkalosis
- Due to extrarenal loss
  - Gastrointestinal (GI)—vomiting, diarrhea, tubes, fistula
  - Sweat
  - Third-spacing—pancreatitis, burns, muscle trauma, peritonitis, effusions, ascites
- Euvolemic hyponatremia:
  - Syndrome of inappropriate antidiuretic hormone secretion (SIADH)
    - Tumors
    - Chest disorders
    - Central nervous system (CNS) disorders—infection, trauma, shunt failure
    - Drugs—vincristine, vinblastine, diuretics, carbamazepine, amitriptyline, morphine, isoproterenol, nicotine, adenine arabinoside, colchicine, barbiturates
  - Glucocorticoid deficiency
  - Hypothyroidism
  - Water intoxication due to intravenous (IV) therapy, tap water enema, or psychogenic (excess) water drinking

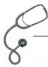

Hyponatremia can be factitious in the presence of high plasma lipids or proteins; consider the presence of another osmotically active solute in the ECF such as glucose or mannitol when hypotonicity is absent.

Signs and Symptoms

- Symptoms may occur at serum concentrations of ≤ 125 mEq/L.
- Cerebral edema—more pronounced in acute.
  - Early—anorexia, nausea, headache
  - Mental status changes
  - Later—beware of brain herniation: posturing, autonomic dysfunction, respiratory depression, seizures, coma
- Cerebral pontine myelinolysis can occur if hyponatremia corrected too quickly.

SIADH:
- Euvolemia
- Low urine output
- High urinary sodium loss
- Treat with fluid restriction

Diagnosis

- Volume status
- Acute versus chronic
- Serum and urine osmolality and sodium concentration, blood urea nitrogen (BUN), creatinine, other labs (glucose, aldosterone, thyroid-stimulating hormone [TSH], etc.)

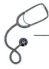

The rise in serum Na^+ in the correction of chronic hyponatremia should not exceed 2 mEq/L/hr or cerebral pontine myelinosis may occur secondary to fluid shifts from the intracellular fluid.

Treatment

- Na^+ deficit = (Na^+ desired − Na^+ observed) × body weight (kg) × 0.6.
- One half of the deficit is given in the first 8 hours of therapy, and the rest is given over the next 16 hours.
- Deficit and maintenance fluids are given together.
- If serum Na^+ is < 120 mEq/L and CNS symptoms are present, a 3% NaCl solution may be given IV over 1 hour to raise the serum Na^+ over 120 mEq/L.

HYPERNATREMIA

In hypertonic (hypernatremic) dehydration, serum Na^+ > 150 mEq/L.

Etiology

- Decreased water or increased sodium intake.
- Decreased sodium or increased water output.

The fluid deficit plus maintenance calculations generally approximate 5% dextrose with 0.45% saline. 6 mL/kg of 3% NaCl will raise the serum Na^+ by 5 mEq/L.

Look for a low urine specific gravity (< 1.010) in diabetes insipidus. These patients appear euvolemic because most of the free water loss is from intracellular and interstitial spaces, not intravascular.

A hypervolemic hypernatremic condition can be caused by the administration of improperly mixed formula, or this may present as a primary hyperaldosteronism. Always demonstrate the proper mixing of formula to parents who use powdered preparations.

If the serum Na⁺ falls rapidly, cerebral edema, seizures, and cerebral injury may occur secondary to fluid shifts from the ECF into the CNS.

- Diabetes insipidus (either nephrogenic or central) can cause hypernatremic dehydration secondary to urinary free water losses.
- Hypovolemic hypernatremia:
    - Extrarenal or renal fluid losses.
    - Adipsic hypernatremia is secondary to decreased thirst—behavioral or damage to the hypothalamic thirst centers.
- Hypervolemic hypernatremia:
    - Hypertonic saline infusion
    - Sodium bicarbonate administration
    - Accidental salt ingestion
    - Mineralocorticoid excess (Cushing syndrome)
- Euvolemic hypernatremia:
    - Extrarenal losses—increased insensible loss
    - Renal free water losses—central diabetes insipidus (DI), nephrogenic DI

Signs and Symptoms

- Anorexia, nausea, irritability
- Mental status changes
- Muscle twitching, ataxia

Treatment

- The treatment of elevated serum Na⁺ must be done gradually at a rate of decrease around 10 to 15 mEq/L/day.
- Usually, a 5% dextrose with 0.2% saline solution is used to replace the calculated fluid deficit over 48 hours after initial restoration of adequate tissue perfusion using isotonic solution.
- If the serum Na⁺ deficit is not correcting, the free water deficit may be given as 4 mL/kg of free water for each milliequivalent of serum Na⁺ over 145, given as 5% dextrose water over 48 hours.
- Too rapid correction of hypernatremia can result in cerebral edema.

HYPOKALEMIA

Can be considered at K⁺ < 3.5 mEq/L, but is extreme when K⁺ < 2.5 mEq/L.

Etiology

Excess renin, excess mineralocorticoid, Cushing's syndrome, renal tubular acidosis (RTA), Fanconi syndrome, Bartter syndrome, diuretic use/abuse, GI losses, skin losses, diabetic ketoacidosis (DKA).

Signs and Symptoms

Decreased peristalsis or ileus, hyporeflexia, paralysis, rhabdomyolysis, and arrhythmias including premature ventricular contractions (PVCs), atrial nodal or ventricular tachycardia, and ventricular fibrillation.

Diagnosis

- Serum value
- ECG may demonstrate flattened T waves, shortened PR interval, and U waves

Treatment

- Consider cardiac monitor.
- **If potassium is dangerously low and patient is symptomatic, IV potassium must be given.**

- Do not exceed the rate of 0.5 mEq/kg/hr.
- Oral potassium may be given to replenish stores over a longer period of time. Common forms of potassium include the chloride, phosphate, citrate, and gluconate salts.

HYPERKALEMIA

- Mild to moderate is K^+ = 6.0 to 7.0.
- Severe is K^+ > 7.0.

Etiology

Renal failure, hypoaldosteronism, aldosterone insensitivity, K^+-sparing diuretics, cell breakdown, metabolic acidosis, transfusion with aged blood.

Signs and Symptoms

Muscle weakness, paresthesias, tetany, ascending paralysis, and arrhythmias including sinus bradycardia, sinus arrest, atrioventricular block, nodal or idioventricular rhythms, and ventricular tachycardia and fibrillation.

Diagnosis

- Serum value
- ECG may demonstrate peaked T waves and wide QRS.

Treatment

- If hyperkalemia is severe or symptomatic, give calcium chloride or gluconate (10%) solution to stabilize the cardiac cellular membrane and place on cardiac monitor.
- Sodium bicarbonate, albuterol nebulizer, or glucose plus insulin can be given to shift K^+ to the intracellular compartment.
- Kayexalate resin can be given to bind K^+ in the gut (works the slowest).
- Furosemide can be given to enhance urinary K^+ excretion.
- In extreme cases, hemo- or peritoneal dialysis may be necessary.

VITAMIN AND MINERAL SUPPLEMENTS

Fluoride

- Supplement after age 6 months if the water is not fluorinated sufficiently (particularly well water).
- If < 3.3 ppm, supplement with 0.25 mg per day.
- Deficiency—dental caries.
- Excess—fluorosis: mottling, staining, or hypoplasia of the enamel.

Vitamin D

- Deficiency can occur if breast-feeding infant's mother has insufficient intake, infant's sun exposure is inadequate, or the infant is fed on whole cow's milk.
- Supplementation is with 400 IU per day.
- Deficiency—rickets, tetany.
- Vitamin D deficiency can lead to hypocalcemia.

Iron

- Newborn iron stores are sufficient for 6 months in a term infant.

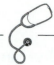

Hypokalemia can precipitate digitalis toxicity.

For every 0.1-unit reduction in serum pH, there is an increase in serum K^+ of about 0.2 to 0.4 mEq/L.

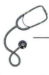

Because of the increased risk for fluorosis, don't give fluoride supplements before age 6 months!

Most bottled water is not fluorinated.

Dark-skinned kids are more likely to have inadequate sun exposure.

- Therefore, breast-fed infants need iron supplementation (i.e., iron-fortified cereals and baby foods), beginning at 4 to 6 months. Preterm breast-fed infants should start at 2 months of age.
- Deficiency—anemia (hypochromic microcytic) and growth failure.

Vitamin K

- Human breast milk is deficient in vitamin K.
- Therefore, it is necessary to administer a 1-mg vitamin K shot at birth. Recommended for every newborn, not just breast-fed.
- Deficiency—thought to contribute to hemorrhagic disease of the newborn.

Zinc

- Deficiency-associated intestinal malabsorption, nutritional intake limited to breast milk.
- Deficiency used to be associated with total parenteral nutrition (TPN); now formulas have zinc in them.
- Deficiency manifests as acrodermatitis, alopecia, and growth failure.

Typical Scenario

A 5-week-old infant feeding poorly on standard formula switched to whole cow's milk has an afebrile grand mal seizure and tremulousness. *Think:* Hypocalcemia, secondary to insufficient vitamin D.

Vitamin A

- Hypervitaminosis A
  - Congenital absence of enzymes needed to convert provitamin A carotenoids to vitamin A
  - Excessive ingestion of carotenoid-containing foods, especially fruits and vegetables
  - Acute:
    - Pseudotumor cerebri—bulging fontanelle, drowsiness, cranial nerve palsies
    - Nausea, vomiting
  - Chronic:
    - Poor weight gain
    - Irritability
    - Tender swelling of bones—hyperostosis of long bones, craniotabes; decreased mineralization of skull
    - Pruritus, fissures, desquamation

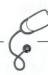

Breast milk has less iron than cow's milk, but the iron it does have is more bioavailable.

Other Supplements

- If mother is a strict vegetarian, supplement thiamine and vitamin B_{12}.
- Thiamine deficiency causes beriberi (weakness, irritability, nausea, vomiting, pruritus, tremor, possible CHF).
- Human milk will have adequate vitamin C only if mother's intake is sufficient.
- Commercial formula is often modified from cow's milk and fortified with vitamins and minerals so that no additional supplements are needed for the full-term infant.

Typical Scenario

A 14-month-old infant presents with anorexia, pruritus, and failure to gain weight; has a bulging anterior fontanelle and tender swelling over both tibias. Mother buys all food at a natural foods store. *Think:* Hypervitaminosis A.

OBESITY

DEFINITION

- Generalized and excessive accumulation of fat in subcutaneous tissues.
- Obese patients have actual body weight 20% greater than their ideal body weight for age, gender, and height.

RISK FACTORS

- Excessive intake of high-energy foods
- Inadequate exercise in relation to age and activity, sedentary lifestyle
- Low metabolic rate relative to body composition and mass
- Increased respiratory quotient in resting state
- Increased insulin sensitivity
- Genetics: strong relationship between body mass index (BMI) of patients and their biologic parents:
  - If one parent is obese, risk of obesity as an adult is 40%.
  - If two parents are obese, risk of obesity as an adult is 80%.
- Certain genetic disorders (Alström syndrome, Carpenter's syndrome, Cushing's syndrome, Fröhlich's syndrome, hyperinsulinism, Laurence–Moon–Bardet–Biedl syndrome, muscular dystrophy, myelodysplasia, Prader–Willi syndrome, pseudohypoparathyroidism, Turner's syndrome)

EPIDEMIOLOGY

Most often presents at ages 1 year, 4 to 5 years, and adolescence.

COMPLICATIONS

- Negative social attitudes—embarrassment, harassment
- Respiratory—sleep apnea
- Orthopedic—slipped capital femoral epiphysis (SCFE)
- Metabolic—Type 2 diabetes mellitus
- Cardiovascular—hypertension, hyperlipidemia

PREVENTION

- Early awareness and starting good eating and exercise habits early may hinder the development of overeating and obesity.
- Newborns need all the nourishment they can get. They need to be fed on a continuous schedule and on demand.
- Within the first year, offer food only when child is hungry.
- Avoid overeating by implementing regimental feeding times.
- Avoid using food as reward or punishment.

DIAGNOSIS

BMI is the most useful index for screening for obesity. It correlates well with subcutaneous fat, total body fat, blood pressure, blood lipid levels, and lipoprotein concentrations in adolescents.

TREATMENT

- Adherence to well-organized program that involves both a balanced diet and exercise.
- Behavioral modification.
- Involvement of family in therapy.
- Surgery and pharmacotherapy are contraindicated in children.
- Very-low-calorie diets are detrimental to growth and development—all nutritional needs should be met.
- Avoid rapid decreases in weight.
- Goal of effective weight reduction is not so much to lose pounds but to maintain weight through growth spurt.

Vitamin A deficiency is the number 1 worldwide most common cause of blindness in young children.

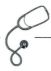

There is a direct relationship between degree of obesity and severity of medical complications.

Obesity makes **SHADE:**
SCFE
Hypertension
Apnea (sleep)
Diabetes
Embarrassment

HIGH-YIELD FACTS

Nutrition

Health Supervision and Prevention of Illness and Injury in Children and Adolescents

MORBIDITY AND MORTALITY

- The leading cause of death in children **under 1 year of age** is grouped under the term *perinatal conditions*, which include:
  - Low birth weight
  - Respiratory distress syndrome
  - Complications of pregnancy
  - Perinatal infections
  - Intrauterine or birth hypoxia
- From **1 year to 24 years of age** the leading cause of death is injury.

PREVENTION

Prevention is of primary importance in caring for the pediatric patient and is promoted through:
- Parental guidance
- Appropriate lab tests
- Vaccines

PARENTAL GUIDANCE

Age-appropriate anticipatory guidance is provided to parents at various well-child visits.

First Week to 1 Month

- Place infant to sleep on back to prevent sudden infant death syndrome (SIDS).
- Use of a car seat.
- Knowing signs of an illness.
- Maintaining a smoke-free environment (associated with SIDS and ear infections).
- Maintain water temperature at < 120°F (48.8°C).
- Do not give honey to a child under 1 year of age (botulism).

Be aware of social services and financial assistance available to parents and patients.

Any child with a rectal temperature > 101.4°F (38.5°C) in the first 6 months of life should be seen immediately.

2 Months to 1 Year

- Childproof home to keep children safe from poisons, household cleaners, medications, plastic bags, electrical outlets, hot liquids, matches, small and sharp objects, guns, and knives.
- Explain proper use of syrup of ipecac for poisonings, and give telephone number to local poison control hotline.
- No solid food until 4 to 6 months.
- Avoid baby walkers.
- Do not put baby to bed with bottle, as it can cause dental caries.
- Breast-feed or give iron-fortified formula, but no whole milk until after 1 year of age.
- Avoid choking hazards such as peanuts, popcorn, carrot sticks, hard candy, whole grapes, and hot dogs.
- May start using cup at 6 to 9 months.

1 to 5 Years

- Use toddler car seat if proper weight.
- Brush teeth.
- Wean from bottle.
- Make sure home is childproof again.
- Allow child to eat with hands or utensils.
- Use sunscreen.
- Wear bicycle helmet.
- Provide close supervision, especially near dogs, driveways, streets, and lawnmowers.
- Make appointment with dentist by 2 years of age.
- Ensure child is supervised when near water; build fence around swimming pool.

6 to 10 Years

- Reinforce personal hygiene.
- Teach stranger safety.
- Provide healthy meals and snacks.
- Keep matches and guns out of children's reach.
- Use seat belt always.

11 to 21 Years

- Continue to support a healthy diet and exercise.
- Wear appropriate protective sports gear.
- Counsel on safe sex and avoiding alcohol and drugs.
- Promote a healthy social life.
- Ask about mood or eating disorders (see below).

SCREENING

Metabolic screening may vary from region to region.

Metabolic Screening

In the first month of life the neonate should receive screening for various metabolic disorders including hypothyroidism, phenylketonuria (PKU), sickle cell disease, and adrenal cortex abnormalities.

Lead Screening

- Exposure increased by:
  - Living in or visiting a house built before 1960 with peeling or chipped paint
  - Plumbing with lead pipes or lead solder joints
  - Living near a major highway where soil may be contaminated with lead
  - Contact with someone who works with lead
  - Living near an industrial site that may release lead into the environment
  - Taking home remedies that may contain lead
  - Having friends/relatives who have had lead poisoning
- Done at 9 to 12 months

Hematocrit

Done at 9 to 12 months of age where certification is needed for WIC (Women, Infants, and Children) or if the appropriate risk factors are present.

Hyperlipidemia

- Screening may be considered in children with the appropriate risk factors:
  - Family history of coronary or peripheral vascular disease before the age of 55 years in parents or grandparents
  - Obesity
  - Hypertension
  - Diabetes mellitus
- Screening may also be considered in children with inactivity, also in adolescents who smoke.

Risk factors for anemia include low socioeconomic status, birth weight under 1,500 g, whole milk received before 6 months of age, low-iron formula given, low intake of iron-rich foods.

Vision and Hearing

- A hearing screen is recommended shortly after birth.
- Vision screening may begin at age 3 years, sooner if concerns.
- Suspect hearing loss earlier if child's speech is not developing appropriately.
- A child's cooperation is essential to obtaining a valuable screening.

Car Seats

- Car seats should be used for travel in automobiles for children from birth until the child reaches at least 40 pounds.
- Children under 20 pounds should be in an infant car seat, which belongs in the back seat and is rear-facing.
- Children from 20 pounds to 40 pounds belong in a car seat that is in the back seat but that is forward facing.
- Never place a car seat in front of an air bag.
- Make sure parents understand the proper use of car seats.

Newborns should not leave the hospital without a car seat.

See pocket card.

Hepatitis B

- First given at birth or within first 2 months of life IM (intramuscularly)
- Second dose given 1 month after first dose
- Third dose given 4 months after first dose and 2 months after second dose, but not before 6 months of age
- Must give at birth if baby exposed transplacentally or if maternal status is unknown along with HBIG (hepatitis B immune globulin)

CONTENT

Adsorbed recombinant hepatitis B surface antigen proteins.

SIDE EFFECTS

- Pain at injection site
- Fever > 99.9°F (37.7°C) in 1–6%

CONTRAINDICATIONS

Anaphylactic reaction to vaccine, yeast, or another vaccine constituent.

Diphtheria, Tetanus, and Pertussis

- Given at 2, 4, and 6 months of age, then another between 12 and 18 months of age.
- Given IM.
- Allow 6 months between third and fourth doses.

CONTENT

- DTaP is diphtheria and tetanus toxoids with acellular pertussis.
- DTP contains a whole-cell pertussis.

SIDE EFFECTS

- Erythema, pain, and swelling at injection site
- Fever > 100.9°F (38.3°C) in 3–5%
- Anaphylaxis in 1/50,000

CONTRAINDICATIONS

- Anaphylactic reaction to vaccine or another vaccine constituent
- Encephalopathy not attributable to another cause within 7 days of a prior dose of pertussis vaccine

Haemophilus influenzae Type B

- Given at 2, 4, and 6 months of age, then again between 12 and 15 months of age
- Given IM

CONTENT

Consists of a capsular polysaccharide antigen conjugated to a carrier.

SIDE EFFECTS

Erythema, pain, and swelling at injection site in 25%.

CONTRAINDICATIONS

Anaphylactic reaction to vaccine or vaccine constituent.

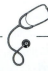

Fever is not a contraindication to receiving immunization. Moderate/severe illness is a contraindication. This holds true for all vaccines.

DTaP is the preferred for children under 7 years of age. Td is given after 7 years of age.

DTP has greater risks of side effects than DTaP.

DTaP is not a substitute for DTP if a contraindication to pertussis exists.

Measles, Mumps, and Rubella

- First dose given at 12 to 15 months of age, then again at 4 to 6 years of age.
- Given SC (subcutaneously).
- Second dose may be given at any time after 4 weeks from first dose if necessary.
- Must be at least 12 months old to ensure a sufficient response.

CONTENT

Composed of live attenuated viruses.

SIDE EFFECTS

- Fever > 102.9°F (39.4°C) 7 to 12 days after immunization in 10%
- Transient rash in 5%

CONTRAINDICATIONS

- Anaphylactic reaction to prior vaccine
- Anaphylactic reaction to neomycin or gelatin
- Immunocompromised states
- Pregnant women

Poliomyelitis

- Given at 2 and 4 months, then again between 6 and 18 months, then a fourth between 4 and 6 years of age
- IPV given SC
- OPV given orally

CONTENT

- Inactivated poliovirus vaccine (IPV) contains inactivated poliovirus types 1, 2, and 3.
- Live oral poliovirus vaccine (OPV) contains live attenuated poliovirus types 1, 2, and 3.

SIDE EFFECTS

- Vaccine associated paralytic polio (VAPP) with OPV in 1/760,000.
- With prior IPV risk is reduced by 75–90%.

CONTRAINDICATIONS

- Anaphylaxis to vaccine or vaccine constituent
- Anaphylaxis to streptomycin, polymixin B, or neomycin

Varicella

- Given once between 12 and 18 months of age.
- Given SC.
- Susceptible persons > 13 years of age must receive two doses at least 4 weeks apart.

CONTENT

Cell-free live attenuated varicella virus.

SIDE EFFECTS

- Erythema, swelling, and redness in 20–35%
- Fever in 10%
- Varicelliform rash in 1–4%

CONTRAINDICATIONS

- Anaphylactic reaction to vaccine, neomycin, or gelatin
- Patients with altered immunity, including corticosteroid use for > 14 days

MMR is a live virus vaccine.

Febrile seizures and encephalopathy with MMR vaccine are rare. Transient thrombocytopenia may occur 2 to 3 weeks after vaccine in 1/40,000.

An all-IPV schedule is recommended now in the United States to prevent VAPP (vaccine-associated paralytic polio). Under certain circumstances OPV may be used.

OPV is contraindicated in immunodeficiency disorders or when household contacts are immunocompromised.

Varicella vaccine contains live virus.

- Patients on salicylate therapy
- Pregnant women
- Recent blood product or IG administration (defer at least 5 months)

Influenza

- Given to children > 6 months of age yearly beginning in autumn, usually between October and mid-November.
- Given IM.
- All children should receive this vaccine, especially high-risk children.

CONTENT

- Contains three virus strains, usually two type A and one type B, and can be an inactivated whole-virus vaccine or a "split" vaccine containing disrupted virus particles.
- Children < 9 years of age should receive the "split" vaccine only.
- Children without exposure to influenza should receive two vaccines 1 month apart in order to obtain a good response.

SIDE EFFECTS

- Pain, swelling, and erythema at injection site.
- Fever may occur, especially in children < 24 months of age.
- In children > 13 years of age, fever may occur in up to 10%.

CONTRAINDICATIONS

Children with anaphylactic reactions to chicken or egg protein.

Pneumococcus

- Babies receive three doses (shots) 2 months apart starting at 2 months, and a fourth dose when they are 12 to 15 months old.
- Also given to high-risk children ≥ 2 years of age.
- If the child is < 10 years of age, a second dose is recommended 3 to 5 years after the first dose.
- If the child is > 10 years of age, then a second dose is recommended 5 years after the first.

CONTENT

The older PPV-23 vaccine (not indicated under age 2) contains the purified capsular polysaccharide antigens of 23 pneumococcal serotypes. The PPV-23 is usually reserved for high-risk children. The newer PCV-7 is the conjugate vaccine described above.

SIDE EFFECTS

- Erythema and pain at injection site.
- Anaphylaxis reported rarely.
- Fever and myalgia are uncommon.

CONTRAINDICATIONS

Usually deferred during pregnancy.

Respiratory Syncytial Virus (RSV)

- Given once a month at the beginning of RSV season, usually beginning in October and ending in March.
- Given IM.
- Children < 2 years of age with chronic lung disease who have required medical therapy 6 months before the anticipated RSV season should receive the vaccine.

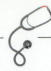

Vaccinating for influenza those with asthma, chronic lung disease, cardiac defects, immunosuppressive disorders, sickle cell anemia, chronic renal disease, and chronic metabolic disease is especially important.

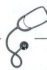

Influenza vaccine does not cause the disease. The vaccine has been associated with an increased risk of Guillain–Barré syndrome (GBS) in older adults, but no such cases have been reported in children.

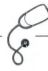

Chemoprophylaxis against influenza is recommended as an alternative means of protection in those who cannot be vaccinated.

Live attenuated vaccines include:
- MMR
- VZV
- Nasal influenza vaccine
- OPV
- Smallpox
- Typhoid

These should be avoided in the immunocompromised.

- Children born at 32 weeks' gestation or earlier with other risk factors for lung disease should receive the vaccine.

CONTENT

- Palivizumab consists of a monoclonal antibody.
- RSV–immune globulin intravenous (RSV-IGIV) consists of RSV neutralizing antibodies collected from donors selected for high serum titers.

Tuberculosis (TB)

The Mantoux test contains five tuberculin units of purified protein derivative (PPD).

SCREENING

The test is placed intradermally in:
- Children having contact with persons with confirmed or suspected disease
- Children with radiographic or clinical findings of TB
- Children from endemic countries
- Children with travel history to endemic countries
- Children with HIV

MEDICATIONS

Only 25% of Food and Drug Administration (FDA)-approved drugs have been approved for pediatric use.

Differences Between Children and Adults

ABSORPTION

- Infants have thinner skin; therefore, topical substances can more likely cause systemic toxicity.
- Children do not have the stomach acidity of adults until age 2, and gastric emptying time is slower and less predictable, leading to increased absorption of some medications.

DISTRIBUTION

- Less predictable in children.
- Total body water decreases from 90% in infants to 60% in adults.
- Fat stores are similar to adults in term infants, but much less in preterm infants.
- Newborns have smaller protein concentration, therefore less binding of substances in the blood.
- Infants have an immature blood–brain barrier.

METABOLISM

Infants metabolize drugs more slowly than adults and may create a different proportion of active metabolites.

ELIMINATION

Kidney function increases with age, so younger children may clear drugs less efficiently.

DOSAGE

Pediatric medications are generally dosed by milligrams per kilogram (mg/kg).

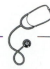

The pneumococcal vaccine helps to protect against meningitis, bacteremia, pneumonia, and otitis media caused by serotypes of *Streptococcus pneumoniae*.

Palivizumab is more commonly used than RSV-IVIG for RSV vaccine.

Controls with *Candida*, measles, or diphtheria can be placed along with the PPD to test for anergy, although opinion may vary in practice.

EPIDEMIOLOGY

More often accidental in younger children and suicide gestures or attempts in older children/adolescents.

SIGNS AND SYMPTOMS

- See Table 6-1.

PREVENTION

- Child-proof home including cabinets and containers.
- Store toxic substances in their orignal containers and out of children's reach.
- Supervise children appropriately.
- Have poison control center number easily accessible.

MANAGEMENT

- Frequently, ingested substances are nontoxic, but if symptoms arise or there is any question, a physician and/or poison control center should be contacted.
- History taking—precise name of product (generic, brand, chemical—bring container or extra substance/pills); estimate amount of exposure; time of exposure; progression of symptoms; other medical conditions (e.g., pregnancy, seizure disorder).
- Gastric decontamination—emesis (induced by syrup of ipecac) and gastric lavage remove only one third of stomach contents and are not generally recommended, though the combination of the latter with activated charcoal may be most effective.
- Activated charcoal is effective for absorbing many drugs and chemicals, though it does not bind metals, many alcohols, some acids, most organic solvents, and certain insecticides. It may be used in conjunction with cathartics such as magnesium sulfate.

TABLE 6-1. "Toxidromes," symptoms, and some causes.

	Anticholinergic	Cholinergic	Extra-pyramidal	Hypermetabolic	Opiates	Withdrawal	Sympathomimetic
Symptoms	Hyposecretion, thirst, urinary retention Flushed skin, dilated pupils Tachycardia, respiratory insufficiency Delirium, hallucinations	Hyper-secretion Muscle fasciculation, weakness Bronchospasm, arrhythmias Convulsions, coma	Tremor, rigidity	Fever Tachycardia Hyperpnea Restlessness Convulsions Metabolic acidosis	CNS depression Dilated pupils Hypothermia Hypotension	Abdominal cramps, diarrhea Lacrimation, sweating Tachycardia, restlessness Hallucinations	Hyperthermia, hypertension, tachypnea Dilated pupils Psychosis, convulsions
Causes	Belladonna Some mushrooms Antihistamines Tricyclic antidepressants	Organo-phosphates (insecticides) Some mushrooms, Black widow spider bites Tobacco	Haloperidol Meto-clopramide	Salicylates	Lomotil Propoxyphene Heroin Methadone Codeine Morphine Demerol	Cessation of: Alcohol Benzo-diazepines Barbiturates Opiates	Amphetamines Cocaine Theophylline Caffeine

HIGH-YIELD FACTS

Health Supervision

- Dilution of stomach contents with milk has limited value except in the case of ingestion of caustic materials.
- Skin decontamination—remove clothing, use gloves, flood area with water for 15 minutes, use other mild material such as petroleum or alcohol to remove substances not removed by water.
- Ocular decontamination—rinse eyes with water, saline, or lactated Ringer's for > 15 minutes; consider emergency ophthalmologic exam.
- Respiratory decontamination—move to fresh air; bronchodilators may be effective, inhaled dilute sodium bicarbonate may help acid or chlorine inhalation.
- Antidotes—see Table 6-2.
- Treat seizures, respiratory distress/depression, hemodynamics, and electrolyte disturbances as they arise.

ADOLESCENCE

- Adolescence comprises the ages between 10 and 21 years.
- The most common health problems seen in this age group include unintended pregnancies, sexually transmitted diseases, mental health disorders, physical injuries, and substance abuse.

PREVENTION

- Be on the lookout for adolescents at high risk for health problems, including physical, mental, and emotional health.
- Look for decline in school performance, excessive school absences, cutting class; frequent psychosomatic complaints; changes in sleeping or eating habits; difficulty in concentrating; signs of depression, stress, or anxiety; conflict with parents; social withdrawal; sexual acting-out; conflicts with the law; suicidal thoughts; preoccupation with death; and substance abuse.

SCREENING

- Routine health care should involve audiometry and vision screening, blood pressure checks, exams for scoliosis.
- Breast and pelvic exams in females may also be necessary, and self-exams should be emphasized.
- Likewise, examination for scrotal masses is necessary in males with emphasis on self-examination.
- Sexually transmitted diseases (STDs) including HIV should be considered in those adolescents with high-risk behaviors.

PHYSICAL EXAM

Sexual maturity should be assessed at each visit.

Pregnancy

EPIDEMIOLOGY

- Over 1 million teenage girls become pregnant in the United States each year.
- Over half of these pregnancies result in teen birth, one third result in abortion, and the remainder end in miscarriage.
- The 1997 birth rate for teenagers ages 15 to 19 years old was 94.3 per 1,000.
- Eighty percent of teen pregnancies are unintended.

The leading causes of death for adolescents are accidents and homicide.

One percent of adolescents have made at least one suicide gesture.

An increase in the number of years of schooling for a woman delays the age at which a woman marries and has her first child.

TABLE 6-2. Drug toxicities.

Drug	Signs and Symptoms	Treatment/Antidote
Sulfonamides	Kernicterus in infants	
Chloramphenicol	Gray baby syndrome—vomiting, ashen color, cardiovascular collapse	
Quinolones	May cause cartilage defects in children	
Tetracycline	Gray enamel of permanent teeth, affects bone growth (avoid in children < 9 years old)	Not necessary unless massive ingestion
Salicylate	Reye's syndrome—hepatic injury, hypoglycemia, vomiting—in children with viral illnesses Hypermetabolic	
Acetaminophen	Generalized malaise, nausea, vomiting Latent period Jaundice and bleeding (direct hepatocellular necrosis) Metabolic acidosis, renal and myocardial damage, coma	*N*-acetylcysteine (Mucomyst)
Tricyclic antidepressants	Anticholinergic Widened QRS, flattened T waves	Intubation and activated charcoal if altered sensorium Sodium bicarbonate IV
Prednisone	Growth retardation Cataracts	
Organophosphates	Cholinergic	Atropine Pralidoxime
Heavy metals (e.g., arsenic, mercury, lead, chromium, copper, gold, nickel, zinc)		Dimercaperol Dimercaptosuccinic acid (succimer, DMSA), EDTA
Iron	Abdominal pain	Deferoxamine
Methanol, ethylene glycol	Intoxication blindness (methanol)	Ethanol Fomepizol
Benzodiazepines	Sedation	Flumenazil (recommended only in cases of iatrogenic overdose)
Opiates	Respiratory depression Pinpoint pupils	Naloxone
Anticholinergics	"Mad as a hatter; Dry as a bone; Blind as a bat; Red as a beet; Hot as Hades"	

Contraception

EPIDEMIOLOGY

- According to the Centers for Disease Control and Prevention (CDC), 66.4% of high school seniors report having ever had intercourse.

- 49.7% report being currently sexually active.
- 36.9% of 9th graders report having had sex
- 23.6% report being sexually active.
- Boys reported being sexually active more often than girls.

RISK FACTORS

Factors associated with early sexual activity include lower expectations for education, poor perception of life options, low school grades, and involvement in other high-risk behaviors such as substance abuse.

FORMS OF CONTRACEPTION

- Abstinence, condoms (male and female), diaphragm, cervical cap, spermicides, or some combination of these.
- Hormonal methods include oral contraceptive pills and injectable or implantable hormones.

COMBINATION ORAL CONTRACEPTIVES

Usually consist of either 50, 35, 30, or 20 μg of an estrogenic substance such as mestranol or ethinyl estradiol plus a progestin.

SIDE EFFECTS

- Short-term effects may include nausea and weight gain.
- Other possible effects include thrombophlebitis, hepatic adenomas, myocardial infarction, and carbohydrate intolerance.

POTENTIAL BENEFITS

Long-range benefits include decreased risks of benign breast disease and ovarian disease.

HIV/AIDS

See chapter on infectious diseases.

EPIDEMIOLOGY

- HIV/AIDS is the sixth leading cause of death among adolescents age 15 to 24 years.
- One in four new infections is acquired by a person younger than 22 years old.

SCREENING

Screening should include adolescents with risk factors such as previous STD, unprotected sex, practicing insertive or receptive anal sex, trading sex for money or drugs, homelessness, intravenous drug or crack cocaine use, being the victim of sexual abuse.

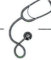

Adolescents who smoke may increase their risk for side effects from oral contraceptives.

In light of the long latency period between contraction of HIV and progression to AIDS, many cases in young adults were most likely contracted during adolescence.

CHILD ABUSE

DEFINITION

Child maltreatment encompasses a spectrum of abusive actions, and lack of action, that result in morbidity or death. Forms of child abuse include:
- Physical abuse
- Sexual abuse
- Neglect

RISK FACTORS

- Parental risk factors:
  - History of being abused as a child

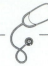

If the story doesn't make sense, suspect abuse.

Mongolian spots can be confused with bruises.

Sometimes abusive parents "punish" their children for enuresis or resistance to toilet training by forcibly immersing their buttocks in hot water.

Skeletal injuries suspicious of abuse: "**S**ome **P**arents **A**re **M**aliciously **M**ean" (or **P**arents **S**hould **M**anage **A**nger)

A child who presents with multiple fractures at multiple sites and in various stages of healing should be considered abused until proven otherwise.

- Alcoholism, drug use, psychosis
- Social isolation
- Child risk factors:
  - Handicapped children (chronic illness, congenital malformation, mental retardation)
  - Age < 3 years
  - "Difficult" children

Physical Abuse

Suspect if injury is:
- Unexplained
- Unexplainable
- Inconsistent with mechanism suggested by history
- History changes each time it is told
- Repeated "accidents"
- Delay in seeking care

SKIN MANIFESTATIONS

Bruises
Most common manifestation of physical abuse
- Suspicious if:
  - Seen on nonambulatory infants
  - Have geometric pattern (belt buckles, looped-cord marks)

Burns
- Suspicious if:
  - Involve both hand or feet in stocking-glove distribution or buttocks with sharp demarcation line (forced immersion in hot water)
  - Cigarette burns—if nonaccidental, usually full-thickness, sharply circumscribed
  - "Branding" injuries (inflicted by hot iron, radiator cover, etc.)

SKELETAL INJURIES

Suspicious if:
- **S**piral fractures of lower extremities in nonambulatory children (see Figure 6-1A and B)
- **P**osterior rib fractures (usually caused by squeezing the chest)
- Fractures of different **A**ges
- **M**etaphyseal "chip" fractures (usually caused by wrenching)
- **M**ultiple fractures

CENTRAL NERVOUS SYSTEM (CNS) INJURIES

- Most common cause of death in child abuse: "shaken baby syndrome"
- Occurs due to violent shakes and slamming against mattress or wall while an infant is held by the trunk or upper extremities
- Findings include:
  - **M**etaphyseal "chip" fractures
  - **R**etinal hemorrhages
  - **S**ubdural hematoma (from rupturing of bridging veins between dura mater and brain cortex)
- Symptoms include:
  - Lethargy or irritability
  - Vomiting
  - Seizures
  - Bulging fontanelle

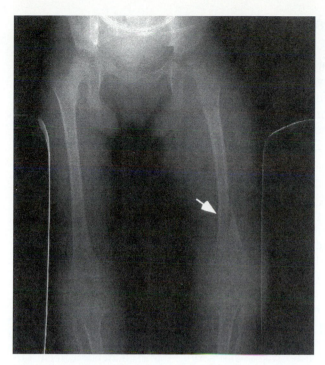
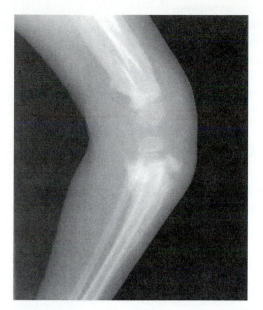

FIGURE 6-1. A. Spiral fracture (arrow) of the femur in a nonambulatory child, consistent with nonaccidental trauma. **B.** Same child 2 months later. Note the exuberant callus formation at all the fracture sites in the femur and proximal tibia and fibula.

ABDOMINAL INJURIES

- Second most common cause of death in child abuse.
- Usually no external marks. Most commonly, liver or spleen is ruptured.
- Symptoms include:
  - Vomiting
  - Abdominal distention
  - Shock

Sexual Abuse

- Includes genital, anal, oral contact; fondling; and involvement in pornography
- Most common perpetrators—fathers, stepfathers, mother's boyfriend(s) (adults known to child)
- Suspect if:
  - Genital trauma
  - Sexually transmitted disease in small children
  - Sexualized behavior toward adults or children
  - Unexplained decline in school performance
  - Runaway
  - Chronic somatic complains (abdominal pain, headaches)
- Symptoms include:
  - May be totally absent
  - Tears/bleeding in female or male genitalia
  - Anal tears
  - Hymenal tears (last two are not very reliable symptoms)

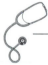

Epiphyseal–metaphyseal injury is virtually diagnostic of physical abuse in an infant, since an infant cannot generate enough force to fracture a bone at the epiphysis.

Children too young to talk about what has happened to them (generally younger than 2) should have a complete skeletal survey if you suspect abuse.

CNS injuries suspicious of abuse: "**M**others, **R**efuse **S**haking!" (**M**etaphyseal fractures, **R**etinal hemorrhages, **S**ubdural hematoma)

Shaken baby syndrome can mimic meningitis or sepsis.

Management of abuse:
Suspect
↓
Report
↓
Disposition
↓
Family counseling

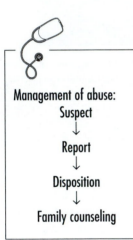

Baron von Munchausen was an 18th-century nobleman who became famous because of his incredible stories, which included travel to the moon and flying atop a cannonball over Constantinople, as well as visiting an island made of cheese. His name became a synonym for gross confabulations.

Evaluation of Suspected Abuse

PHYSICAL ABUSE

- Bleeding disorders must be ruled out in case of multiple bruises.
- X-ray skeletal survey (skull, chest, long bones) in children < 2 years of age (to look for old/new fractures).
- Computed tomographic (CT) scans of the head/abdomen as indicated.
- Ophthalmology consult.

SEXUAL ABUSE

Cultures for STD, test for presence of sperm, if indicated (usually within 72 hours of assault).

Management

- If abuse is suspected, it must be reported to child protective services (CPS) (after medical stabilization, if needed).
- All siblings need to be evaluated for abuse, too (up to 20% of them might have signs of abuse).
- Disposition of the child (i.e., whether to discharge the patient back to parents or to a CPS worker if medically cleared) has to be decided by CPS in conjunction with treating physician.
- Family must receive intensive social services' and, if needed, legal authorities' intervention.
- *Remember:* If sent back to abusive family without intervention, up to 5% of children can be killed and up to 25% seriously reinjured.

Neglect

DEFINITION

Neglect to meet nutritional and/or developmental needs of a child can present as:
- Failure to thrive
- Poor hygiene (severe diaper rash, unwashed clothing, uncut nails)
- Developmental/speech delay
- Delayed immunizations

MANAGEMENT

If nonorganic (i.e., due to insufficient feeding), failure to thrive is suspected:
- Patient should be hospitalized and given unlimited feedings for 1 week; 2 oz/24 hours of weight gain is expected.
- All suspected cases of neglect must be reported to CPS.

Munchausen Syndrome by Proxy

DEFINITION

- Illness that is inflicted or fabricated by a parent/caretaker.
- Psychiatrically disturbed parent(s) gain satisfaction from attention and empathy from hospital personnel or their own family because of problems created.

EPIDEMIOLOGY

- Affected children are usually < 6 years old.
- Parent (usually mother) has some medical knowledge.

- Vomiting (induced by ipecac)
- Chronic diarrhea (from laxatives)
- Recurrent abscesses or sepsis (usually polymicrobial, from injecting contaminated fluids)
- Apnea (from choking the child)
- Fever (from heating thermometers)
- Bloody vomiting or diarrhea (from adding blood to urine or stool specimens)

DIAGNOSIS

Diagnosis is difficult, but is initiated by removing child from parent via hospitilization. Usually, child without access to parent will have all/most symptoms resolve; testing will also usually be normal.

MANAGEMENT

- Admission to the hospital for observation, possibly using hidden video cameras.
- All cases of suspected Munchausen syndrome by proxy must be reported to CPS.

Sudden Infant Death Syndrome (SIDS)

DEFINITION

Sudden death of an infant (< 1 year old) that remains unexplained after thorough case investigation, autopsy, and review of the clinical history.

ETIOLOGY

Apnea hypothesis.

DIAGNOSIS

Difficult to differentiate from intentional harm.

PREVENTION

- There has been a vast decrease in the number of cases since the trend of having infants sleep on their backs (supine).
- The number one preventive measure to date is parental education, though the use of cardiorespiratory monitoring in the home is being debated.

HIGH-YIELD FACTS

Health Supervision

Congenital Malformations and Chromosomal Anomalies

INTRODUCTION

It is important for all pediatricians in all fields to recognize signs and symptoms of congenital disorders, including dysmorphologic features. It is also important to involve genetics in the patient's care, for appropriate screening and treatment of conditions associated with genetic syndromes, genetic testing, if available and appropriate, and counseling regarding siblings and possible future offspring of the patient. Lastly, physicians strive for a unifying diagnosis and usually one is sufficient, but patients can have more than one thing going on *and* children with genetic disorders can also get the diseases children without genetic conditions get!

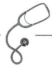

Trisomies:
- Age 13, Puberty: **Patau's**
- Age 18, can vote — "Elect": **Edwards'**
- Age 21, can Drink: **Down's**

AUTOSOMAL TRISOMIES

Trisomy 21 (Down's Syndrome)

ETIOLOGY

- 95% complete trisomy (meiotic nondisjunction of homologous chromosomes)
- 4% Robertsonian translocation (to chromosome 14)
- 1% mosaicism

EPIDEMIOLOGY

One in 600 births.

RISK FACTORS

Advanced maternal age.

SIGNS AND SYMPTOMS

- Varying degrees of mental retardation
- Generalized hypotonia (of central nervous system [CNS] origin)
- Balding scalp hair pattern
- Upslanted eyes with epicanthal folds (see Figure 7-1)
- Flat nasal bridge
- Prominent tongue
- Extra neck skin folds (sometimes visible on prenatal ultrasound)
- Transverse palmar (simian) creases (secondary to edema)
- Small ears
- Short stature
- Joint laxity
- Hypoplastic nipples
- Brushfield's spots on irises

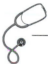

Patients with Down's syndrome develop Alzheimer's dementia early, around age 35.

Typical Scenario

A female infant has slanted palpebral fissures, epicanthal folds, and some delayed development. *Think:* Down's syndrome.

Chromosome 21 encodes two of the three proteins needed to assemble the triple helix of collagen VI, which is found to be abnormal in people with Down's syndrome. Collagen VI is important in scaffolding during embryologic development of nervous and connective tissue.

One can understand many of the defects of Down's in terms of a developmental connective tissue disturbance: cardiac septal defects, duodenal atresia, imperforate anus, facial dysmorphisms, joint laxity, nuchal folds, transverse palmar creases (palmar edema secondary to loose connective tissue), atlantoaxial instability, even mental retardation and Hirschsprung's disease when its role in nervous system development is considered. Note: This is a mnemonic, not accepted pathophysiology.

Every patient with Down's must have a cervical spine x-ray before being cleared to participate in sports, due to risk of atlantoaxial dislocation.

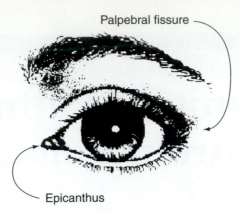

Palpebral fissure

Epicanthus

FIGURE 7-1. Location of epicanthus and palpebral fissure. In Down's syndrome, there are epicanthal folds and upwardly slanted palpebral fissures. (Artwork by S. Matthew Stead)

- Subendocardial cushion defect (atrial/ventricular septal defect [ASD/VSD], atrioventricular [AV] canal)
- Duodenal atresia, Hirschsprung's disease, imperforate anus
- Hypothyroidsim
- Amyloid plaques and neurofibrillary tangles in brain—early-onset dementia
- Increased risk of leukemia (acute lymphocytic leukemia [ALL], acute myelogenous leukemia [AML], acute megakaryocytic leukemia)
- Increased risk of neonatal leukemoid reactions
- Atlantoaxial instability becomes an issue later in life

DIAGNOSIS

Karyotype.

TREATMENT

- Early childhood intervention to maximize social and intellectual capacity
- Life skills training
- Surgery for correction of cardiac and duodenal defects
- At risk for atlantoaxial dislocation and cervical cord compression
- Increased risk for leukemia and respiratory tract infections

Trisomy 18 (Edwards' Syndrome)

ETIOLOGY

- Most common type is complete trisomy.
- Small percentage are due to mosaicism.

EPIDEMIOLOGY

One in 8,000 live births.

SIGNS AND SYMPTOMS

- Prominent occiput
- Low-set ears
- Small mouth
- Short sternum
- Thumb and radius agenesis/hypoplasia
- Camptodactyly (little finger fixed in flexion)
- Redundancy of cardiac valve leaflets
- Hypertonia
- Seizures

TREATMENT

- Supportive.
- Few survive the newborn period. Most common cause of death is apnea.
- Those who survive are severely mentally retarded.

Trisomy 13 (Patau's Syndrome)

ETIOLOGY

- 75% complete trisomy
- 23% Robertsonian translocation (to chromosome 14)
- 4% mosaicism

EPIDEMIOLOGY

One in 10,000 live births.

SIGNS AND SYMPTOMS

- Holoprosencephaly (failure of telencephalon to divide into two hemi-spheres, resulting in large central ventricle; brain assumes configuration of a fluid-filled ball)
- Microphthalmia
- Midline facial cleft
- Polydactyly
- Scalp cutis aplasia
- Cystic kidneys
- Rocker bottom feet
- VSD

TREATMENT

- Supportive
- Similar prognosis to Edwards' syndrome

SEX CHROMOSOME ANOMALIES

Turner's Syndrome

ETIOLOGY

45,XO—missing one X chromosome.

EPIDEMIOLOGY

One in 2,000 to 5,000 live female births.

RISK FACTORS

Not related to advanced maternal age.

SIGNS AND SYMPTOMS

- Short stature
- Phenotypically female
- Pterygium colli (webbed neck)
- Small mandible
- Narrow maxilla
- Epicanthal folds
- Increased distance between nipples
- Pedal edema
- Cubitus valgus
- Impaired hearing
- Delay in motor skill development
- Coarctation of the aorta
- Ovarian dysgenesis

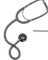

Turner's syndrome is the most common cause of primary amenorrhea.

Typical Scenario

A newborn infant has lymphedema of the hands and feet, extra skin folds at a short neck, widely spaced nipples, and decreased femoral pulses. *Think:* Gonadal dysgenesis (45,X) Turner's syndrome, and do a chromosomal analysis to confirm the diagnosis.

- May consider exogenous growth hormone to promote growth.
- Monitor for autoimmune hypothyroidism.
- Refer to an endocrinologist for induction of puberty at an appropriate age.
- Resection of any intra-abdominal gonads to prevent malignancy.

Klinefelter's Syndrome

ETIOLOGY

- Presence of an extra X chromosome in males
- 47,XXY most common
- 48,XXXY or more also seen

EPIDEMIOLOGY

One in 3,000 males.

RISK FACTORS

Advanced maternal age.

SIGNS AND SYMPTOMS

- Hypogonadism
- Azoospermia (absence of sperm)
- Tall stature (eunuchoid)
- Female hair distribution
- Learning disabilities
- Delay of motor skill development
- Presence of inactivated X chromosome (Barr body)

TREATMENT

- Administration of testosterone during puberty to improve secondary sex characteristics.
- Interventions for developmental delays/learning disabilities.

Angelman's Syndrome

ETIOLOGY

- 75% due to **maternal** deletion 15q11 → q13 (see Prader–Willi syndrome)
- 23% chromosome 15 mutations

EPIDEMIOLOGY

One in 20,000.

SIGNS AND SYMPTOMS

- Happy, laughing disposition—previously known as the "happy puppet" or "marionette joyeuse" syndrome, because of this and stereotyped flapping of hands
- Often strikingly attractive children with lighter pigmentation than other family members (often blond-haired, blue-eyed)
- Mental retardation
- Microcephaly
- Ataxia
- Hypotonia (ataxia and hypotonia create the characteristic "puppet"-like gait)
- Epilepsy (80%) with characteristic electroencephalographic (EEG) findings
- Complete absence of speech
- Unusual facies characterized by a large mandible and open-mouthed expression revealing tongue
- Strabismus

The same chromosomal deletion causes Angelman's syndrome and Prader–Willi syndrome. The only difference is that in Angelman's the missing genetic material is maternal, and in Prader–Willi, paternal.

- Supportive.
- Seizures are often refractory to anticonvulsant therapy.
- Normal life span.

Prader–Willi Syndrome

ETIOLOGY

- Genetic
  - 75% **paternal** deletion 15q11 → q13 (see Angelman's syndrome)
  - 25% maternal disomy
- Hyperphagia/lack of satiety, decreased caloric requirement secondary to hypotonia/decreased movement, and obsessions/compulsions that focus on food all contribute to the vicious cycle leading to obesity in these patients.

EPIDEMIOLOGY

One in 20,000.

SIGNS AND SYMPTOMS

- Hypotonia and poor feeding
- Precocious puberty
- Micropenis
- Obesity, hyperphagia
- Mild mental retardation
- Sleep disturbances
- Lighter pigmentation than other family members
- Significant behavioral problems (stubborn, manipulative, aggressive)
- Fluent speech
- Obsessive/compulsive traits

TREATMENT

- Strict diet and behavioral interventions to prevent obesity.
- Growth hormone to promote stature, and other timely hormone supplementation to promote secondary sex characteristics.
- Patients develop complications from obesity that limit their life span.
- Early prevention of obesity is the key to quality and quantity of life in these patients.

XYY males

EPIDEMIOLOGY

Increased frequency in inmates of penal institutions (reasons are controversial).

SIGNS AND SYMPTOMS

- Normal or low-normal intelligence
- Phenotypically normal
- Tall
- Severe acne
- Rarely, antisocial behavior

XXX Syndrome

DEFINITION

47,XXX.

ETIOLOGY

More than half the time, this is caused by maternal meiotic nondisjunction.

EPIDEMIOLOGY

Most common X chromosome abnormality in women.

- Phenotypically normal female, with normal sexual development and menarche
- Marked variability in severity of speech and language delays, lack of coordination, and poor academic performance
- May be gangly and tall and have behavior disorders

XXXX or XXXXX

SIGNS AND SYMPTOMS

- Usually mentally retarded, worse with increasing number of X chromosomes
- Associated with epicanthal folds, hypertelorism, clinodactyly, transverse palmar creases, radioulnar synostosis, and congenital heart disease
- Often incomplete sexual maturation
- Often tall with XXXX; short stature with XXXXX

Noonan's Syndrome

DEFINITION

46,XX or 46,XY.

ETIOLOGY

Maps to chromosome 12.

EPIDEMIOLOGY

- Sporadic or autosomal dominant.
- Males = Females

SIGNS AND SYMPTOMS

- Similar characteristics to Turner's syndrome:
  - Facies—triangular-shaped face, hypertelorism, down-slanting eyes, ptosis, strabismus, amblyopia, refractive errors, low-set ears with thickened helices, high nasal bridge, short webbed neck
  - Pectus carinatum/excavatum, scoliosis
  - Cardiac—often pulmonary stenosis, ASD
  - Assorted skeletal abnormalities
  - Skin—lymphedema, prominent pads of digits
  - Neurologic—hypotonia
- Mental retardation (25%)
- Delayed sexual maturation, premature ovarian failure; more than half of male patients have undescended testes

Fragile X Syndrome

ETIOLOGY

X-linked dominant.

EPIDEMIOLOGY

- One in 2,000 births
- Males = females

RISK FACTORS

Family history.

SIGNS AND SYMPTOMS

- Mental retardation
- Macroorchidism in boys
- Protruding ears
- Triangular, elongated facies

Patients with Noonan's syndrome have a normal karyotype, unlike those with Turner's syndrome.

There is a combined neurofibromatosis I/Noonan's syndrome, which maps to the NF1 region on chromosome 17.

HIGH-YIELD FACTS

Congenital Malformations and Chromosomal Anomalies

- Flat malar bones
- Shyness, autistic behavior, avoidance of eye contact

Alport's Syndrome

- Rare, X-linked recessive disorder of basement membranes of the kidney, eye, and ear
- Glomerulonephritis, end-stage renal disease by age 40 (men)
- Hearing loss

Typical Scenario

Male adolescent presents with hematuria, proteinuria, and decreased hearing. *Think:* Alport's syndrome (rare disorder but not rare on shelf exams).

AUTOSOMAL DOMINANT CONDITIONS

- People in every generation are affected.
- Examples include adult polycystic kidney disease, familial hypercholesterolemia, Marfan's syndrome, neurofibromatosis-1 (von Recklinghausen's disease), von Hippel–Lindau, Huntington's disease, familial adenomatous polyposis, and hereditary spherocytosis.

AUTOSOMAL RECESSIVE CONDITIONS

- Skips generations (often a grandparent has had a similar condition).
- Examples include cystic fibrosis and many enzyme deficiencies/metabolic disorders.
- History of early deaths from unknown disorders or multiple miscarriages.
- Consanguinity really increases the odds—you must ask if the parents are blood relatives.

X-LINKED RECESSIVE CONDITIONS

- Only males are affected; females are unaffected or only partially affected (due to lyonization) carriers of the trait.
- Examples include Duchenne and Becker muscular dystrophies, hemophilia A and B, Fabry's disease, glucose-6-phosphate dehydrogenase (G6PD) deficiency, Hunter's syndrome, ocular albinism, red–green color blindness, and Alport's syndrome.

CONGENITAL ANOMALIES

Polydactyly

DEFINITION

Presence of more than five fingers or toes, which may be rudimentary to fully developed.

ETIOLOGY

- May occur as an isolated defect (whether genetic, toxic, or mechanical) or in conjunction with syndromes such as:
  - Ellis–van Creveld syndrome—with congenital heart disease
  - Bardet–Biedl syndrome—with obesity, pigmentary retinopathy, mental retardation, hypogonadism, and renal failure
  - Meckel–Gruber syndrome—triad of occipital encephalocele, large polycystic kidneys, and postaxial polydactyly. Associated abnormalities include oral clefting, genital anomalies, CNS malformations, fibrosis of the liver, and pulmonary hypoplasia.

The X chromosome lyonizes randomly early in embryogenesis when there are relatively few cells. Since all daughter cells lyonize the same X, the odds that a significantly disproportionate inactivation of the "good" X will occur in carrier females, while small, are not infinitesimal. When this occurs, the carrier is affected, and the mechanism is termed *unfortunate lyonization*.

DIAGNOSIS
Observation, x-ray, fetal sonogram.

TREATMENT
Surgery, usually at 1 year of age.

Syndactyly

DEFINITION
Webbing or fusing of two or more fingers or toes. May be bony and/or cutaneous. Often looked for between the second and third toes.

PATHOPHYSIOLOGY
Failure of cell apoptosis between digits during development.

TREATMENT
Surgery.

Craniosynostosis

DEFINITION
- Premature closing of one or more cranial sutures due to abnormalities of skull development
- Can be primary skull/bone defect or a result of failure of brain growth

ETIOLOGY
May occur alone or in conjunction with syndromes such as:
- Apert's syndrome
- Chotzen's syndrome
- Pfeiffer's syndrome
- Carpenter's syndrome
- Crouzon's syndrome

SIGNS AND SYMPTOMS
Early closure of fontanels and sutures.

COMPLICATIONS
- Hydrocephalus
- Increased intracranial pressure (ICP)
- Developmental delay

TREATMENT
- Craniotomy to prevent intracranial and ophthalmologic complications
- Multidisciplinary approach—genetics, psychology, pediatrics, surgery, neurology
- Genetic counseling
- Long-term follow-up

Amniotic Bands

DEFINITION
Fibrous strands of membrane stretching across chorionic cavity.

EPIDEMIOLOGY
Not associated with problems in future pregnancies.

ETIOLOGY
- Spontaneous

- Associated with abdominal trauma
- May be associated with chorionic villus sampling (CVS)

PATHOPHYSIOLOGY

Caused by early amnion rupture and leakage of chorionic fluid.

SIGNS AND SYMPTOMS

- May be innocent and not cause any harm to the fetus
- Can lead to limb or other body part constriction or amputation
- May be associated with oligohydramnios and decreased fetal movement

DIAGNOSIS

Ultrasound.

TREATMENT

Most bands disappear on their own, not appearing on follow-up ultrasound.

Cleft Palate/Lip

DEFINITION

- Spectrum of defects of the upper lip, philtrum, and hard and soft palates
- Cleft lip, cleft palate, or both
- Unilateral or bilateral

EPIDEMIOLOGY

- Fourth most common birth defect
- Occur more often in infants of Asian, Latino, or Native American descent

ETIOLOGY

- Teratogens—ethanol, anticonvulsants, steroids, chemotherapy, maternal vitamin A excess
- Gestational factors—maternal diabetes, amniotic bands
- Chromosomal abnormalities
- Idiopathic

PATHOPHYSIOLOGY

- Clefting of lip and anterior (primary) palate due to defect in fusing of both maxillary processes with the frontonasal process during weeks 5 and 6.
- Clefting of posterior (secondary) palate due to defect in fusion of palatal shelves during weeks 7 and 8.

SIGNS AND SYMPTOMS

Can affect feeding, speech, illness (colds and ear infections), teething, hearing, and emotional coping.

DIAGNOSIS

Physical exam of lips, palate, and oropharynx.

TREATMENT

- Infants with cleft palate may require assistance with feeding.
- Surgical repair of lip within first months of life; palate around 1 year of life; potential for final repairs and scar revisions in adolescence.
- Cleft team can include plastic and oral surgeons; geneticist; ear, nose, and throat (ENT) specialist; dentist; speech pathologist; audiologist; social worker or psychologist; and nurse coordinator.
- Genetic counseling.

Omphalocele

DEFINITION

Herniation of abdominal contents (usually only intestine, though can include liver and/or spleen) through umbilical root, which is covered only by peritoneum.

EPIDEMIOLOGY

May be associated with other congenital defects, including chromosomal anomalies, heart defects, and diaphragmatic hernia.

DIAGNOSIS

Some may be detected on prenatal ultrasounds.

TREATMENT

- Until any other, more serious conditions have been taken care of, the extruded contents are covered.
- Serial reductions of intestines back into abdomen until skin closure is possible.

Oligohydramnios

DEFINITION

Abnormally small amount of amniotic fluid (amniotic fluid index [AFI] < 5.0 cm or single pocket of fluid < 2 cm).

ETIOLOGY

- Premature rupture of membranes (PROM)
- Intrauterine growth retardation (IUGR)
- Postdates pregnancy
- Renal anomalies (e.g., bilateral renal agenesis, multicystic dysplastic kidneys, posterior urethral valves)
- Other congenital anomalies (e.g., aneuploidy)
- Placental abruption
- Twin–twin transfusion
- Iatrogenic—nonsteroidal prostaglandin synthetase inhibitors, first-trimester chorionic villus sampling, second-trimester amniocentesis; amniotic fluid level may return to normal
- Idiopathic

PATHOPHYSIOLOGY

Amniotic fluid is regulated by fetal urine, as well as fetal oral secretions and respiratory secretions. Any process disrupting this exchange of fluid can lead to pathological amniotic fluid levels.

COMPLICATIONS

- Fetal demise
- Pulmonary hypoplasia
- Facial deformities
- Skeletal deformities (e.g., compressed thorax, twisted feet)

Potter's Syndrome

- Potter's syndrome specifically refers to bilateral renal agenesis, though other renal anomalies leading to oligohydramnios have also used the eponym.

In a normal pregnancy, there are approximately 600 mL of amniotic fluid surrounding the baby at 40 weeks' gestation.

Isolated third-trimester oligohydramnios is not necessarily associated with poor perinatal outcome.

- Potter's syndrome includes pulmonary hypoplasia, skeletal anomalies, and characteristic facies (sloping forehead; flattened nose; recessed chin; and lowset, floppy ears).
- It is incompatible with neonatal life.

DIAGNOSIS

- Amniotic fluid index (AFI)—sum of the maximum vertical pocket of amniotic fluid in each quadrant of the uterus
- Best to use average of three readings

TREATMENT

- Depends on etiology.
- First goal is to remove the inciting cause or correct the underlying problem (e.g., discontinue prostaglandin inhibitor, place a shunt).
- Measures to prepare fetus for possible premature birth (corticosteroids and antibiotics for PROM).
- Antepartum testing to determine appropriate time for delivery in IUGR.

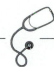

Patients with second-trimester oligohydramnios have a higher prevalence of congenital anomalies and a lower fetal survival rate than those women with oligohydramnios in the third trimester.

Hypospadias

DEFINITION

Improper location of urethral meatus, not at tip of penis, but on underside of penis, even as far back as the scrotum.

ETIOLOGY

Hereditary—if father has, there is a 20% chance that child will.

SIGNS AND SYMPTOMS

- Curvature of penis downwards
- Potentially may have to sit down to urinate

DIAGNOSIS

Clinical, though radiologic studies may be necessary if other congenital defects possibly present.

TREATMENT

- Surgical correction to extend urethra to end of penis before 18 months of age and chordae repair if sexual function will be affected by bent erect penis.
- May require more than one operation.
- Beware of postop bleeding, infections, stenosis, and fistulae.

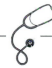

Infants with hypospadias should not be circumcised at birth, as the foreskin may be useful in the repair.

Metabolic Disease

INBORN ERRORS OF METABOLISM

DEFINITION

Inherited biochemical disorders.

PATHOPHYSIOLOGY

Mutations affecting proteins involved in the many metabolic pathways of the body.

EPIDEMIOLOGY

Disorders involving deficiencies of enzymes are often autosomal recessive (please see noted exceptions in this chapter).

SIGNS AND SYMPTOMS

- Often normal at birth, but can show signs early, including metabolic acidosis, poor feeding, vomiting, lethargy, and convulsion.
- Mental retardation, organomegaly, unusual bodily odors, episodic decompensation.

DIAGNOSIS

- Many can be detected in the neonatal period or infancy, and some are included in newborn screening.
- Usually involves laboratory studies.

TREATMENT

- Treatment varies but is often supportive/symptomatic.
- Frequently includes dietary modifications.

DEFECTS OF AMINO ACID METABOLISM

See Table 8-1.

Phenylketonuria (PKU)

DEFINITION

Inherited disorder of amino acid metabolism in which phenylalanine cannot be converted to tyrosine.

ETIOLOGY

Deficiency of phenylalanine hydroxylase (or its cofactor tetrahydrobiopterin).

83

TABLE 8-1. Disorders of amino acid metabolism

Disease	Accumulation	Deficiency	Distinctive Feature	
Phenylketonuria (PKU)	Phenylalanine and metabolites	Usually phenylalanine hydroxylase	Fair hair and skin, blue eyes, mousy odor	AR
Homocystinemia/ Homocystinuria	Homocystine, methionine	Usually cystathionine synthase	Ectopia lentis	AR
Maple syrup urine disease (MSUD)	Branched-chain amino acids: leucine, isoleucine, valine	Branched-chain ketoacid dehydrogenase	Odor of maple syrup in urine, sweat, cerumen	AR
Hartnup's disease	Deficiency of neutral amino acids: tryptophan	Sodium-dependent amino acid transport system in renal tubules and intestines	Most are asymptomatic	AR

Phenylketones: phenyl-acetate, -lactate, and -pyruvate, in urine.

Aspartame (Nutrasweet) contains phenylalanine.

Decreased pigmentation in PKU is secondary to the inhibition of tyrosinase by phenylalanine.

Lethargy, anorexia, anemia, rashes, and diarrhea are signs of tyrosine deficiency.

PATHOPHYSIOLOGY

- Accumulation of phenylalanine and its phenylketone metabolites disrupt normal metabolism and cause brain damage.
- Tyrosine becomes essential amino acid.

EPIDEMIOLOGY

- Autosomal recessive
- One in 10,000 to 20,000 live births

SIGNS AND SYMPTOMS

- Normal at birth
- Mental retardation, fair hair and skin, blue eyes, eczema, mousy/musty body odor

DIAGNOSIS

- Serum tested 72 hours after initiation of first protein feed (test may be negative prior to 72 hours).
- If not screened neonatally, diagnosis usually made at 4 to 6 months of age.
- Prenatal and carrier testing possible.

TREATMENT

Limit dietary phenylalanine (e.g., in artificial sweeteners) and increase tyrosine.

Homocystinemia/Homocystinuria

DEFINITION

Inherited disorder of amino acid metabolism in which homocysteine is present in greater than trace amounts in the urine.

ETIOLOGY

Most commonly a deficiency of cystathionine synthase, but can also be a defect of methylcobalamin formation or deficiency of methyltetrahydrofolate reductase.

PATHOPHYSIOLOGY

Homocysteine is not remethylated to methionine (see Figure 8-1).

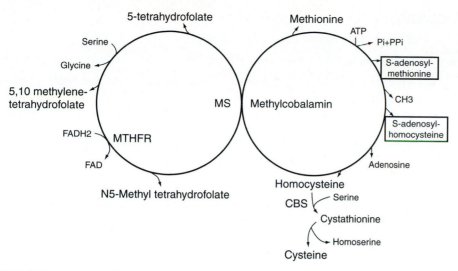

FIGURE 8-1. Homocysteine pathway.

EPIDEMIOLOGY

Autosomal recessive.

SIGNS AND SYMPTOMS

- Depends on particular enzyme deficiency.
- Most commonly normal at birth, with failure to thrive and developmental delay subsequently occurring.
- Later, ectopia lentis, marfanoid body habitus, progressive mental retardation, vaso-occlusive disease, osteoporosis, or fair skin with malar flush can occur.

DIAGNOSIS

- Normal at birth; diagnosis usually made after 3 years of age
- Elevated methionine and homocystine in body fluids
- Prenatal diagnosis possible

TREATMENT

- High-dose vitamin B_6 (may require concurrent folic acid to show response).
- Restriction of methionine intake and supplementation of cysteine.
- Betaine if unresponsive to B_6 therapy.
- Other types may require vitamin B_{12} or methionine supplementation.

Maple Syrup Urine Disease (MSUD)

DEFINITION

Inherited disorder of branched-chain amino acid metabolism in which elevated quantities of leucine, isoleucine, valine, and corresponding oxoacids accumulate in the body fluids.

ETIOLOGY

Deficiency of branched-chain ketoacid dehydrogenase.

PATHOPHYSIOLOGY

Defect in the decarboxylation of leucine, isoleucine, and valine by a branched-chain ketoacid dehydrogenase.

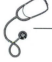

Ectopia lentis is subluxation of the lens, signaled by iridodonesis (quivering of iris) and myopia.
Late complications:
- Astigmatism
- Optic atrophy
- Glaucoma
- Cataracts
- Retinal detachment

Branched-chain amino acids are: leucine, isoleucine, valine.

In MSUD, plasma leucine levels are usually higher than those of the other accumulating branched amino acids.

Correcting the serum glucose level in MSUD does not improve the clinical state.

Urinary proline, hydroxyproline, and arginine remain normal in Hartnup's disease (unlike in other causes of generalized aminoaciduria, such as Fanconi's).

EPIDEMIOLOGY

One in 290,000 live births.

SIGNS AND SYMPTOMS

- Deficiency of different subunits of enzyme account for wide clinical variability.
- Poor feeding, vomiting in first week of life, proceeding to lethargy and coma.
- Alternating hypertonicity and flaccidity, convulsions, hypoglycemia.
- Odor of maple syrup in urine, sweat, cerumen.

DIAGNOSIS

- Elevated plasma and urine levels if leucine, isoleucine, valine, and alloisoleucine; decreased plasma alanine.
- Urine precipitant test.
- Neuroimaging in the acute state shows cerebral edema.

TREATMENT

- Chronically, low branched-chain amino acid diet
- Frequent serum level monitoring
- Acutely, intravenous administration of amino acids other than branched-chain

Hartnup's Disease

DEFINITION

Inherited defect in transport of neutral amino acids by intestinal mucosa and renal tubules.

ETIOLOGY

Deficient activity of a sodium-dependent transport system.

PATHOPHYSIOLOGY

Deficiency of tryptophan results in the clinical manifestations.

EPIDEMIOLOGY

Autosomal recessive.

SIGNS AND SYMPTOMS

- Usually asymptomatic.
- Rarely, cutaneous photosensitivity, episodic psychiatric changes.
- Marginal nutrition results in clinical manifestations in predisposed individuals.

DIAGNOSIS

- Aminoaciduria (neutral: alanine, serine, threonine, valine, leucine, isoleucine, phenylalanine, tyrosine, tryptophan, histidine)
- Normal plasma amino acid levels

TREATMENT

Nicotinic acid/nicotinamide and a high-protein diet in symptomatic patients.

DEFECTS OF LIPID METABOLISM—LYSOSOMAL STORAGE DISEASES

Lipidoses

See Table 8-2.

TABLE 8-2. Lysosomal storage diseases—lipidoses.

Disease	Deficiency/Accumulation	Feature	Inheritance
GM1 gangliosidoses	■ Deficiency of β-galactosidase ■ Accumulation of GM1 ganglioside	■ Infantile, juvenile, adult forms ■ 50% cherry red spot on macula ■ Hepatosplenomegaly ■ Rashes, edema, psychomotor retardation ■ Coarse facial features, skeletal abnormalities ■ Blind and deaf by 1 year, death by 3 to 4 years of age	AR
GM2 gangliosidoses	*Tay–Sachs disease:* ■ Deficiency of hexoseaminidase A ■ Results in accumulation of GM2 ganglioside in brain *Sandhoff disease:* ■ Accumulation of GM2 ganglioside in brain and peripheral organs ■ Defect of hexoseaminidases A + B	■ Infantile and juvenile forms ■ Diagnosis at 5–6 months, death by 3 years of age ■ Cherry red spot on macula ■ Hyperacusis (exaggerated startle response) ■ Froglike position ■ No organomegaly in Tay–Sachs ■ Hepatosplenomegaly in Sandhoff disease	AR Ashkenazi Jews (Tay–Sachs)
Niemann–Pick (six subtypes)	■ Deficiency of sphingomyelinase ■ Accumulation of sphingomyelin and cholesterol in reticuloendothelial and parenchymal cells	■ 50% cherry red spot on macula ■ Hepatosplenomegaly ■ Diagnosis by 4 months, death by 3 years of age ■ Varying neurologic signs/deterioration	AR Ashkenazi Jews
Gaucher's	■ Deficiency of β-glucosidase ■ Accumulation of glucocerebroside in reticuloendothelial system	■ Affects brain, liver, spleen, bone marrow ■ Pancytopenia ■ Bone fractures, pain, avascular necrosis ■ Gaucher cells—"crinkled paper" cytoplasm ■ Infantile form—rapid neurologic deterioration ■ Adult form—more common, normal life span	AR
Fabry's	■ Deficiency of ceramide trihexosidase or α-galactosidase A ■ Accumulation of glycosphingolipids in vascular endothelium, nerves, and organs	■ Angiokeratomas (dark, red, punctate macules that do not blanch, occur in clusters, some become papules, distribution in bilateral and symmetric, naval and buttocks most common) ■ Progressive kidney failure (biopsy shows lipid) ■ Neuropathy, vascular disease ■ Ocular opacities	X-linked recessive
Krabbe's (globoid cell leuko-dystrophy)	■ Deficiency of galactosyl-ceramide β-galactosidase or galacto-cerebrosidase ■ Accumulation of ceramide galactose within lysosomes of brain white matter	■ Progressive central nervous system degeneration ■ Optic atrophy, spasticity, early death ■ Globoid cells in areas of demyelination (distended, multinucleated bodies found in basal ganglia, pontine nuclei, and cerebellar white matter)	AR
Farber's	■ Deficiency of ceramidase ■ Accumulation of ceramide in peripheral organs, joints, and lymph nodes	■ Normal at birth, diagnosis at 1 year ■ Nodules (granulomas containing ceramide) on joints, vocal cords (hoarseness, respiratory complications)	AR

AR, autosomal recessive.

DEFINITION/ETIOLOGY/PATHOPHYSIOLOGY

Inherited deficiencies of lysosomal hydrolases cause lysosomal accumulation of sphingolipids in brain and viscera.

EPIDEMIOLOGY

Most are autosomal recessive.

SIGNS AND SYMPTOMS

- Depends on site of abnormal accumulations:
  - Nervous system—neurodegeneration, ocular findings
  - Viscera—organomegaly, skeletal abnormalities, pulmonary infiltration

DIAGNOSIS

Measurement of specific enzymatic activity in leukocytes or cultured fibroblasts.

TREATMENT

- Usually no specific treatment
- Supportive/symptomatic therapy

Mucopolysaccharidoses (see Table 8-3)

DEFINITION/ETIOLOGY/PATHOPHYSIOLOGY

Inherited deficiencies of lysosomal enzymes needed for the degradation of glycosaminoglycans (GAGs) resulting in widespread lysosomal storage of dermatan and heparan sulfates and severe clinical abnormalities. Keratan sulfates accumulate in other mucopolysaccharidoses not mentioned.

EPIDEMIOLOGY

Most are autosomal recessive.

SIGNS AND SYMPTOMS

- Normal at birth, diagnosis at 1+ years
- "Gargoyle" cells containing lysosomes engorged with mucopolysaccharide
- Excessive urinary excretion of GAGs
- Progressive mental and physical deterioration
- Coarse features
- Corneal clouding
- Stiff joints (abnormal hyalinization of collagen)
- Organomegaly
- Skeletal abnormalities

Fabry's is X-linked recessive.

Gangliosidoses (e.g., GM1 and Tay–Sachs) have cherry red spot on macula in 50% of cases as does Niemann–Pick.

Hepatosplenomegaly occurs in the GM1 gangliosidoses and Sandhoff disease, but not in Tay–Sachs disease.

Hunter's syndrome is X-linked recessive.

TABLE 8-3. Lysosomal storage diseases—mucopolysaccharidoses.

Syndrome	Deficiency	Distinctive Features	Inheritance
Hurler's	α-L-iduronidase	Severe, progressive, death by 10 years of age Mental retardation, heart disease, corneal clouding, organomegaly Dystosis multiplex, obstructive airway disease Enlarged tongue, hearing loss, limited language	AR
Scheie's (milder form of Hurler's)	α-L-iduronidase	Normal intelligence and life span Corneal clouding, stiff joints, aortic regurgitation	AR
Hunter's	Iduronate sulfatase	Mild to severe, death before 15 years in severe form Dystosis multiplex, mental retardation, organomegaly	X-linked recessive

AR, autosomal recessive.

Diagnosis

- Detection of enzyme deficiency in leukocytes or cultured fibroblasts
- Roentgenographic changes consistent with dystosis multiplex
- Urinary excretion of dermatan and heparan sulfates

Treatment

Supportive therapy. Hurler's can be treated with bone marrow transplant.

DEFECTS OF CARBOHYDRATE METABOLISM—GLYCOGEN STORAGE DISEASES

See Table 8-4.

Von Gierke's Disease

Definition

Inherited disorder of glycogen metabolism characterized by deposition of glycogen in the *liver*, *kidney*, and *intestine*.

Etiology

Deficiency of glucose-6-phosphatase.

Pathophysiology

Glycogen-to-glucose metabolism stops at glucose-6-phosphate.

Epidemiology

Autosomal recessive.

Signs and Symptoms

- Massive hepatomegaly
- Hypoglycemia
- Elevated serum levels of lactate, uric acid, cholesterol, triglycerides
- Renal complications (Fanconi's, nephrocalcinosis, focal segmental glomerulosclerosis)

Diagnosis

- Normal at birth, diagnosis usually at 5 months.
- Administration of epinephrine, glucagons, galactose, fructose, or glycerol does not provoke normal hyperglycemic response.
- Tests may precipitate acidosis.
- Liver biopsy demonstrates accumulation of glycogen in cells.

Treatment

- Supportive therapy
- Frequent, high-carbohydrate meals
- Avoid fasting

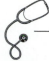

Dystosis multiplex
- Large dolichocephalic skull
- Thickened calvarium
- Ovoid vertebral bodies
- Flared iliac bones
- Shallow acetabulae
- Irregular widening of long bones

— **Typical Scenario** —

A 3-month-old, breast-fed infant has failure to thrive, severe hepatomegaly, thin extremities, fasting hypoglycemia, lipemia, and metabolic acidosis. *Think:* von Gierke's.

TABLE 8-4. Glycogen storage diseases.

Disease	Glycogen Accumulation	Deficiency	Type
Von Gierke's	Liver, kidney, and intestine	Glucose-6-phosphatase	I
McArdle's	Skeletal muscle	Skeletal muscle glycogen phosphorylase	V
Pompe's	Cardiac and skeletal muscle	α-1,4-glucosidase (acid maltase)	II

- Macrophage colony stimulating factors to combat neutropenia and inflammation
- Allopurinol to lower urate levels
- Transplant/hemodialysis for renal failure

McArdle's Disease

DEFINITION

Inherited disorder of glycogen metabolism characterized by deposition of glycogen in skeletal muscle.

ETIOLOGY

Deficiency of muscle glycogen phosphorylase (myophosphorylase).

EPIDEMIOLOGY

Autosomal recessive.

SIGNS AND SYMPTOMS

- Temporary weakness and cramping of skeletal muscles after exercise
- No rise in blood lactate during ischemic exercise
- Characteristic "second wind" with initiation of fatty acid metabolism

DIAGNOSIS

- Asymptomatic during infancy.
- Muscle biopsy and assay show deficiency of enzyme.
- Myoglobinuria, elevated CK after exercise

TREATMENT

Dietary modification (high fat and protein); supportive therapy.

Pompe's Disease

DEFINITION

Inherited disorder of glycogen metabolism characterized by deposition of glycogen in cardiac and skeletal muscle.

ETIOLOGY

Deficiency of acid α-1,4-glucosidase.

PATHOPHYSIOLOGY

- Generalized glycogenesis because the defect is in all cells
- Results in inability to convert mannose to glucose

EPIDEMIOLOGY

Autosomal recessive.

SIGNS AND SYMPTOMS

- Rapid, progressive cardiomyopathy with massive cardiomegaly, macroglossia, hypotonia, hepatomegaly, death by 1 to 2 years
- Juvenile form milder, slowly progressive myopathy, little to no cardiac abnormality

DIAGNOSIS

Electrocardiogram (ECG), electromyogram (EMG).

TREATMENT

No specific treatment; supportive therapy.

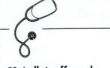

McArdle's affects the Muscles.

Pompe's affects the "Pump."

Galactosemia

DEFINITION

Inborn errors of carbohydrate metabolism that result in elevated galactose and metabolite levels in blood and urine.

ETIOLOGY

Three types:

- Classic: Absence of galactose-1-phosphate uridyltransferase
- Others: Galactokinase, uridine diphosphate galactose-4-epimerase

PATHOPHYSIOLOGY

- Ingestion of galactose leads to increased concentrations in the blood and urine.
- Toxic substances, including galactitol, cause organ damage.

EPIDEMIOLOGY

- Autosomal recessive
- One in 60,000

SIGNS AND SYMPTOMS

Cataracts, hepatosplenomegaly, mental retardation.

DIAGNOSIS

- Should be considered in newborn, infant, or child if jaundice, hepatomegaly, vomiting, hypoglycemia, convulsions, lethargy, irritability, feeding difficulties, poor weight gain, aminoaciduria, cataracts, vitreous hemorrhage, hepatic cirrhosis, ascites, splenomegaly, or mental retardation are noted.
- Demonstrate reducing substance in urine after administration of human or cow's milk.

TREATMENT

Exclude galactose and lactose from diet.

Fructosuria

DEFINITION

Inborn errors of carbohydrate metabolism that result in elevated fructose and metabolite levels in blood and urine.

ETIOLOGY

Deficiency of fructokinase.

PATHOPHYSIOLOGY

- Enzyme is normally found in the liver, kidney, and intestine.
- Ingested fructose is not metabolized.

EPIDEMIOLOGY

Autosomal recessive.

SIGNS AND SYMPTOMS

- Asymptomatic until fructose introduced into diet
- Fructosemia and fructosuria

Lactose = galactose + glucose.

Typical Scenario

A 2-week-old neonate has jaundice, hepatomegaly, and positive urinary-reducing substance. Odor of urine is normal. *Think:* Galactosemia.

When diagnosis of galactosemia is not made at birth, damage to the liver and brain become irreversible.

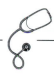

Neonates with galactosemia are at increased risk for *Escherichia coli* sepsis.

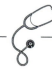

Elimination of galactose from diet in galactosemia does not ensure reversal of cataract formation.

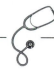

There is almost no renal threshold for fructose.

DIAGNOSIS

Presence of urinary-reducing substrate without clinical symptoms.

TREATMENT

None indicated.

DEFECTS IN PURINE METABOLISM

Lesch–Nyhan Syndrome

DEFINITION

An X-linked disorder of purine metabolism resulting in deposition of purines in tissues and subsequent clinical abnormalities.

ETIOLOGY

Deficiency of *hypoxanthine–guanine phosphoribosyl transferase (HGPRT)*.

SIGNS AND SYMPTOMS

- Retardation of motor development, spastic cerebral palsy, self-injurious behavior
- Hyperuricemia, uricosuria, urinary tract calculi, nephropathy, tophi, gouty arthritis

DIAGNOSIS

- Normal at birth, diagnosis usually made at 3 months when delayed motor development becomes apparent.
- Serum uric acid levels.

TREATMENT

- No specific treatment; supportive therapy
- Allopurinol to reduce serum uric acid levels
- Prevention of self-injury

Self-injurious behavior in Lesch–Nyhan syndrome can include banging head against wall and biting/mutilating one's fingers.

FAMILIAL HYPERCHOLESTEROLEMIAS

See Table 8-5.

Table 8-5. Familial hyperlipidemias.

Disorder	Lipids	Clinical Manifestations	Treatment	Deficiency
Hypercholesterol-emia (type II hyperlipopro-teinemia)	■ Large elevations in serum cholesterol (> 500 mg/dL) ■ Heterozygous form is common: ~1:500 ■ Homozygous form is very rare: ~1:1,000,000	■ Tendinous xanthomata ■ Early atherosclerotic cardiovascular disease (late childhood/early adulthood myocardial infarction)	■ Statins and cholestyramine for heterozygous form ■ Liver transplant for rare homozygous form	Genetic defect in low-density lipoprotein (LDL) receptor
Hyperchylo-micronemia (type I hyperlipo-proteinemia)	■ Accumulation of chylomicrons ■ Low/normal LDL ■ Serum grossly milky	■ Eruptive xanthomata ■ Periodic severe abdominal pain (pancreatitis) starting in infancy (colic) ■ No atherosclerotic disease	■ Very-low-fat diet may resolve xanthomatosis and reduce the risk of painful (and sometimes fatal) crises	AR (rarer than type II) Deficiency of lipoprotein lipase or cofactor apolipoprotein C-II
Dysbetalipo-proteinemia	■ Absent chylomicrons ■ Abnormal very-low-density lipoprotein (VLDL) and LDL ■ Increased cholesterol and triglycerides (TGs) ■ Cholesterol: TG ratio may equal 1	■ Planar xanthomata ■ Peripheral vascular disease	■ Weight loss, diet, exercise ■ Adults with persistent elevations treated with fibric acid derivatives	Abnormal apolipoprotein E
Endogenous hyper-triglyceridemia	■ Increased VLDL	■ Obesity, glucose intolerance ■ Insulin resistance ■ Hyperinsulinemia ■ Hyperuricemia	■ Weight control ■ Dietary modification	Overproduction or reduced clearance of VLDL

Immunologic Disease

IMMUNE SYSTEM

- Primary lymphoid organs—development of lymphocytes: bone marrow, thymus, fetal liver and spleen.
- Secondary lymphoid tissue—mature lymphocytes interact with antigen: lymph nodes, spleen, mucosal-associated lymphoid tissues (MALT), and gut-associated lymphoid tissues (GALT).
- Cell-mediated—B and T lymphocytes.
- Humoral (antibody-mediated)—immunoglobulins A, M, G, and E (IgA, IgM, IgG, IgE).
- Maternal serum antibodies (IgG) transferred across the placenta protect the infant from birth until approximately 6 to 12 months of age.
- Maternal antibodies (IgA) are transferred to the child's intestinal tract through breast milk.
- A child's own antibodies begin developing between about 6 months and 1 year of age.
- Childhood vaccinations are important for preventing infection from youth to adulthood.

HYPERSENSITIVITY REACTIONS

Hypersensitivity (allergic) reactions can range from mild/uncomfortable to severe/life threatening. It is important to differentiate between true allergies and other adverse effects/sensitivities.

Anaphylaxis

DEFINITION

Life-threatening systemic reaction caused by release of mediators from tissue mast cells and blood basophils.

ETIOLOGY

- Foods: Milk, egg, peanuts, shellfish
- Drugs: β-lactam antibiotics, sulfa
- Immunizing agents:
  - Latex (gloves, Foley cathers, and endotracheal tubes)
  - Radiocontrast material
  - Blood products

PATHOPHYSIOLOGY

IgE mediated.

SIGNS AND SYMPTOMS

- Generalized pruritus and urticaria
- Respiratory symptoms—upper airway obstruction (laryngeal edema)
- Hypotension, shock, dysrhythmia

- First immunoglobulin to appear in the bloodstream after the first exposure to an antigen (primary antibody response): **IgM**
- Secretory antibody response — **IgA**
- Major antibody to protein antigens — **IgG**

Transplacental antibodies protect neonates against chickenpox, measles, mumps, and rubella, but *not* chlamydia.

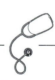

Anaphylactoid Reaction
- Clinically similar to anaphylaxis
- Not IgE mediated
- Does not require previous exposure

DIAGNOSIS

- History of exposure
- Rapid onset of symptoms (usually in minutes)
- Serum tryptase (1, 4, and 8 hours)

TREATMENT

- Airway, breathing, circulation (ABC)
- 100% oxygen
- Epinephrine (1:1,000–0.01 mL/kg subcutaneously). Minimum dose: 0.1 mL. Maximum dose: 0.3. mL
- Diphenhydramine 1 to 2 mg/kg IV, IM, or PO q4–6h
- Cimetidine 5 to 10 mg/kg IV q6h (refractory cases)

Risk factors for severe anaphylactic reaction:
- Asthma
- β Blockade
- Adrenal insufficiency

Monitor vital signs frequently during anaphylaxis.

Viral infections are the most common causes of urticaria in children.

Urticaria (Hives)

DEFINITION

Type 1 hypersensitivity reaction characterized by wheals:

- Most common skin rash.
- Angioedema involves deeper tissues.

ETIOLOGY

- Infections:
  - Viruses (influenza, enterovirus, adenovirus, infectious mononucleosis, hepatitis)
  - Bacteria (group A β-hemolytic streptococci)
- Medications (penicillin, cephalosporin, phenytoin, barbiturate, aspirin)
- Foods
- Insect stings
- Autoimmune diseases
- Malignancies

SIGNS AND SYMPTOMS

Raised pale and pink pruritic areas with annular or serpiginous morphology.

DIAGNOSIS

- Diagnosis is clinical.
- No routine laboratory test.

TREATMENT

- Avoiding the precipitating cause
- Epinephrine (1:1000 at 0.01 mg/kg) if urticaria is severe
- Diphenhydramine

Serum Sickness

DEFINITION

Type III hypersensitivity reaction.

ETIOLOGY

- Anti-gout medications—allopurinol, gold salts
- Antimicrobials—cephalosporins, penicillins, griseofulvin, furazolidone
- Antiarrhythmics—quinidine, procainamide
- Antihypertensives—captopril, hydralazine
- Thyroid medications—thiouracil, iodides
- Other medications—arsenicals and mercurial derivatives, barbiturates, halothane, methyldopa, para-aminosalicylic acid, penicillamine, phenytoin, piperazine, streptokinase, sulfonamides
- Serum/blood products, venom, hormones, vaccines

Incidence in the United States is decreasing due to vaccination programs and refinement of antitoxins.

SIGNS AND SYMPTOMS

- Fever, arthralgia, lymphadenopathy, edema, and skin eruption (serpiginous, erythematous, and purpuric eruption at the junction of the palmar or plantar skin).
- May include renal, cardiovascular, pulmonary, or neurologic manifestations.
- Symptoms occur 6 to 21 days after exposure.
- May occur in 1 to 4 days after second exposure with the same antigen.
- Symptoms usually spontaneously subside in 1 to 2 weeks; long-term sequelae and fatalities are rare.

Drug Reaction

DEFINITION

- Abnormal immunologically mediated hypersensitivity responses
- Relatively rare

ETIOLOGY

Potentially any drug can cause drug reaction.

PATHOPHYSIOLOGY

- Type I: IgE mediated
  - Penicillin, insulin, cephalosporin
- Type II: Cytotoxic antibody mediated
  - Penicillin—hemolytic anemia
  - Quinidine—thrombocytopenia
- Type III: Immune complex mediated
  - Penicillin, sulfonamides, cephalosporin
- Type IV: Cell mediated
  - Neosporin contact dermatitis, topical antihistamines

CLINICAL CRITERIA

- Reactions do not resemble pharmacologic action of the drug.
- Similar to those that may occur with other allergens.
- Induction period: 7 to 10 days.
- Reproduced by minute doses.
- Discontinuation may result in resolution.

SIGNS AND SYMPTOMS

- Mild rash to anaphylaxis
- *Fixed drug eruptions*—recur at the same site after each administration of causative drug (sulfonamides are the most common)

DIAGNOSIS

- Skin test
- Radioallergosorbent test (RAST)

DISPOSITION

- Discontinue likely offending agent.
- Admit if:
  - Stevens–Johnson syndrome
  - Toxic epidermal necrolysis
  - Severe drug reaction
  - Respiratory distress

Typical Scenario

For the past 2 weeks, a 6-year-old boy has had aggressive edema of various sites—puffy cheeks and eyes on awakening and swelling of the feet and abdomen as the day progresses. His history includes an upper respiratory illness and a sting by a yellow jacket. *Think:* Serum sickness.

Most common causes of drug reactions: penicillin, sulfonamide

Drug Reactions:
- Most are afebrile.
- Eruption may worsen before improving after discontinuation of the drug.

The most common site for the manifestation of drug reactions is the skin.

HIGH-YIELD FACTS

Immunologic Disease

Penicillin Allergy

TYPES

Wide variety of allergic reactions:
- Type I: anaphylaxis
- Type II: hemolytic anemia
- Type III: serum sickness

AMPICILLIN RASH

- Not urticarial
- Seen with:
  - Infectious mononucleosis
  - Hyperuricemia

Food Allergy/Sensitivity

Most adverse reactions to food do not have an immunologic basis.

DEFINITION

- Adverse food reaction—food hypersensitivity (IgE mediated)
- Food intolerance—adverse physiologic response (e.g., vomiting, gas, diarrhea, dizziness)

ETIOLOGY

- Food allergy
- Enzyme deficiencies
- Immunologic (celiac disease)
- Nonimmunologic

SIGNS AND SYMPTOMS

- With true allergies:
  - Generalized anaphylaxis
  - Urticaria
  - Atopic dermatitis

TREATMENT

- Avoidance of offending agent
- Treatment directed at the clinical manifestation

Stevens–Johnson Syndrome (SJS) (Erythema Multiforme Major)

Mild EM does not progress to SJS.

DEFINITION

Extreme variant of erythema multiforme (EM) with systemic toxicity and involvement of the mucous membranes.

ETIOLOGY

- Drugs: sulfonamides and anticonvulsants
- *Mycoplasma pneumoniae*

SIGNS AND SYMPTOMS

The oral cavity is almost always involved in erythema mulitforme major.

- Classic triad:
  - Conjunctivitis
  - Oral ulceration
  - Urethritis
- Prodromal phase (1–14 days): Fever, headache, malaise
- Dermatologic manifestations:
  - Erythematous blistering rash (target lesions)
  - Inflamed bullous lesions

- Criteria:
  - Cutaneous lesion plus at least two mucosal surfaces involved: conjunctivitis, rhinitis, keratitis, proctitis, balanitis, vulvovaginitis
- See chapter on dermatologic disease.

DIAGNOSIS

Skin biopsy—perivascular mononuclear cell infiltrate.

TREATMENT

- Hospitalization
- Supportive care:
  - Intravenous (IV) hydration
  - Hyperalimentation
  - Intensive skin care

IMMUNODEFICIENCIES

See Table 9-1.

Severe Combined Immunodeficiency (SCID)

DEFINITION

Abnormalities of both humoral and cellular immunity.

ETIOLOGY

- Defect in stem cell maturation
- Decreased adenosine deaminase

SIGNS AND SYMPTOMS

- Presents within first 6 months with diarrhea, pneumonia, otitis, sepsis, failure to thrive, and skin rashes
- Frequency and severity of infections
- Persistent infection with opportunistic organisms

Oral candidiasis at 10 months of age should arouse suspicion for the presence of an immunodeficiency.

TABLE 9-1. Immunodeficiencies.
Combined Immunodeficiencies
SCID
T-cell Deficiency
DiGeorge syndrome
Chronic mucocutaneous candidiasis
Humoral Deficiency
Bruton's agammaglobulinemia
IgA deficiency
CVID
Phagocytosis
Chronic granulomatous disease
Chédiak–Higashi syndrome
Job syndrome
Other
Wiskott–Aldrich syndrome
Ataxia–telangiectasia

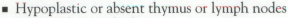

- Hypoplastic or absent thymus or lymph nodes
- Absent thymic shadow

DIAGNOSIS

- Lymphopenia
- Decreased serum IgG, IgA, and IgM

TREATMENT

- True pediatric emergency
- Bone marrow transplantation

PROGNOSIS

Death within first 2 years if untreated.

Letterer–Siwe Disease

DEFINITION

- Acute disseminated form of Langerhans' cell histiocytosis
- Manifestation of complex immune dysregulation

SIGNS AND SYMPTOMS

- Skeleton involved (80%)—skull, vertebrae
- Skin (50%)—seborrheic dermatitis
- Lymphadenopathy (33%)
- Hepatosplenomegaly (20%)
- Exophthalmos
- Pituitary dysfunction—growth retardation, diabetes insipidus
- Systemic manifestations—fever, weight loss, irritability, failure to thrive
- Bone marrow involvement—anemia, thrombocytopenia

LAB

- Complete blood count (CBC)
- Liver function tests (LFTs)
- Coagulation profile
- Chest x-ray
- Skeletal survey
- Urine osmolality
- Tissue biopsy (skin or bone lesions)

TREATMENT

- Single system disease—generally benign
- Treatment directed at arresting the progression of lesion (low-dose local radiation)
- Multisystem disease
- Systemic multiagent chemotherapy
- Spontaneous remission

Ataxia–Telangiectasia (AT)

DEFINITION

- Telangiectasia
- Ataxia
- Variable immunodeficiency
- Autosomal recessive

ETIOLOGY

Defective chromosome repair.

Measures to be taken in SCID:
- Protective isolation
- Irradiation of all blood products

HIGH-YIELD FACTS

Immunologic Disease

- Progressive cerebellar ataxia
  - Usually presents during first 6 years
  - Confined to wheelchair by 10 to 12 years
- Both humoral and cellular immunodeficiency
- Oculocutaneous telangiectasias
- Chronic sinopulmonary infection
- Increased risk of malignancy
  - Hodgkin's disease
  - Leukemia
  - Lymphoma
  - Lymphosarcoma

LAB

Increased serum α-fetoprotein + carcinoembryonic antigen.

TREATMENT

- Supportive therapy
- Improve pulmonary function
- Improve immunologic status

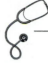

Earliest site of telangiectasia in ataxia–telangectasia is bulbar conjunctivae.

Chronic Mucocutaneous Candidiasis

DEFINITION

T-cell disorder.

SIGNS AND SYMPTOMS

- Superficial candidal infections of mucous membranes, skin, and nails
- Often associated with endocrinopathy
  - Hypoparathyroidism
  - Hyperthyroidism
  - Polyendocrinopathy

Typical Scenario

A 10-year-old girl has a persistent, unresponsive infection of the oral cavity and nails. *Think:* Chronic mucocutaneous candidiasis.

Wiskott–Aldrich Syndrome

DEFINITION

- Thrombocytopenia, eczema, and increased susceptibility to infection
- X-linked recessive (classic symptoms occur only in males)

ETIOLOGY

Inability to form antibody to bacterial capsular polysaccharide antigens.

SIGNS AND SYMPTOMS

- Atopic dermatitis/eczema
- Thrombocytopenic purpura
- Recurrent infections in infancy
- Pneumococci
- Impaired humoral and cell-mediated immunity
- Excessive bleeding from circumcision site
- At risk for sepsis and hemorrhage

Triad of thrombocytopenia, eczema, and recurrent bacterial infections in males. *Think:* Wiskott–Aldrich syndrome.

LAB

- Decreased IgM
- Increased IgA

HIGH-YIELD FACTS

Immunologic Disease

Common Variable Hypogammaglobulinemia (CVID)

DEFINITION

- Inherited disorder of hypogammaglobulinemia
- Infections less severe than SCID
- Involves the formation of autoantibodies

SIGNS AND SYMPTOMS

- Clinically similar to Bruton's agammaglobulinemia
- Sprue-like syndrome
- Thymoma
- Alopecia areata
- Achlorhydria
- Pernicious anemia
- Lymphoid interstitial pneumonia
- Pseudolymphoma
- Noncaseating sarcoid-like granulomas of lungs, spleen, skin, and liver

Bruton's Congenital Agammaglobulinemia

DEFINITION

- Profound defects in B lymphocytes (both function and number)
- Severe hypogammaglobulinemia
- X-linked

ETIOLOGY

- Gene defect in Xq22
- Defective protein tyrosine kinase on B cell

SIGNS AND SYMPTOMS

- Increased susceptibility to infections with *Streptococcus*, *Haemophilus influenzae*, and echovirus meningoencephalitis
- Hypoplasia of tonsils, adenoids, and peripheral lymph nodes

DIAGNOSIS

- Very low or absent immunoglobulins
- Very low or absent mature B lymphocytes

Selective IgA Deficiency

DEFINITION

Deficiency of IgA–predominant immunoglobulin on mucosal surfaces.

EPIDEMIOLOGY

Most common humoral antibody deficiency.

SIGNS AND SYMPTOMS

- Respiratory tract infections
- Urinary tract infections
- Gastrointestinal (GI) infections—*Giardia*
- Autoimmune diseases

DIAGNOSIS

- IgA < 5 mg/dL
- Normal levels of other immunoglobulin
- Normal cell-mediated immunity

Infants with Bruton's congenital agammaglobulinemia remain well for the first 6 to 9 months because of maternal transmitted IgG antibodies.

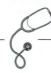

Most common immunoglobulin deficiency: selective IgA deficiency. Avoid X-ray exposure.

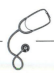

Selective IgA deficiency can lead to fatal anaphylactic reaction to blood products and intravenous immunoglobulin (IVIG). Immunoglobulin therapy is contraindicated.

IgA is the major immunoglobulin within the upper airway.

DiGeorge's Syndrome

DEFINITION

Primary disorder of T-cell function.

ETIOLOGY

- Chromosome 22, q11 deletion
- Abnormal development of third and fourth branchial pouches
- Absent T lymphocytes—thymic hypoplasia

SIGNS AND SYMPTOMS

- Congenital heart disease (atrial septal defect, ventricular septal defect)
- Right-sided aortic arch
- Hypocalcemic tetany
- Esophageal atresia
- Hypoparathyroidism
- Abnormal facies (short philtrum, hypertelorism, low-set ears)

TREATMENT

- Thymic tissue transplant.
- Bone marrow transplant—at risk for graft versus host disease (GVHD).
- Use irradiated blood products only.

Chédiak–Higashi Syndrome

DEFINITION

- Abnormal neutrophil function
- Autosomal recessive

SIGNS AND SYMPTOMS

- Increased susceptibility to infection of skin and respiratory tract (*Staphylococcus aureus*, β-hemolytic strep)
- Mild bleeding diathesis
- Partial oculocutaneous albinism
- Progressive peripheral neuropathy
- Lymphoma-like syndrome
- Pancytopenia

DIAGNOSIS

Large inclusions in all nucleated cells.

TREATMENT

- High-dose ascorbic acid
- Antibiotics for acute infections
- Bone marrow transplant (does not prevent or cure peripheral neuropathy)

Chronic Granulomatous Disease

DEFINITION

- Neutrophil dysfunction
- Chemotaxis and phagocytosis intact
- Defective killing
- Most common inherited disorder of phagocytosis

ETIOLOGY

- Defect in generation of microbial oxygen metabolites
- Inability to kill catalase-positive microorganisms

> **Typical Scenario**
>
> A 2-month-old infant with congenital heart disease is hospitalized with cough and tachypnea. X-ray films of the chest show diffuse infiltrates and no thymic shadow. Serum calcium is 6.5 mg/dL (low). *Think:* DiGeorge's syndrome.

> Recognized functions of T lymphocytes include: cytotoxicity against virus-infected cells, mediation of delayed-type hypersensitivity, production of interleukin-2 (IL-2), and production of lymphokines.

Typical Scenario

A 14-year-old boy has had lifelong skin infections. His leukocytes are unable to reduce nitroblue tetrazolium. *Think:* Chronic granulomatous disease.

Impaired intracellular bactericidal activity is the definitive test for chronic granulomatous disease.

Hypocomplimentemia occurs in patients with lupus nephritis and poststreptococcal glomerulonephritis, not in Henoch–Schönlein purpura or minimal change disease.

SIGNS AND SYMPTOMS

- Severe recurrent infections of skin and lymph nodes
- Pneumonitis → pneumatocele
- Osteomyelitis
- Hepatosplenomegaly

DIAGNOSIS

- Leukocytosis
- Increased erythrocyte sedimentation rate (ESR)
- Abnormal chest x-ray
- Hypergammaglobulinemia

Complement Deficiency

COMPLEMENT

Complex system of nine serum proteins (C1–C9).

FUNCTIONS OF COMPLEMENT

- Opsonization
- Mediation of inflammation
- Cell lysis
- Modulation of immune response

ASSOCIATED DISEASES

- C1q deficiency—systemic lupus erythematosus (SLE)
- C1r, C1r/C1s, C4, C2, and C3 deficiency
  - Vasculitis—SLE
- C5–C8 deficiency—neisserial infection
- C3 deficiency—pneumococci
- C1 esterase inhibitor (C1 INH) deficiency—hereditary angioedema

DIAGNOSIS

CH_{50} screening test.

Asplenia

DEFINITION

Missing blood filter.

ETIOLOGY

- Associated with some congenital syndromes.
- Functional asplenia may be secondary to sickle cell disease or other hemoglobinopathies.
- Hyposplenia may be secondary to SLE, rheumatoid arthritis (RA), inflammatory bowel disease (IBD), GVHD, nephrotic syndrome, or prematurity.
- Splenectomy may be indicated in trauma, Hodgkin's lymphoma, and hereditary spherocytosis.

DIAGNOSIS

- Decreased IgM antibodies, alternate complement pathway, and tuftsin
- Increased requirement for opsonic antibodies
- Howell–Jolly bodies in erythrocytes

COMPLICATIONS

Sepsis with encapsulated organisms:
- 0 to 6 months—gram-negative enteric (*Klebsiella*, *Escherichia coli*).

- After 6 months of age—*S. pneumoniae, H. influenzae* type B; *Neisseria meningitidis* is less common.
- Malaria, babesiosis, and certain viral infections may also be more severe.

TREATMENT
- Penicillin prophylaxis
- Pneumococcal immunization

Job Syndrome (Hyper IgE)

DEFINITION
- Neutrophil chemotactic defect
- Autosomal recessive

SIGNS AND SYMPTOMS
- Recurrent staph infections
- Resistant to therapy
- Pruritic eczematoid dermatitis
- Coarse facial features

DIAGNOSIS
- Increased IgE (> 10,000 IU/mL)
- Eosinophilia

TREATMENT
- Penicillinase-resistant antibiotics
- IVIG

X-linked Lymphoproliferative Disease (Duncan's Disease)

DEFINITION
Inadequate immune response to Epstein–Barr virus (EBV).

EPIDEMIOLOGY
- Mean age < 5 years
- X-linked recessive trait

SIGNS AND SYMPTOMS
- Healthy until acquire EBV infection
- High mortality due to extensive liver necrosis

Graft Versus Host Disease (GVHD)

DEFINITION
- Donor lymphocytes detect host as foreign.
- Complication of bone marrow transplant.

ETIOLOGY
Engraftment by immunocompetent donor lymphocytes in an immunologically compromised host.

PATHOPHYSIOLOGY
Donor T-cell activation by antibodies against host major histocompatibility complex antigens.

Requirements for Graft Versus Host Disease:
- Graft must contain immunocompetent cells.
- Host must be immunocompromised.
- Histocompatibility differences must exist.

SIGNS AND SYMPTOMS

- **Acute** (5–40 days)
  - Erythroderma
  - Cholestatic hepatitis—abnormal LFTs
  - Enteritis—diarrhea
  - Increased susceptibility to infections
- **Chronic** (weeks to months—average 100 days)
  - Sjögren's syndrome—dry eyes and mouth
  - SLE
  - Scleroderma
  - Lichen planus
  - Primary biliary cirrhosis
  - Increased susceptibility to infections
  - Possible lung and GI disorders

TREATMENT

- High-dose corticosteroids
- Second-line—antibodies to T cells
- Prevention—ABO- and human lymphocyte antigen (HLA)-compatible donors, family members preferable

Infectious Disease

OCCULT BACTEREMIA

DEFINITION
Positive blood culture with no signs of infection and well appearance.

ETIOLOGY
Neonates
- Group B streptococci
- *Escherichia coli*
- *Staphylococcus aureus*
- *Listeria monocytogenes*
- Coagulase-negative *Staphylococcus* (preterm infants)
- *Candida albicans* (preterm infants)

Children
- *Streptococcus pneumoniae*
- *Neisseria meningitidis*
- *Salmonella typhimurium*
- *S. aureus*
- Group A streptococci

SIGNS AND SYMPTOMS
- Fever
- Leukocytosis
- No obvious focus of infections

PREDISPOSING FACTORS
- Loss of external defenses (burns, ulceration, catheter)
- Inadequate phagocytic or immune function
- Impaired reticuloendothelial function
- Overwhelming inoculum

DIAGNOSTIC WORKUP
- Blood and urine cultures
- Complete blood count (CBC)
- Chest x-ray (CXR)
- Lumbar puncture if < 28 days old, altered mental status, or meningeal signs

TREATMENT
- Treat to prevent progression to septicemia.
- See Table 10-1 for age-based criteria.

Group B strep is the most common cause of neonatal septicemia.

TABLE 10-1. Age-based management of occult bacteremia.	
Age	**Management**
< 28 days	▪ All considered for hospitalization and parenteral antibiotics. Ampicillin and gentamicin most appropriate.
29–90 days	▪ Low risk: previously healthy, no focal infection, negative laboratory screen (WBC < 15,000, normal urinalysis); manage as outpatient if good follow-up.
	▪ High risk: ceftriaxone if no meningitis, parental ampicillin if invasive disease (enterococcus or *Listeria monocytogenes*).
3–36 months	▪ If fever > 102.2°F (39°C): get WBC; cultures of blood, urine, and stool; chest x-ray if lower respiratory signs.
	▪ Ceftriaxone if WBC > 15,000 or septic appearance; follow-up extremely important.

SEPSIS

DEFINITION

- Life-threatening bacterial invasion of intravascular compartment
- May or may not be associated with a focus of infection

ETIOLOGY

Same as for occult bacteremia above.

SIGNS AND SYMPTOMS

- General
  - Fever, temperature instability
  - "Not doing well"
  - Poor feeding
  - Edema
- Gastrointestinal system
  - Abdominal distention
  - Vomiting
  - Diarrhea
  - Hepatomegaly
- Respiratory system
  - Apnea, dyspnea
  - Tachypnea, retractions
  - Flaring, grunting
  - Cyanosis
- Renal system
  - Oliguria
- Cardiovascular system
  - Pallor; mottling; cold, clammy skin
  - Tachycardia
  - Hypotension
  - Bradycardia
- Central nervous system
  - Irritability, lethargy
  - Tremors, seizures
  - Hyporeflexia, hypotonia
  - Abnormal Moro reflex
  - Irregular respirations
  - Full fontanelle
  - High-pitched cry

- Hematologic system
  - Jaundice
  - Splenomegaly
  - Pallor
  - Petechiae, purpura
  - Bleeding

DIAGNOSIS
- Same as for occult bactermia
- 10% will have negative cultures

RISK FACTORS
- Younger at greater risk
- Prematurity
- Immunodeficiency
- Catheters
- Contact with known *N. meningitidis* or *Haemophilus influenzae* infection

┌─ **Typical Scenario** ─┐

A 5-year-old boy presents with sudden onset of high fever and reddish-purple spots. He is rapidly progressing to shock. *Think:* Meningiococcemia.

Septic Shock

Sepsis with hypotension despite fluid resuscitation.

Meningococcemia (Figure 10-1)
- Presents nonspecifically but progresses rapidly (hours to days).
- Most progress to septic shock due to large amounts of menigococcal endotoxin.
- First petechiae, then purpura, and finally ecchymoses (one of the rashes seen on palms and soles).
- Failure to perfuse distal extremeties.
- Adrenal hemorrhage (Waterhouse–Friedrichsen syndrome) and insufficiency common.
- Establish diagnosis by culture of blood, cerebrospinal fluid (CSF), and skin lesions.
- Intravenous penicillin is treatment of choice.
- Vaccine available.

TREATMENT
- Hospital admission.
- Broad-spectrum antibiotic initiated and changed when susceptibility is known (vancomycin and gentamicin generally first course).
- Manage shock with supportive therapy to maintain blood pressure, perfusion, and oxygenation.

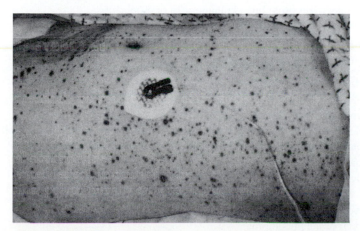

FIGURE 10-1. Meningococcemia. (Reproduced, with permission, from Knoop et al. *Atlas of Emergency Medicine*. New York: McGraw Hill, 1997:404)

ETIOLOGY

- Infants: Vertical transmission from mother either perinatally or through breast milk (preventable with antiretroviral prophylaxis)
- Adolescents: Sexual transmission or intravenous drug use

DIAGNOSIS

- Most high-risk mothers are screened so infection is known before clinically apparent.
- Presence of opportunistic infection.
- Immunodeficiency.
- See Table 10-2 for clinical classifications.

TREATMENT

- Three classes:
  - Nucleoside reverse transcriptase inhibitors (NRTIs)
  - Non-nucleoside reverse transcriptase inhibitors (NNRTIs)
  - Protease inhibitors
- HIV rapidly becomes resistant; therefore, multidrug therapy is necessary.

TABLE 10-2. 1993 Centers for Disease Control and Prevention clinical classification of HIV infection in children < 13 years.

Clinical Category	Diagnostic Criteria
Not symptomatic	If two positive results on separate occasions
Mildly symptomatic	Two or more of following conditions: ■ Lymphadenopathy ■ Hepatomegaly ■ Splenomegaly ■ Dermatitis ■ Parotitis ■ Recurrent or persistent upper respiratory infections, sinusitis, or otitis media
Moderately symptomatic	■ Anemia, neutropenia, or thrombocytopenia persisting for 30 days ■ Bacterial meningitis, pneumonia, or sepsis ■ Candidiasis persisting > 2 months in child > 6 months ■ Cardiomyopathy ■ Cytomegalovirus infection ■ Hepatitis ■ Herpes zoster: two episodes in more than one dermatome ■ Disseminated varicella ■ Herpes simplex virus bronchitis, pneumonitis, or esophagitis ■ Nephropathy ■ Persistent fever (> 1 month) ■ Toxoplasmosis
Severely symptomatic	■ Serious bacterial infection (two in 2 years' time) ■ Disseminated coccidioidomycosis ■ Extrapulmonary cryptococcosis ■ Encephalopathy: more than one finding for > 2 months with no illness to explain ■ Disseminated histoplasmosis ■ Kaposi sarcoma ■ Primary lymphoma in brain ■ Tuberculosis ■ Other mycobacterium infection ■ *Pneumocystis carinii* pneumonia ■ Polymorphonuclear leukocytes ■ Wasting syndrome

Toxoplasmosis

See chapter on gestation and birth.

ETIOLOGY

- Caused by *Toxoplasma gondii* (intracellular protozoan)
- See TORCH infections (toxoplasmosis, other [hepatitis B, syphilis, varicella-zoster virus], rubella, cytomegalovirus, herpes simplex virus/HIV) in chapter on gestation and birth.

PATHOPHYSIOLOGY

- Cats excrete cysts in feces.

SIGNS AND SYMPTOMS

- Mononucleosis syndrome including fever, lymphadenopathy, and hepatosplenomegaly
- Disseminated infection—myocarditis, pneumonia, and encephalitis

DIAGNOSIS

Serologic antibody tests, biopsy, visualization of parasites in CSF.

TREATMENT

Pyrimethamine and sulfadiazine used concurrently (both inhibit folic acid synthesis, so replace folic acid).

PREVENTION

Pregnant women should avoid contact with cat litter/litterbox.

Cryptococcosis

DEFINITION

Fungal infection.

SIGNS AND SYMPTOMS

- Primary infection in lungs.
- Disseminates to brain, meninges, skin, eyes, and skeletal system.
- Subacute or chronic meningitis is the most common presentation in acquired immune deficiency syndrome (AIDS).
- Typically presents with fever, headache, and malaise.
- Postinfectious sequelae common including:
  - Hydrocephalus
  - Change in visual acuity
  - Deafness
  - Cranial nerve palsies
  - Seizures
  - Ataxia

DIAGNOSIS

- Serology: can be detected by latex particle agglutination or enzyme-linked immunosorbent assay (ELISA)
- Microscopy: encapsulated yeast seen as white halos when CSF is mixed with India ink
- Can be grown in culture (takes up to 3 weeks)
- May also see cryptococcomas on head CT

TREATMENT

- Relapse rate is > 50%.
- Treat with combination therapy using amphotericin B and flucytosine.
- High rate of recurrence necessitates induction and maintenance therapy.

HIGH-YIELD FACTS

Infectious Disease

Pneumocystis carinii is now known as *Pneumocystis jiroveci* and is classified as a fungus rather than a protozoan. (*Source:* Centers for Disease Control and Prevention)

Pneumocystis carinii Pneumonia (PCP)

EPIDEMIOLOGY

- Peak incidence 3 to 6 months of age
- Highest mortality rate under 1 year

SIGNS AND SYMPTOMS

- Acute onset of fever, tachypnea, dyspnea, nonproductive cough, and progressive hypoxemia
- Chest x-ray—interstitial bilateral infiltrates or diffuse alveolar disease, which rapidly progresses

DIAGNOSIS

Diagnosis by methenamine silver staining of bronchoalveolar fluid lavage (BAL) to identify cyst walls or Giemsa staining to identify nuclei of trophozoites.

TREATMENT

- First-line treatment is trimethoprim–sulfamethoxazole (TMP-SMZ) (TMP: 15–20 mg/kg/24 hr; SMZ: 75–100 mg/kg/24 hr) q6h for 5 to 7 days.
- Alternative regimens: pentamidine, TMP-SMZ plus dapsone, atovaquone, primaquine plus clindamycin.

PROPHYLAXIS

TMP-SMZ if CD4 < 200.

Atypical Mycobacterial Infections

ETIOLOGY

- *Mycobacterium avium* complex (MAC).
- *Mycobacterium intracellulare* (MAI).
- *Mycobacterium kansasii*.
- These atypical mycobacterial infections are considered AIDS-defining illnesses. Patients with CD4 counts < 50/mm are at highest risk.

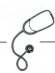

Rifabutin decreases serum levels of azidothymidine (AZT) and clarithromycin.

SIGNS AND SYMPTOMS

Disseminated disease:

- Fever
- Malaise
- Weight loss
- Night sweats
- May have abdominal symptoms

Fluconzole can decrease the level of rifabutin by 80%.

DIAGNOSIS

Diagnosis by culture from blood, bone marrow, or tissue.

TREATMENT

Two-drug regimen:

- Either clarithromycin *or* azithromycin
- *Plus* ethambutol, rifabutin, rifampin, ciprofloxacin, *or* amikacin

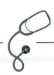

Rifabutin can color body secretions such as urine, sweat, and tears a bright orange (similar to pyridium).

PROPHYLAXIS

- For CD4 < 50
- Rifabutin
- Clarithromycin
- Azithromycin

Cytomegalovirus (CMV)

ETIOLOGY

Herpesvirus.

PATHOPHYSIOLOGY

Lung, liver, kidney, gastrointestinal (GI) tract, and salivary glands are most common organs infected.

SIGNS AND SYMPTOMS

- CMV infection in most immunocompetent hosts is a subclinical infection that is self-limiting. It is mostly an issue in pregnant women, transplant recipients, and the immunocompromised (because it reactivates a dormant infection).
- Pneumonitis.
- Retinitis (can cause blindness).
- May cause mononucleosis-like symptoms.

DIAGNOSIS

- Serology: most commonly by ELISA
- Microscopy: enlarged cells with large intranuclear inclusions

TREATMENT

- No routine treatment.
- Vaccine research underway.
- For sight or life-threatening infections, intravenous (IV) foscarnet or ganciclovir is used.
- Transplant recipients are given oral ganciclovir CMV prophylaxis.

CMV is the most frequently transmitted virus to a child before birth.

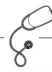

CMV is a major cause of death in immunocompromised persons.

VIRAL EXANTHEMS

Varicella (Chickenpox)

DEFINITION

Highly contagious, self-limited viral infection characterized by multiple pruritic vesicles (Figure 10-2).

ETIOLOGY

Varicella-zoster virus (herpesvirus).

EPIDEMIOLOGY

- Ninety percent of patients are < 10 years old.
- Incidence is decreasing with introduction of vaccine.

PATHOPHYSIOLOGY

- Transmitted by respiratory secretions and fluid from the skin lesions.
- Virus replicates in respiratory tract.
- Establishes latent infection in sensory ganglia cells.
- Reactivation of latent infection causes herpes zoster.

SIGNS AND SYMPTOMS

- Papular lesions evolve into small, clear vesicles on an erythematous base.
- Within days, vesicles become turbid and crusted (see Figure 10-2).
- New crops continue to appear for 3 to 5 days.

Herpes zoster is the reactivation of varicella-zoster virus and occurs in dermatomal distribution.

"Dew drops on a rose petal" and multiple crops of lesions in various stages are typical for varicella.

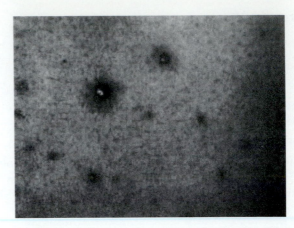

FIGURE 10-2. Varicella (chickenpox). Note dew drop appearance of lesion and that there are lesions in multiple stages of eruption.

Smallpox generally presents with all lesions in the same stage (versus chickenpox).

- Lesions initially appear on face and spread to trunk and extremities, sparing palms and soles.
- After crusts clear within 1 to 3 weeks, a punched-out white scar may remain.
- May be preceded by a prodrome of fever, malaise, anorexia, headache, and abdominal pain 24 to 48 hours before the onset of the rash.
- Usually has a history of exposure to infected individual.

DIAGNOSIS

Clinical, supported by evidence of multinucleated giant cells on Tzanck preparation.

COMPLICATIONS

- Skin lesions may be complicated by secondary bacterial infections (generally *Streptococcus pyogenes* or *Staphylococcus aureus*)
- Pneumonia
- Encephalitis
- Reye's syndrome (associated with aspirin use)

VACCINE

- Live-attenuated vaccine given between 12 and 18 months of age.
- Children older than 12 need two vaccinations at least 1 month apart.

TREATMENT

- For most immunocompetent children: oral antihistamines, topical calamine lotion, oatmeal baths, cool compress to alleviate pruritus
- For varicella zoster virus (VZV) pneumonia and immunocompromised individuals:
  - Acyclovir:
    - IV: 30 mg/kg/24 hr 7 to 10 days
    - PO: 80 mg/kg/24 hr QID 5 days
    - Max dose: 3,200 mg/24 hr
- Varicella-zoster immune globulin (VZIG) used for postexposure prophylaxis in immunocompromised or newborns exposed to maternal varicella

Congenital Varicella Syndrome

Caused by maternal varicella infection in first 20 weeks of pregnancy.

- Growth retardation
- Cicatricial skin lesions
- Limb hypoplasia
- Neurologic deficits

Rubeola (Measles)

ETIOLOGY

Paramyxovirus (RNA virus).

SIGNS AND SYMPTOMS

- High fever.
- Runny nose.
- Dry cough.
- Coryza.
- Conjunctivitis.
- Rash starts as faint macules on upper lateral neck, behind ears, along hairline, and on cheeks.
- Lesions become increasingly maculopapular and spreads quickly to entire face, neck, upper arms, and chest.
- May have lymphadenopathy or splenomegaly.
- Koplik spots: irregularly shaped spots with grayish white centers inside mouth (pathognomonic) (see Figure 10-3).

DIAGNOSIS

- Clinical
- Laboratory rarely needed

VACCINE

- Live-attenuated vaccine included in measles–mumps–rubella (MMR) vaccine.
- Generally given at 12 to 15 months with a booster given at 4 to 6 years.

TREATMENT

- Generally supportive
- Immunoglobulin available

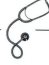

Children under the age of 6 to 8 months do not usually get measles due to passive immunity they still have from mother.

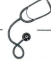

Measles vaccine should not be given to pregnant women, persons with tuberculosis (TB) or immunocompromise, or those allergic to eggs or neomycin.

HIGH-YIELD FACTS

Infectious Disease

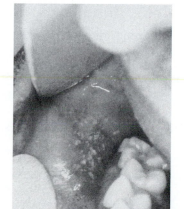

FIGURE 10-3. Rubeola. (Reproduced, with permission, from Knoop et al. *Atlas of Emergency Medicine.* New York: McGraw Hill, 1997:174)

COMPLICATIONS

- Otitis media
- Pneumonia
- Encephalitis

Fifth Disease

ETIOLOGY

Parvovirus B19.

PATHOPHYSIOLOGY

- Attacks red cell line
- Transmitted in respiratory secretions

SIGNS AND SYMPTOMS

- "Slapped cheek" rash.
- Rash spreads rapidly to trunk and extremities.
- Prodrome consisting of low-grade fever, headache, and mild upper respiratory symptoms.

DIAGNOSIS

- Clinical
- Serology for parvovirus B19 available, but not especially useful in acute setting

TREATMENT

Supportive (antipyretics, increase oral fluid intake, rest).

COMPLICATIONS

- Arthropathy
- Transient aplastic crisis in patients with chronic hemolysis including sickle cell disease, thalassemia, hereditary spherocytosis, and pyruvate kinase deficiency

Roseola

ETIOLOGY

Human herpesvirus types 6 and 7.

SIGNS AND SYMPTOMS

- High fever.
- Mild upper respiratory symptoms.
- Mild cervical lymphadenopathy.
- Rash consists of discrete small raised lesions on trunk that spreads to the neck, face, and proximal extremities.

TREATMENT

Supportive (antipyretics, increase oral fluid intake, rest).

Rubella

ETIOLOGY

RNA virus.

SIGNS AND SYMPTOMS

- Mild fever prodrome for 1 to 2 days.
- Then mild lymphadenopathy (retroauricular, posterior cervical, and postoccipital).

The high fever seen with roseola infantum can trigger febrile seizures in young children.

Typical Scenario

A 2-year-old boy is brought in by his mother for evaluation of a rash. She is worried because for the last 3 days the boy had a high fever. Today, the fever has completely resolved, but he broke out into a diffuse rash. *Think:* Roseola infantum.

Rubella is contagious from 1 week before the rash appears to 1 week after it fades.

- Rash begins on face and spreads quickly to trunk. As it spreads to trunk, it clears on face.
- Rash does not itch.
- Can also be associated with a mild conjunctivitis.

COMPLICATIONS

- Progressive panencephalitis (very rare)
  - Insidious behavior change
  - Deteriorating school performance
  - Later dementia and multifocal neurologic deficits

TREATMENT

- Supportive; usually lasts about 3 days
- Immunoglobulin prophylaxis available

VACCINE

- Live-attenuated vaccine included in MMR vaccine
- Generally given at 12 to 15 months with a booster given at 4 to 6 years

Mumps

ETIOLOGY

Paramyxovirus (RNA virus).

PATHOPHYSIOLOGY

- Spread via respiratory secretions.
- Incubation period of 14 to 24 days.
- Early viremia may account for multiple complications.

SIGNS AND SYMPTOMS

- Swelling in one or both parotid glands
- Rare viral prodrome

COMPLICATIONS

- Orchitis and epididymitis
- Meningoencephalomyelitis (rare)
- Oophoritis
- Pancreatitis
- Thyroiditis
- Myocarditis
- Deafness
- Arthritis

VACCINE

- Live-attenuated vaccine included in MMR vaccine
- Generally given at 12 to 15 months with a booster given at 4 to 6 years.

> **Typical Scenario**
>
> A 10-year-old boy who originally presented with fever and swollen parotid gland presents 8 days later with a swollen tender testis. *Think:* Mumps orchitis.

BACTERIAL INFECTIONS

Lyme Disease

DEFINITION

- A multisystem disease transmitted by the bite of an *Ixodes* deer tick infected with a spirochetal bacteria.
- Characterized by three stages of disease: localized, disseminated, and chronic.
- Patients are often unaware of tick bite.

ETIOLOGY

Borrelia burgdorferi.

EPIDEMIOLOGY

- More frequent in late May through early fall.
- Increased prevalence in Northeast and North Central regions, primarily Connecticut, Rhode Island, New York, New Jersey, Delaware, and Pennsylvania.

SIGNS AND SYMPTOMS

- History—acute onset of fever, chills, myalgia, weakness, headache, and photophobia.
- First manifestation (7–14 days after bite):
  - Target-shaped rash known as erythema chronicum migrans (ECM) (see Figure 10-4) develops at site of tick bite in 75% of patients within 1 month (an expanding erythematous annular plaque with a central clearing).
  - Usually affects the trunk, proximal extremities, axilla, and inguinal area.
  - May have multiple ECM lesions if multiple tick bites are present.
  - Fifteen percent of patients develop secondary annular lesions that resemble ECM but are smaller and migrate less.
- Early disease (several days after first lesion):
  - Migrating erythematous rash
  - Fever
  - Myalgia
  - Headache
  - Malaise
- Late disease (months after initial manifestation):
  - Arthritis
  - Carditis
  - Neurologic problems

> **Treatment of Lyme Disease**
> If untreated, lesions fade within 28 days. If treated adequately, lesions fade within days and the late manifestations of the disease are prevented. If delayed diagnosis, may have permanent neurologic or joint disabilities.

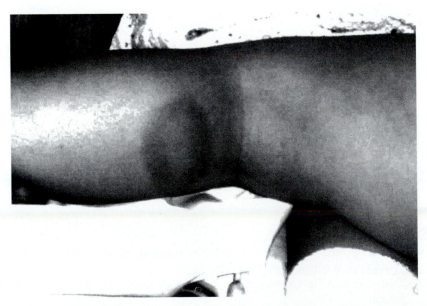

FIGURE 10-4. Erythema chronicum migrans rash characteristic of Lyme disease.

DIAGNOSIS

- Clinical, confirmed by serology.
- Immunoglobulin M (IgM) titers are elevated in acute disease and peak 3 to 6 weeks after exposure.
- IgG levels peak when arthritis develops.
- An elevated IgG titer in absence of an elevated IgM indicates prior exposure as opposed to recent infection.
- May have false-negative results in first 2 to 4 weeks and false-positive results with other spirochetal infection and in patients with some autoimmune disorders (systemic lupus erythematosus [SLE], rheumatoid arthritis [RA]).
- Polymerase chain reaction (PCR) can detect spirochete DNA in CSF and synovial fluid. Forty percent of skin biopsies reveal spirochetes.

COMPLICATIONS

- Sixty percent of untreated cases with disseminated infection develop arthritis (mediated by immune complex formation) 4 to 6 weeks following tick bite.
- May also develop neurologic (meningitis, encephalitis, or Bell's palsy) and cardiac involvement (carditis, atrioventricular block).

TREATMENT

Amoxicillin or doxycycline.

Typhoid Fever

ETIOLOGY

Salmonella typhi.

PATHOPHYSIOLOGY

- Fecal–oral transmission
- Incubation period of 7 to 14 days
- Time of incubation dependent on inoculum size

SIGNS AND SYMPTOMS

- Diarrhea later changing to constipation
- Fever
- Malaise
- Anorexia
- Myalgia
- Headache
- Abdominal pain
- Rose-colored spots on trunk
- Hepatosplenomegaly

COMPLICATIONS

- Intestinal hemorrhage
- Intestinal perforation
- Pneumonia caused by superinfection by other organisms

DIAGNOSIS

- Culture.
- PCR is becoming available.
- Anemia due to blood loss.

TREATMENT

Amoxicillin or TMP-SMZ.

VACCINE

Available for travelers to endemic areas (not routinely recommended).

Hand–Foot–Mouth Disease

ETIOLOGY

Coxsackievirus A16.

SIGNS AND SYMPTOMS

- Summer and fall seasonal pattern
- GI discomfort (usually not vomiting)
- Ulcerative mouth lesions
- Hand and foot lesions tender and vesicular
- Hands more commonly involved than feet
- Usually dorsal surfaces but may occur on palms and soles

COMPLICATIONS

- Aseptic meningitis
- Encephalitis
- Paralytic disease

Rocky Mountain Spotted Fever (RMSF)

DEFINITION

- A potentially life-threatening disease following a tick bite.
- The infected tick adheres to vascular endothelium, resulting in vascular necrosis and extravasation of blood.

ETIOLOGY

- *Rickettsia rickettsii.*
- Transmitted by tick bites.
- Dogs and rodents are hosts.
- One-week incubation.

EPIDEMIOLOGY

- Endemic to almost every state in the United States.
- Highest incidence in children aged 5 to 10 years old.
- Ninety-five percent of cases occur from April through September.
- Occurs only in the western hemisphere, primarily in southeastern states and most often in Oklahoma, North and South Carolina, and Tennessee.
- Rarely occurs in the Rocky Mountains.
- Only 60% of patients report a history of a tick bite.

RMSF rash spreads from extremities to trunk.

SIGNS AND SYMPTOMS

- Sudden onset of high fever, myalgia, severe headache, rigors, nausea, and photophobia within first 2 days of tick bite.
- Fifty percent develop rash within 3 days. Another 30% develop the rash within 6 days.
- Rash consists of 2- to 6-mm pink **blanchable macules** that first appear peripherally on wrists, forearms, ankles, **palms,** and **soles.**
- Within 6 to 18 hours the exanthem spreads centrally to the trunk, proximal extremities, and face (centrifugal).

- Within 1 to 3 days the macules evolve to deep red papules, and within 2 to 4 days the exanthem is hemorrhagic and no longer blanchable.
- Up to 15% have no rash.
- Many patients have exquisite tenderness of the gastrocnemius muscle.

DIAGNOSIS

- Indirect fluorescent antibody (IFA) assay.
  - Titer > 1:64 is diagnostic.
  - Most sensitive and specific test.
- Other, less sensitive tests include: indirect hemagglutinin, Weil–Felix, complement fixation, and latex agglutination tests.
- Biopsy would demonstrate necrotizing vasculitis.

TREATMENT

- Tetracycline: 25 to 50 mg/kg/24 hr PO q6h (not in children < 8 years old)
- Chloramphenicol: 50 to 75 mg/kg/24 hr q6h

COMPLICATIONS

- Fulminant infection in glucose-6-phosphate dehydrogenase (G6PD) deficiency
- Noncardiogenic pulmonary edema
- Meningoencephalitis
- Multiorgan damage due to vasculitis

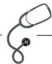

In real time, RMSF is a clinical diagnosis (because current diagnostic tests aren't back fast enough). It is important not to delay treatment.

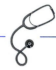

RMSF is one of the few indications these days to use chloramphenicol. It is seldom used anymore due to potential for hepatotoxicity and associated complication of gray baby syndrome.

Toxic Shock Syndrome

DEFINITION

Acute, multisystemic disease characterized by high fever, hypotension, and erythematous rash.

ETIOLOGY

- Toxins from *Staphylococcus* spp. function as superantigens activating entire subsets of T cells, resulting in massive release of cytokines, which has profound physiologic consequences (i.e., fever, vasodilation, hypotension, and multisystem organ involvement).
- Source may be tampon, nasal packing, wound packing, or abscess.

SIGNS AND SYMPTOMS

- High fever.
- Vomiting.
- Diarrhea.
- Myalgias.
- Headache.
- Malaise.
- Diffuse sunburn-like macular rash appears within 24 hours.
- Rash is associated with hyperemia of pharyngeal, conjunctival, and vaginal mucous membranes.
- Altered level of consciousness.
- Generally accompanied by desquamation of palms and soles, hair and nail loss.

LABORATORY

- Coagulopathy
- Hypocalcemia
- Hypoalbuminemia
- Leukocytosis
- Elevated blood urea nitrogen (BUN), creatinine
- Elevated creatine phosphokinase (CPK)

TREATMENT

- Recovery in 7 to 10 days
- Aggressive fluid replacement
- Eradication of source
- Parenteral β-lactamase–resistant antibiotic

FUNGAL INFECTIONS

Coccidioidomycosis

PATHOPHYSIOLOGY

Three forms:

- Benign, self-limited (60% no clinical manifestations)
- Residual pulmonary lesions
- Rare disseminating disease

EPIDEMIOLOGY

Southwestern United States.

SIGNS AND SYMPTOMS

- Usually benign self-limited disease with:
  - Malaise, chills, and fever
  - Chest pain
  - Night sweats and anorexia
- Fatal disseminated form also occurs, but rare.

TREATMENT

- Same as for histoplasmosis below.
- Surgery for chronic pulmonary coccidioidal disease that is unresponsive to IV azole or amphotericin B therapy

DIAGNOSIS

- Tissue culture
- Coccidioidin skin test
- May see nodules on chest x-ray
- Elevated erythrocyte sedimentation rate (ESR), and alkaline phosphatase
- Marked eosinophilia

Histoplasmosis

PATHOPHYSIOLOGY

Three forms:

- Acute pulmonary infection
- Chronic pulmonary infection (adults with centrilobular emphysema; rare in children)
- Progressive disseminated disease (infants and immunosuppressed) Usually under age 2.

EPIDEMIOLOGY

- Ohio and Mississippi River valleys
- History of exposure to bird droppings

SIGNS AND SYMPTOMS

- Generally asymptomatic
- Flulike prodrome
- Hepatosplenomegaly in younger children

DIAGNOSIS

- Mediastinal granulomas may be seen on CXR.
- Elevated liver function tests.
- Radioimmunoassay for dectection of *Histoplasma* antigen.
- Sputum culture yield is variable.
- Blood cultures negative in acute cases.

TREATMENT

- Supportive therapy only for immunocompetent and asymptomatic children.
- Oral itraconazole for those who fail to improve after 1 month.
- IV amphotericin B for severe cases.

PROTOZOAL INFECTIONS

Schistosomiasis

ETIOLOGY

- Caused by trematodes (flukes)
- *Schistosoma haematobium:* bladder
- *Schistosoma interclatum* and *Schistosoma mekongi:* mesenteric vessels
- *Schistosoma mansoni* and *Schistosoma japonicum:* liver

PATHOPHYSIOLOGY

Transmission due to infected water containing immature form, which penetrates the skin.

SIGNS AND SYMPTOMS

- Within 3 to 12 weeks: fever, malaise, cough, abdominal pain, and rash (due to worm maturing).
- Hematuria.
- Bladder granulomas lead to renal failure and bladder cancer (*S. haematobium*).
- Ulceration of intestine and colon, abdominal pain, and bloody diarrhea (*S. interclatum* and *S. mekongi*).
- Hepateosplenomegaly, portal hypertension, ascites, and hematemesis (*S. mansoni* and *S. japonicum*).

DIAGNOSIS

Eggs in stool or urine.

TREATMENT

Praziquantel.

Visceral Larva Migrans

PATHOPHYSIOLOGY

- Ingestion of dog or cat tapeworms.
- Ingested eggs hatch and penetrate the GI tract, migrating to the liver, lung, eye, central nervous system, and heart, where they die and calcify.

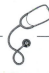

Differentiate eye lesions of visceral larva migrans from retinoblastoma.

SIGNS AND SYMPTOMS

- Most individuals are asymptomatic.
- May have fever, cough, wheezing, and seizures.
- Physical findings: hepatomegaly, rales, rash, and adenopathy.
- May have visual symptoms.
- Granulomatous lesion near macula or disc.

DIAGNOSIS

Eosinophilia and confirmation by serology.

TREATMENT

Generally self-limited.

TRAUMATIC INFECTIONS

Animal Bites/Scratches

- Antibiotic prophylaxis for human, cat, and dog bites (amoxicillin/clavulanate).
- Cleaning, debridement, and irrigation are most important treatment.
- X-ray to check for bone involvement if deep wound.
- Most wounds should not be sutured; if deep wounds, surgical consult is best.
- Assess risk for rabies.
- Ensure tetanus immunization is up to date.

Abrasions and Lacerations

- Cleaning, debridement, and irrigation are most important initial treatment. Suturing indicated if no obvious signs of infection.
- If secondarily infected, debride and drain.
- Initial antibiotic given based on most likely organism; Gram stain and culture to determine best antibiotic in chronic or complex wounds.
- *Staphylococcus* and *Streptococcus* are the most common pathogens, so first-generation cephalosporin such as cephalexin is commonly given as empiric treatment.

Gastrointestinal Disease

ESOPHAGEAL ATRESIA

DEFINITION

- The esophagus ends blindly approximately 10 to 12 cm from the nares.
- Occurs in 1/3,000 to 1/4,500 live births.
- In 85% of cases the distal esophagus communicates with the posterior trachea (distal tracheoesophageal fistula [TEF]).

SIGNS AND SYMPTOMS

- History of maternal polyhydramnios
- Newborn with increased oral secretions
- Choking, cyanosis, coughing during feeding (more commonly aspiration of pharyngeal secretions)
- Esophageal atresia with fistula
  - Aspiration of gastric contents via distal fistula—**life threatening** (chemical pneumonitis)
  - Tympanitic distended abdomen
  - Esophageal atresia without fistula
  - Recurrent coughing with aspiration pneumonia (delayed diagnosis)
  - Aspiration of pharyngeal secretions common
  - Airless abdomen on abdominal x-ray

DIAGNOSIS

- Usually made at delivery
- Unable to pass nasogastric tube (NGT) into stomach (see coiled NGT on chest x-ray)
- May also use contrast radiology, videoesophagram, or bronchoscopy
- Chest x-ray (CXR) demonstrates air in upper esophagus (see Figure 11–1)

TREATMENT

Surgical repair (may be done in stages).

Esophageal atresia can be associated with the **VACTERL** sequence
Vertebral
Anorectal
Cardiac
Tracheal
Esophageal
Renal
Limb anomalies

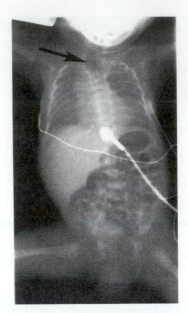

FIGURE 11-1. Esophageal atresia. Radiograph demonstrating air in the upper esophagus (arrow) and GI tract, consistent with esophageal atresia.

GERD is the etiology for Sandifer's syndrome (reflux, back arching, stiffness, and torticollis). Sandifer's syndrome is most often confused with a neurologic or apparent life-threatening event.

ESOPHAGEAL FOREIGN BODY

See Figure 11–2.

GASTROESOPHAGEAL REFLUX DISEASE (GERD)

DEFINITION

- Passive reflux of gastric contents due to incompetent lower esophageal sphincter (LES).
- Approximately 1/300 children suffer from significant reflux and complication.

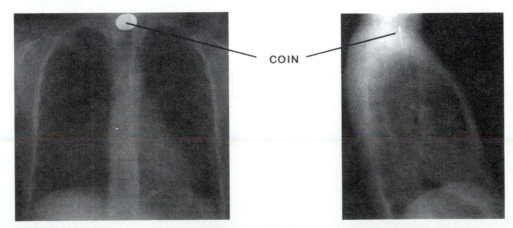

COIN

FIGURE 11-2. Esophageal foreign body. A coin in the esophagus will be seen flat or *en face* on an AP radiograph, and on its edge on a lateral view. (Photo courtesy of Dr. Julia Rosekrans.)

SIGNS AND SYMPTOMS

- Excessive spitting up in the first week of life (in 85% of affected).
- Symptomatic by 6 weeks (10%).
- Symptoms resolve without treatment by age 2 (60%).
- Forceful vomiting (occasional).
- Aspiration pneumonia (30%).
- Chronic cough, wheezing, and recurrent pneumonia (later childhood).
- Rarely may cause laryngospasm, apnea, and bradycardia.

DIAGNOSIS

- Clinical assessment in mild cases
- Esophageal pH probe studies and barium esophagography in severe cases
- Esophagoscopy with biopsy for diagnosis of esophagitis

TREATMENT

- Positioning following feeds—keep infant upright up to an hour after feeds.
- In older children, mealtime more than 2 hours before sleep and sleeping with head elevated.
- Thickening formula with rice cereal.
- Medications:
  - Antacids, histamine-2 (H_2) blockers (ranitidine) and proton pump inhibitors (PPIs) (omeprazole)
  - Motility agents such as metoclopramide and erythromycin (stimulate gastric emptying)
- Surgery—Nissen fundoplication.

The most common cause of esophagitis is *Candida*.

Typical Scenario

An 8-month-old infant has been hospitalized for 4 months in the chronic care unit. In the last 2 weeks, the nurses have noted that he is regurgitating several times an hour. He makes chewing movements preceding these episodes of regurgitation. *Think:* Rumination.

PEPTIC ULCER

DEFINITION

Includes primary and secondary (related to stress).

SIGNS AND SYMPTOMS

- Primary—pain, vomiting, and acute and chronic gastrointestinal (GI) blood loss
  - **First month of life:** GI hemorrhage and perforation
  - **Neonatal–2 months:** recurrent vomiting, slow growth, and GI hemorrhage
  - **Preschool:** periumbilical and postprandial pain (with vomiting and hemorrhage)
  - **> 6 years:** epigastric abdominal pain, acute/chronic GI blood loss with anemia
- Secondary
  - Stress ulcers secondary to sepsis, respiratory or cardiac insufficiency, trauma, or dehydration in infants
  - Related to trauma or other life-threatening events (older children)
  - Stress ulcers and erosions associated with burns (Curling ulcers)
  - Ulcers following head trauma or surgery usually Cushing ulcers
  - Drug related—nonsteroidal anti-inflammatory drugs (NSAIDs) or steroids

DIAGNOSIS

- Upper GI endoscopy.
- Barium meal not sensitive.
- Plain x-rays may diagnose perforation of acute ulcers.
- Angiography can demonstrate bleeding site.

TREATMENT

- Antacids, sucralfate, and misoprostol.
- H_2 blockers and PPIs.
- Give prophylaxis for peptic ulcer when child is NPO or is receiving steroids.
- Endoscopic cautery.
- Surgery (vagotomy, pyloroplasty, or antrectomy) for extreme cases.

COLIC

DEFINITION

- Frequent complex of paroxysmal abdominal pain, severe crying
- Usually in infants < 3 months old
- Etiology unknown

SIGNS AND SYMPTOMS

- Sudden-onset loud crying (paroxysms may persist for several hours)
- Facial flushing
- Circumoral pallor
- Distended, tense abdomen
- Legs drawn up on abdomen
- Feet often cold
- Temporary relief apparent with passage of feces or flatus

TREATMENT

- No single treatment provides satisfactory relief.
- Careful exam is important to rule out other causes.
- Passage of flatus or fecal material by aid of enema or suppository may work.
- Improve feeding techniques (burping).
- Avoid over- or underfeeding.

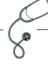

Parents and caretakers of children with colic are often very stressed out, putting the child at risk for child abuse.

PYLORIC STENOSIS

DEFINITION

- Most common etiology is idiopathic.
- Not usually present at birth.
- Associated with exogenous administration of erythromycin, eosinophilic gastroenteritis, epidermolysis bullosa, trisomy 18, and Turner's syndrome.

SIGNS AND SYMPTOMS

- Nonbilious vomiting (projectile or not)
- Usually progressive, after feeding
- Usually after 3 weeks of age, may be as late as 5 months

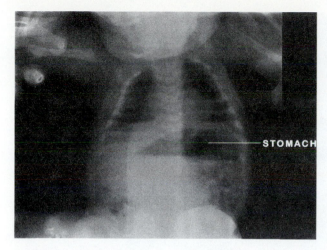
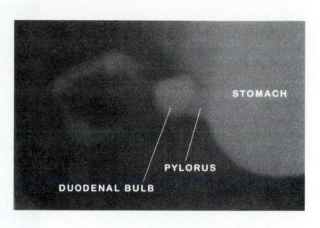

FIGURE 11-3. Abdominal x-ray on the left demonstrates a dilated air-filled stomach with normal caliber bowel, consistent with gastric outlet obstruction. Barium meal figure on the right confirms diagnosis of pyloric stenosis. The dilated duodenal bulb is the "olive" felt on physical exam. Note how there is a paucity of contrast traveling through the duodenum. (Photo courtesy of Drs. Julia Rosekrans and James E. Colletti.)

- Hypochloremic, hypokalemic metabolic alkalosis (rare these days due to earlier diagnosis)
- Palpable pyloric olive-shaped mass in midepigastrium (difficult to find)

DIAGNOSIS

- Ultrasound (90% sensitivity)
  - Elongated pyloric channel (> 14 mm)
  - Thickened pyloric wall (> 4 mm)
- Radiographic contrast series (Figure 11-3)
  - **String sign**—from elongated pyloric channel
  - **Shoulder sign**—bulge of pyloric muscle into the antrum
  - **Double tract sign**—parallel streaks of barium in the narrow channel

TREATMENT

Surgery—pyloromyotomy is curative.

DUODENAL ATRESIA

DEFINITION

- Failure to recanalize lumen after solid phase of intestinal development
- Several forms

SIGNS AND SYMPTOMS

- Bilious vomiting without abdominal distention (first day of life).
- History of polyhydramnios in 50% of pregnancies.
- Down's syndrome seen in 20–30% of cases.
- Associated anomalies include malrotation, esophageal atresia, and congenital heart disease.

DIAGNOSIS

- Clinical
- X-ray findings: **Double bubble sign (Figure 11-4)**

> **Typical Scenario**
>
> A 4-week-old male infant has a 5-day history of vomiting after feedings. Physical exam shows a hungry infant with prominent peristaltic waves in the epigastrium. *Think:* Hypertrophic pyloric stenosis.

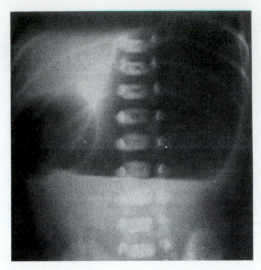

FIGURE 11-4. Duodenal atresia. Gas-filled and dilated stomach show the classic "double bubble" appearance of duodenal atresia. Note no distal gas is present. (Reproduced, with permission, from *Rudolph's Pediatrics,* 20th ed., Appleton & Lange, 1996.)

TREATMENT

- Initially, nasogastric and orogastric decompression with intravenous (IV) fluid replacement.
- Treat life-threatening anomalies.
- Surgery.
- Duodenoduodenostomy.

VOLVULUS

DEFINITION

- Gastric and intestinal:
  - Gastric: sudden onset of severe epigastric pain; intractable retching with emesis; inability to pass gastric tube
  - Intestinal: associated with malrotation (Figure 11-5)

SIGNS AND SYMPTOMS

- Vomiting in infancy
- Emesis
- Abdominal pain
- Early satiety

DIAGNOSIS

- Plain abdominal films: characteristic bird-beak appearance
- May also see air–fluid level without beak

TREATMENT

- Gastric: emergent surgery
- Intestinal: surgery or endoscopy

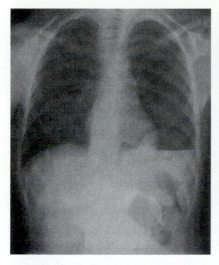
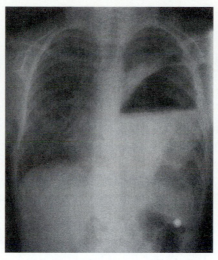
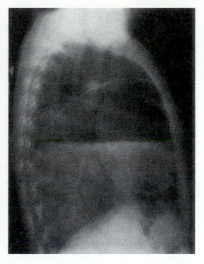

FIGURE 11-5. Volvulus. 1st AP view done 6 weeks prior to the 2nd AP and corresponding lateral view. Note the markedly dilated stomach above the normal level of the left hemidiaphragm, in the thoracic cavity. Also present is a large left-sided diaphragmatic hernia. (Photo courtesy of Dr. Julia Rosekrans.)

INTUSSUSCEPTION

DEFINITION

Invagination of one portion of the bowel into itself. The proximal portion is usually drawn into the distal portion by peristalsis.

EPIDEMIOLOGY

- Incidence: 1 to 4 in 1,000 live births
- Male-to-female ratio: 2:1 to 4:1
- Peak incidence: 5 to 12 months
- Age range: 2 months to 5 years

CAUSES

- Most common etiology is idiopathic.
- Other causes:
  - Viral (enterovirus in summer, rotavirus in winter)
  - A "lead point" (or focus) is thought to be present in older children 2–10% of the time. These lead points can be caused by:
    - Meckel's diverticulum
    - Polyp
    - Lymphoma
    - Henoch–Schönlein purpura
    - Cystic fibrosis

SIGNS AND SYMPTOMS

Classic Triad
- Intermittent colicky abdominal pain
- Bilious vomiting
- Currant jelly stool

Neurologic signs
- Lethargy
- Shock-like state

- Most common cause of acute intestinal obstruction under 2 years of age
- Most common site is ileocolic (90%)

Intussusception is the most common cause of bowel obstruction in children ages 2 months to 5 years.

Intussusception and link with rotavirus vaccine led to withdrawal of vaccine from the market.

- Seizure activity
- Apnea

Right Upper Quadrant Mass
- Sausage shaped
- Ill defined
- Dance's sign—absence of bowel in right lower quadrant

DIAGNOSIS

Abdominal X-Ray
- Paucity of bowel gas (Figure 11-6)
- Loss of visualization of the tip of liver
- "Target sign"—two concentric circles of fat density

Ultrasound
- Test of choice
- "Target" or "donut" sign—single hypoechoic ring with hyperechoic center
- "Pseudokidney" sign—superimposed hypoechoic (edematous walls of bowel) and hyperechoic (areas of compressed mucosa) layers

Barium Enema
- Not useful for ileoileal intussusceptions
- Requires ingestion of barium, so more invasive than ultrasound
- May note cervix-like mass
- Coiled spring appearance on the evacuation film
- Contraindications
  - Peritonitis
  - Perforation
  - Profound shock

Air Enema
Often provides the same diagnostic and therapeutic benefit of a barium enema without the barium

Intussusception
- Classic triad is present in only 20% of cases.
- Absence of currant jelly stool does not exclude the diagnosis.
- Neurologic signs may delay the diagnosis.

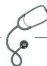

Contrast enema for intussusception can be both diagnostic and therapeutic. Rule of threes:
- Barium column should not exceed a height of 3 feet.
- No more than 3 attempts.
- Only 3 minutes/attempt.

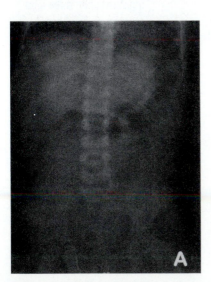
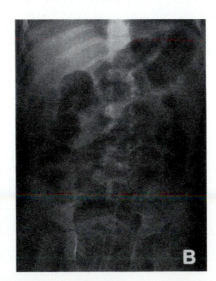
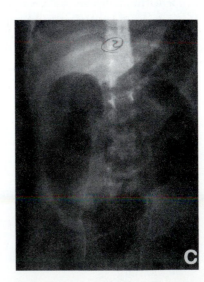

FIGURE 11-6. Intussusception. Note the paucity of bowel gas in film A. Air enema partially reduces it in film B and then completely reduced it in film C.

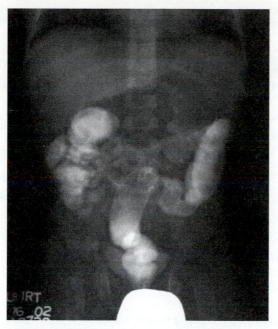

FIGURE 11-7. Abdominal x-ray following barium enema in a 2-month-old boy, consistent with intussusception. Note paucity of gas in right upper quadrant and near obscuring of liver tip.

TREATMENT

- Correct dehydration
- NG tube for decompression
- Hydrostatic reduction
- Barium/air enema (see Figure 11–7)

RECURRENCE

- With radiologic reduction: 7–10%
- With surgical reduction: 2–5%

MECKEL'S DIVERTICULUM

DEFINITION

Persistence of the omphalomesenteric (vitelline) duct (should disappear by seventh week of gestation).

SIGNS AND SYMPTOMS

Usually in first 2 years:
- Intermittent painless rectal bleeding
- Intestinal obstruction
- Diverticulitis

DIAGNOSIS

Meckel's scan (scintigraphy) has 85% sensitivity and 95% specificity. Uptake can be enhanced with cimetidine, glucagons, or gastrin.

TREATMENT

Surgical: diverticular resection with transverse closure of the enterotomy.

Meckel's Rules of 2
- 2% of population
- 2 inches long
- 2 feet from the ileocecal valve
- Patient is usually under 2 years of age
- 2% are symptomatic

Meckel's diverticulum may mimic acute appendicitis and also act as lead point for intussusception.

133

DEFINITION

- Most common cause for emergent surgery in childhood.
- Perforation rates are greatest in youngest children (can't localize symptoms).
- Occurs secondary to obstruction of lumen of appendix.
- Three phases:
  1. Luminal obstruction, venous congestion progresses to mucosal ischemia, necrosis, and ulceration.
  2. Bacterial invasion with inflammatory infiltrate through all layers.
  3. Necrosis of wall results in perforation and contamination.

SIGNS AND SYMPTOMS

- Classically: pain, vomiting, and fever.
- Initially, pain periumbilical; emesis infrequent.
- Anorexia.
- Low-grade fever.
- Diarrhea infrequent.
- Pain radiates to right lower quadrant.
- Perforation rate > 65% after 48 hours.
- Rectal exam may reveal localized mass or tenderness.

DIAGNOSIS

- History and physical exam is key to rule out alternatives first.
- Pain usually occurs before vomiting, diarrhea, or anorexia.
- Labs helpful to rule other diagnosis.
- Computed tomographic (CT) scan (Figure 11-8) indicated for patients in whom diagnosis is equivocal—*not* a requirement for all patients.

TREATMENT

- Surgery as soon as diagnosis made.
- Antibiotics are controversial in nonperforated appendicitis.

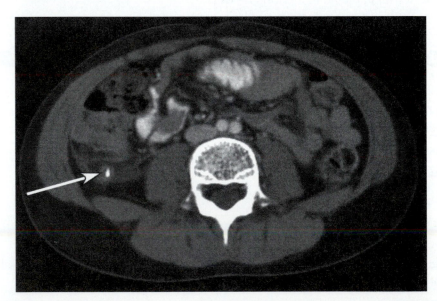

FIGURE 11-8. Abdominal CT of a 10-year-old girl demonstrating enlargement of the appendix, some periappendiceal fluid, and an appendicolith (arrow), consistent with acute appendicitis.

- Broad-spectrum antibiotics needed for cases of perforation (ampicillin, gentamicin, clindamycin, or metronidazole × 7 days).
- Laparoscopic removal associated with shortened hospital stay (nonperforated appendicitis).

CONSTIPATION

DEFINITION/SIGNS AND SYMPTOMS

- Passage of bulky or hard stool at infrequent intervals.
- During the neonatal period usually caused by Hirschsprung disease, intestinal pseudo-obstruction, or hypothyroidism.
- Other causes include organic and inorganic (e.g., cow's milk protein intolerance, drugs).
- May be metabolic (dehydration, hypothyroidism, hypokalemia, hypercalcemia, psychiatric).

TREATMENT

- Increase PO fluid and fiber intake.
- Stool softeners (e.g., mineral oil).
- Glycerin suppositories.
- Cathartics such as senna or docusate.
- Nonabsorbable osmotic agents (polyethylene glycol) and milk of magnesia for short periods only if necessary—can cause electrolyte imbalances.

HIRSCHSPRUNG'S MEGACOLON

DEFINITION

- Abnormal innervation of bowel (i.e., absence of ganglion cells in bowel)
- Increase in familial incidence
- Occurs in males more than females
- Associated with Down's syndrome

SIGNS AND SYMPTOMS

- Delayed passage of meconium at birth
- Increased abdominal distention → decreased blood flow → deterioration of mucosal barrier → bacterial proliferation → enterocolitis
- Chronic constipation and abdominal distention (older children)

DIAGNOSIS

- Rectal manometry: measures pressure of the anal sphincter
- Rectal suction biopsy: must obtain submucosa to evaluate for ganglionic cells

TREATMENT

Surgery is definitive (usually staged procedures).

HIGH-YIELD FACTS

Gastrointestinal Disease

IMPERFORATE ANUS

DEFINITION

- Rectum is blind; located 2 cm from perineal skin
- Sacrum and sphincter mechanism well developed
- Prognosis good

TREATMENT

Surgery (colostomy in newborn period).

> Imperforate anus is frequently associated with Down's syndrome and VACTERL.

ANAL FISSURE

DEFINITION

Painful linear tears in the anal mucosa below the dentate line induced by constipation or excessive diarrhea.

SIGNS AND SYMPTOMS

Pain with defecation, bright red blood on toilet tissue, markedly increased sphincter tone, extreme pain on digital examination, visible tear upon gentle lateral retraction of anal tissue.

DIAGNOSIS

History and physical exam.

TREATMENT

Sitz baths, fiber supplements, increased fluid intake.

> **Typical Scenario**
>
> A well-nourished 3-month-old infant is brought to the emergency department because of constipation, blood-streaked stools, and excessive crying on defecation. *Think:* Anal fissure.

INFLAMMATORY BOWEL DISEASE

DEFINITION

Idiopathic chronic diseases include Crohn's disease and ulcerative colitis (UC).

EPIDEMIOLOGY

- Common onset in adolescence and young adulthood.
- Bimodal pattern in patients 15 to 25 and 50 to 80 years of age.
- Genetics: increased concordance with monozygotic twins versus dizygotic (increased for Crohn's versus UC).

SIGNS AND SYMPTOMS (SEE TABLE 11–1)

- Crampy abdominal pain
- Extraintestinal manifestations greater in Crohn's than UC
- Crohn's: perianal fistula, sclerosing cholangitis, chronic active hepatitis, pyoderma gangrenosum, ankylosing spondylitis
- UC: bloody diarrhea, anorexia, weight loss, pyoderma gangrenosum, sclerosing cholangitis, marked by flare-ups

TREATMENT

- Crohn's: corticosteroids, aminosalicylates, methotrexate, azathioprine, cyclosporine, metronidazole (for perianal disease), sitz baths, anti–tumor necrosis factor-α, surgery for complications
- UC: aminosalicylates, oral corticosteroids, colectomy

> **Typical Scenario**
>
> A 14-year-old girl has a 2-month history of crampy and diffuse abdominal pain with anorexia and a 4.5-kg weight loss. The pain is unrelated to meals, and there is no diarrhea or constipation. Appropriate initial management would include all of the following: rectal exam; stool exam for ova, cysts, and parasites; complete blood count (CBC) and erythrocyte sedimentation rate (ESR); review of family emotional stress, *except* referral to an eating disorder clinic.

Table 11-1. Crohn's disease versus ulcerative colitis.

Feature	Crohn's Disease	Ulcerative Colitis (UC)
Depth of involvement	Transmural	Mucosal
Ileal involvement	Common	Unusual
Ulcers	Common	Unusual
Cancer risk	Lower	Higher
Pyoderma gangrenosum	Slightly increased	Greatly increased
Skip lesions	Common	Unusual
Fistula	Common	Unusual
Rectal bleeding	Sometimes	Common

IRRITABLE BOWEL SYNDROME

DEFINITION

- Abdominal pain associated with intermittent diarrhea and constipation without organic basis
- Approximately 10% in adolescents

SIGNS AND SYMPTOMS

- Abdominal pain
- Diarrhea alternating with constipation

DIAGNOSIS

- Difficult to make, exclude other pathology
- Obtain CBC, ESR, stool occult blood

TREATMENT

- None specific
- Supportive with reinforcement and reassurance
- Address any underlying psychosocial stressors

ACUTE GASTROENTERITIS AND DIARRHEA

DEFINITION

- **Diarrhea** is the excessive loss of fluid and electrolytes in stool, usually secondary to disturbed intestinal solute transport. Technically limited to lower GI tract.
- **Gastroenteritis** is an inflammation of the entire (upper and lower) GI tract, and thus involves both vomiting and diarrhea.

EPIDEMIOLOGY

- Increased susceptibility seen in young age, immunodeficiency, measles, malnutrition, travel, lack of breast-feeding, and contaminated food or water.
- Most common cause of diarrhea in children is viral—often rotavirus.
- Children in developing countries often also get infected by bacterial and parasitic pathogens.

SIGNS AND SYMPTOMS

- Important to obtain information regarding frequency and volume.

Acute diarrhea is usually caused by infectious agents, whereas chronic persistent diarrhea may be secondary to infectious agents, infection of immunocompromised host, or residual symptoms due to intestinal damage.

- Diarrhea and emesis → noninflammatory
- Diarrhea and fever → inflammatory process
- Diarrhea and tenesmus → large colon involvement

Typical Scenario

A 9-month-old infant who attends day care has a temperature of 104°F (40°C) rectally and diarrhea × 2 days. The stools are blood-streaked and contain mucus. WBC count is 23,000 with 40% segmented neutrophils and 20% band forms. Sixty minutes earlier, the patient had a brief generalized seizure. Physical and neurologic exams are normal. *Think:* Shigella sonnei.

Diarrhea is a characteristic finding in children poisoned with bacterial toxin of *Escherichia coli, Salmonella, Staphylococcus aureus,* and *Vibrio parahemolyticus,* but **not** *Clostridium botulinum.*

- General patient appearance important (well appearing versus lethargic).
- Associated findings include cramps, emesis, malaise, and fever.
- May see systemic manifestations, GI tract involvement, or extraintestinal infections.
    - Extraintestinal findings include vulvovaginitis, urinary tract infection (UTI), and keratoconjunctivitis.
    - Systemic manifestations: fever, malaise, and seizures.
- Inflammatory diarrhea—fever, severe abdominal pain, tenesmus.
- Noninflammatory diarrhea—emesis, fever usually absent, crampy abdominal pain, watery diarrhea.

DIAGNOSIS

- Examine stool for mucus, blood, and leukocytes (colitis).
- Fecal leukocyte—presence of invasive cytotoxin organisms (*Shigella, Salmonella*).
- Patients with enterohemorrhagic *Entamoeba coli* and *Entamoeba histolytica*—minimal to no fecal leukocytes.
- Obtain stool cultures early.
- *Clostridium difficile* toxins—test if recent antibiotic use.
- Proctosigmoidoscopy—diagnosis of inflammatory enteritis.

TREATMENT

- Rehydration
    - Oral electrolyte solutions (e.g., Pedialyte).
    - Oral hydration for all but severely dehydrated (IV hydration).
    - Rapid rehydration with replacement of ongoing losses during first 4 to 6 hours.
- Do not use soda, fruit juices, jello, or tea. High osmolality may exacerbate diarrhea.
- Start food with BRAT diet.
- Antidiarrheal compounds are not indicated for use in children.
- See Table 11-2 for antibiotic treatment of enteropathogens.

TABLE 11-2. Antimicrobial treatment for bacterial enteropathogens.

Bacteria	Treatment	Comments
Aeromonas	Trimethoprim–sulfamethoxazole (TMP-SMZ)	Prolonged diarrhea
Campylobacter	Erythromycin	Early in course of illness
Clostridium difficile	Metronidazole or vancomycin	Moderate to severe diagnosis
Enterotoxigenic *Escherichia coli*	TMP-SMZ	Severe or prolonged illness
Enteropathogenic	TMP-SMZ	Nursery epidemics
Enteroinvasive	TMP-SMZ	All cases
Salmonella	Ampicillin or chloramphenicol or TMP-SMZ	Infants < 3 months, immunodeficient patients, bacteremia
Shigella	TMP-SMZ, ceftriaxone	All susceptible organisms
Vibrio cholerae	Tetracycline or doxycycline	All cases

PREVENTION

- Hospitalized patients should be placed under contact precautions (handwashing, gloves, gowns, etc.).
- Education.
- Exclude infected children from child care centers.
- Report cases of bacterial diarrhea to local health department.
- Vaccines for cholera and *Salmonella typhi* are available.

INTESTINAL WORMS

See Table 11-3 for common intestinal worm infestations.

PSEUDOMEMBRANOUS COLITIS

DEFINITION

- Major cause of nosocomial diarrhea.
- Rarely occurs without antecedent antibiotics (usually) penicillins, cephalosporins, or clindamycin.
- Antibiotic disrupts normal bowel flora and predisposes to C. *difficile* diarrhea.

SIGNS AND SYMPTOMS

Classically, blood and mucus with fever, cramps, abdominal pain, nausea, and vomiting days or weeks after antibiotics.

DIAGNOSIS

- Recent history of antibiotic use
- C. *difficile* toxin in stool of patient with diarrhea
- Sigmoidoscopy or colonoscopy

TREATMENT

- Discontinue antibiotics.
- Oral metronidazole × 7 to 10 days.

ABDOMINAL HERNIAS

Umbilical

DEFINITION

- Occurs because of imperfect closure of umbilical ring
- Common in low-birth-weight, female, and African-American infants
- Soft swelling covered by skin that protrudes while crying, straining, or coughing
- Omentum or portions of small intestine involved
- Usually 1 to 5 cm

TREATMENT

- Most disappear spontaneously by 1 year of age.
- Strangulation rare.
- "Strapping" ineffective.
- Surgery not indicated unless symptomatic, strangulated, or grows larger after age 1 or 2.

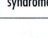

BRAT Diet for Diarrhea
Bread
Rice
Applesauce
Toast

Do not treat *E. coli* 0157:H7 with antibiotics as there is a higher incidence of hemolytic uremic syndrome with treatment.

The most frequent symptom of infestation with *Enterobius vermicularis* is perineal pruritus. Can diagnose with transparent adhesive tape to area (worms stick).

HIGH-YIELD FACTS

Gastrointestinal Disease

TABLE 11-3. Common intestinal worms.

Intestinal Nematodes	Mode of Transmission	Disease, Symptoms and Signs	Treatment
Enterobius vermicularis (pinworm)	Hand to mouth	Perianal itching, especially at night	Albendazole or mebendazole or pyrantel pamoate 11 mg/kg (max. dose, 1 g PO × 1)
Trichuris trichuria (whipworm)	Fecal–oral	■ Usually asymptomatic ■ Mild anemia ■ Abdominal pain ■ Diarrhea, tenesmus ■ Perianal itching	Albendazole or mebendazole
Ascaris lumbricoides	Fecal–oral	■ Pneumonia ■ Loeffler's pneumonitis ■ Intestinal infection/obstruction ■ Liver failure	Albendazole or mebendazole
Necator Americanus (new world hookworm) and *Ancylostoma duodenale* (old world hookworm)	Skin penetration	■ Intense dermatitis ■ Loeffler's pneumonitis ■ Significant anemia ■ GI symptoms ■ Developmental delay in children (irreversible)	Albendazole or mebendazole
Strongyloides stercoralis	Skin penetration	Same as for *Necator*, plus: ■ Diarrhea × 3–6 weeks ■ Superimposed bacterial sepsis	Ivermectin 200 µg/kg/day × 2 days
Trichinella spiralis	Infected pork	Trichinosis ■ Myalgias ■ Facial and periorbital edema ■ Conjunctivitis ■ Pneumonia, myocarditis, encephalitis, nephritis, meningitis	Albendazole 400 mg PO bid × 14 days + prednisone 40–60 mg PO qd

Usual albendazole dose is 400 mg PO × 1; usual mebendazole dose is 100 mg PO × 1 for 3 days.

Adapted, with permission, from Stead L. BRS Emergency Medicine. Lippincott Williams & Wilkins, 2000.

Inguinal

DEFINITION

- Most common diagnosis requiring surgery
- 10 to 20/1,000 live births (50% < 1 year)
- Indirect > direct (rare) > femoral (even more rare)
- Indirect secondary to patent processus vaginalis
- Increased incidence with positive family history

SIGNS AND SYMPTOMS

- Infant with scrotal/inguinal bulge on straining or crying.
- Do careful exam to distinguish from hydrocele (see Figure 11-9).

TREATMENT

- Surgery (elective).
- Avoid trusses or supports.

In inguinal hernia, processus vaginalis herniates through abdominal wall with hydrocele into canal.

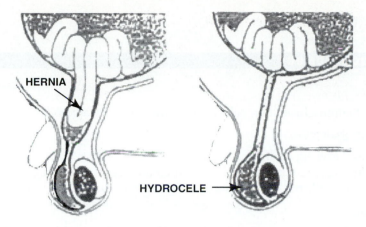

FIGURE 11-9. Inguinal hernia (slippage of bowel through inguinal ring) vs. hydrocele (collection of fluid in scrotum adjacent to testes).

- Contralateral hernia occurs in 30% after unilateral repair.
- Antibiotics only in at-risk children (e.g., congenital heart disease).
- Prognosis excellent (recurrence < 1%, complication rate approximately 2%, infection approximately 1%).
- Complications include incarceration.

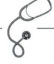

Inguinal hernia increases with straining, hydrocele remains unchanged.

PEUTZ–JEGHERS SYNDROME

DEFINITION

- Mucosal pigmentation of lips and gums with hamartomas of stomach, small intestine, and colon
- Rare; low malignant potential

SIGNS AND SYMPTOMS

- Deeply pigmented freckles on lips and buccal mucosa at birth
- Bleeding and crampy abdominal pain

DIAGNOSIS

Genetic and family studies may reveal history.

TREATMENT

Excise intestinal lesions if significantly symptomatic.

Typical Scenario

A 15-year-old girl with spots on her lips has some crampy abdominal pain associated with bleeding. *Think:* Peutz–Jeghers syndrome.

GARDNER'S SYNDROME

DEFINITION

Multiple intestinal polyps, tumors of soft tissue and bone (especially mandible).

SIGNS AND SYMPTOMS

- Dental abnormalities
- Pigmented lesions in ocular fundus
- Intestinal polyps (usually early adulthood) with high malignant potential

DIAGNOSIS

- Genetic counseling
- Colon surveillance in at-risk children

TREATMENT

Aggressive surgical removal of polyps.

CARCINOID TUMORS

DEFINITION

Tumors of enterochromaffin cells in intestine—usually appendix.

SIGNS AND SYMPTOMS

- May cause appendicitis
- May cause carcinoid syndrome (increased serotonin, vasomotor disturbances, or bronchoconstriction) if metastatic to the liver

TREATMENT

Surgical excision.

FAMILIAL POLYPOSIS COLI

DEFINITION/ETIOLOGY

- Autosomal dominant
- Large number of adenomatous lesions in colon
- Secondary to germ-line mutations in adenopolyposis coli (APC) gene

SIGNS AND SYMPTOMS

- Highly variable
- May see hematochezia, cramps, or diarrhea
- Extracolonic manifestations possible

DIAGNOSIS

- Consider family history (strong).
- Colonoscopy with biopsy (screening annually after 10 years old if positive family history).

TREATMENT

Surgical resection of affected colonic mucosa.

JUVENILE POLYPOSIS COLI

DEFINITION

- Most common childhood bowel tumor (3–4% of patients < 21 years)
- Characteristically, mucus-filled cystic glands (no adenomatous changes, no potential for malignancy)

EPIDEMIOLOGY

Most commonly between 2 and 10 years; less common after 15 years; rarely before 1 year.

SIGNS AND SYMPTOMS

- Bright red painless bleeding with bowel movement
- Iron deficiency

DIAGNOSIS

- Colonoscopy
- May use barium enema (not best test)

TREATMENT

Surgical removal of polyp.

Short Bowel Syndrome

DEFINITION

- Occurs with loss of at least 50% of small bowel (with or without loss of large bowel)
- Decreased absorptive surface and bowel function

ETIOLOGY

- May be congenital (malrotation, atresia, etc.)
- Most commonly secondary to surgical resection

SIGNS AND SYMPTOMS

- Malabsorption and diarrhea
- Steatorrhea (fatty stools): voluminous foul smelling stools that float
- Dehydration
- Decreased sodium and potassium
- Acidosis (secondary to loss of bicarbonate)

TREATMENT

- Total parenteral nutrition (TPN).
- Give small feeds orally.
- Metronidazole empirically to treat bacterial overgrowth.

Celiac Disease

DEFINITION

- Sensitivity to gluten in diet
- Most commonly occurs between 6 months and 2 years

ETIOLOGY

- Factors involved include cereals, genetic predisposition, and environmental factors.
- Associated with HLA-B8, -DR7, -DR3, and DQW2.

SIGNS AND SYMPTOMS

- Diarrhea
- Failure to thrive
- Vomiting
- Pallor
- Abdominal distention
- Large bulky stools

DIAGNOSIS

- Antiendomysial and antitissue transglutaminase antibodies
- Biopsy: most reliable test

TREATMENT

- Dietary restriction of gluten
- Corticosteroids used rarely (very ill patients with profound malnutrition, diarrhea, edema, and hypokalemia)

Tropical Sprue

DEFINITION

- Generalized malabsorption associated with diffuse lesions of small bowel mucosa
- Seen in people who live or have traveled to certain tropical regions— some Caribbean countries, South America, Africa, or parts of Asia

---

Typical Scenario

A 5-year-old girl presents with a protuberant abdomen and wasted extremities. *Think:* Gluten-induced enteropathy.

SIGNS AND SYMPTOMS

- Fever, malaise, and watery diarrhea, acutely
- After 1 week, chronic malabsorption and signs of malnutrition including night blindness, glossitis, stomatitis, cheliosis, muscle wasting

DIAGNOSIS

Biopsy shows villous shortening, increased crypt depth, and increased chronic inflammatory cells in lamina propia of small bowel.

TREATMENT

- Antibiotics × 3 to 4 weeks
- Folate
- Vitamin B_{12}
- Prognosis excellent

Lactase Deficiency

DEFINITION

Decreased or absent enzyme that breaks down lactose in the intestinal brush border.

ETIOLOGY

- Congenital absence reported in few cases
- Usual mechanism relates to developmental pattern of lactase activity
- Autosomal recessive
- Also decreases because of diffuse mucosal disease (can occur post viral gastroenteritis)

SIGNS AND SYMPTOMS

- Seen in response to ingestion of lactose (found in dairy products)
- Explosive watery diarrhea with abdominal distention, borborygmi, and flatulence
- Recurrent, vague abdominal pain
- Episodic mid-abdominal pain (may or may not be related to milk intake)

TREATMENT

- Eliminate milk from diet.
- Oral lactase supplement (Lactaid) or lactose-free milk.
- Yogurt (with lactase enzyme producing bacteria tolerable in such patients).

HYPERBILIRUBINEMIA

Physiology—see chapter on gestation and birth.

DEFINITION

Elevated serum bilirubin

EPIDEMIOLOGY

- Common and in most cases benign
- If untreated, severe indirect hyperbilirubinemia neurotoxic
- Jaundice in first week of life in 60% of term and 80% of preterm infants—results from accumulation of unconjugated bilirubin pigment

SIGNS AND SYMPTOMS

- Jaundice at birth or in neonatal period
- May be lethargic and feed poorly

DIAGNOSIS

- Direct and indirect bilirubin fractions
- Hemoglobin
- Reticulocyte count
- Blood type
- Coombs' test
- Examine peripheral smear

TREATMENT

- Goal is to prevent neurotoxic range.
- Phototherapy.
- Exchange transfusion.
- Treat underlying cause.

Gilbert's Syndrome

Benign condition caused by missense mutation in transferase gene resulting in low enzyme levels with unconjugated hyperbilirubinemia.

Crigler–Najjar I Syndrome

DEFINITION

- Autosomal recessive, secondary to mutations in glucuronyl transferase gene.
- Parents of affected children show partial defects but normal serum bilirubin concentration.

SIGNS AND SYMPTOMS

- In homozygous infants, will see unconjugated hyperbilirubinemia in first 3 days of life.
- Kernicterus common in early neonatal period.
- Some treated infants survive childhood without sequelae.
- Stools pale yellow.
- Persistence of increased levels of indirect bilirubin after first week of life in absence of hemolysis suggests this syndrome.

DIAGNOSIS

- Based on early age of onset and extreme level of bilirubin in absence of hemolysis
- Definitive diagnosis made by measuring glucuronyl transferase activity in liver biopsy specimen
- DNA diagnosis available

TREATMENT

- Maintain serum bilirubin < 20 mg/dL for first 2 to 4 weeks of life.
- Repeated exchange transfusion.
- Phototherapy.
- Treat intercurrent infections.
- Hepatic transplant.

Crigler–Najjar II Syndrome

DEFINITION

- Autosomal dominant with variable penetrance
- May be caused by homozygous mutation in glucuronyl transferase iso-form I activity

- Indirect hyperbilirubinemia, reticulosis, and red cell destruction suggest hemolysis.
- Direct hyperbilirubinemia may indicate hepatitis, cholestasis, inborn errors of metabolism, cystic fibrosis or sepsis.
- If reticulocyte count, Coombs', and direct bilirubin are normal, then physiologic or pathologic indirect hyperbilirubinemia is suggested.

Children with cholestatic hepatic disease need replacement of vitamins A, D, E, and K (fat soluble).

SIGNS AND SYMPTOMS

- Unconjugated hyperbilirubinemia in first 3 days of life.
- Concentration remains increased after third week of life.
- Kernicterus unusual.
- Stool normal.
- Infants asymptomatic.

DIAGNOSIS

- Concentration of bilirubin nearly normal.
- Decreased bilirubin after 7- to 10-day treatment with phenobarbital may be diagnostic.

TREATMENT

Phenobarbital for 7 to 10 days.

Alagille Syndrome

DEFINITION

- Absence or reduction in number of bile ducts
- Results from progressive destruction of the ducts

SIGNS AND SYMPTOMS

- Variably expressed
- Unusual facies (broad forehead, wide-set eyes, underdeveloped mandible)
- Ocular abnormalities
- Cardiovascular abnormalities (peripheral pulmonic stenosis)
- Tubulointerstitial nephropathy
- Vertebral defect

PROGNOSIS

Long-term survival good but may have pruritis, xanthomas, and increased cholesterol and neurologic complications.

Zellweger Syndrome

DEFINITION

- Rare autosomal recessive condition causing progressive degeneration of liver and kidneys
- 1/100,000 births

SIGNS AND SYMPTOMS

- Usually fatal within 6 to 12 months
- Severe generalized hypotonia
- Impaired neurologic function with psychomotor retardation
- Abnormal head and unusual facies
- Hepatomegaly
- Renal cortical cysts
- Ocular abnormalities
- Congenital diaphragmatic hernia

DIAGNOSIS

- Absence of peroxisomes in hepatic cells (on biopsy)
- Genetic testing available

Extrahepatic Biliary Atresia

DEFINITION

Distal segmental bile duct obliteration with patent extrahepatic ducts up to porta hepatis

EPIDEMIOLOGY

- Most common form (85%): obliteration of entire extrahepatic biliary tree at/above porta
- 1/10,000 to 1/15,000 live births

SIGNS AND SYMPTOMS

- Acholic stools
- Increased incidence of polysplenia syndrome with heterotaxia, malrotation, levocardia, and intra-abdominal vascular anomalies

DIAGNOSIS

- Ultrasound
- Hepatobiliary scintigraphy
- Liver biopsy

TREATMENT

- Exploratory laparotomy and direct cholangiography to determine presence and site of obstruction
- Direct drainage—if lesion correctable
- Surgery—if lesion not correctable (liver transplant)

HEPATITIS

- Continues to be major problem worldwide.
- Six known viruses cause hepatitis as their primary manifestation—A (HAV), B (HBV), C (HCV), D (HDV), E (HEV), and G (HGV).
- Many others cause hepatitis as part of their clinical spectrum—herpes simplex virus (HSV), cytomegalovirus (CMV), Epstein–Barr virus (EBV), rubella, enteroviruses, parvovirus.
- HBV is a DNA virus, whereas HAV, HCV, HDV, HEV, and HGV are RNA viruses.
- HAV and HEV are not known to cause chronic illness, but HBV, HCV, and HDV cause important morbidity and mortality through chronic infection.
- HAV causes most cases of hepatitis in children.
- HBV causes one third of all cases; HCV found in 20%.

Hepatitis A

DEFINITION

- RNA-containing member of the Picornavirus family
- Found mostly in developing countries
- Causes acute hepatitis only
- More likely symptomatic in children
- Transmission by person-to-person contact; spread by fecal–oral route
- Percutaneous transmission rare, maternal–neonatal not recognized
- Increased risk in child care centers, contaminated food or water, or travel to endemic areas
- Mean incubation 4 weeks (15–50 days)

- Abrupt onset with fever, malaise, nausea, emesis, anorexia, and abdominal discomfort.
- Diarrhea common.
- Almost all recover but may have relapsing course over several months.
- Jaundice.

DIAGNOSIS

- Consider when history of jaundice in family contacts or child care playmates or travel history to endemic region
- Serologic criteria:
  - IgM anti-HAV present at onset of illness and disappears within 4 months. May persist for more than 6 months (acute infection). IgG is detectable at this point.
  - Increased alanine transaminase (ALT), aspartate transaminase (AST), bilirubin, and gamma-glutamyl transpeptidase (GGT).

TREATMENT

- Careful handwashing
- Vaccines available (preferred over immunoglobulin in children > 2 years)

Hepatitis B

DEFINITION

- DNA virus from the Hepadnaviridae family.
- Most important risk factor for infants is perinatal exposure to hepatitis B surface antigen (HbsAg)-positive mother.

SIGNS AND SYMPTOMS

- Many cases asymptomatic
- Increased ALT prior to lethargy, anorexia, and malaise (6–7 weeks post exposure)
- May be preceded by arthralgias or skin lesions and rashes
- May see extrahepatic conditions, polyarteritis, glomerulonephritis, aplastic anemia
- Jaundice—icteric skin and mucous membranes
- Hepatosplenomegaly and lymphadenopathy common

DIAGNOSIS

- Routine screening requires assay of two serologic markers: HbsAg (all infected persons, increased when symptomatic) and hepatitis b core antigen (HbcAg) (present during acute phase, highly infectious state).
- HbsAg fall prior to symptom resolution; IgMAb to HbcAg also required because it is increased early after infectivity and persist for several months before being replaced by immunoglobulin G (IgG) anti-HbcAg.
- HbcAg most valuable; it is present as early as HbsAg and continues to be present later when HBsAg disappears.
- Only anti-HbsAg detected in immunized persons with hepatitis B vaccine whereas anti-HbsAb and anti-HBcAG seen in persons with resolved infection.

TREATMENT

- No available medical treatment effective in majority of cases.
- Interferon-alpha (INF-α) is approved treatment in children.
- Liver transplant for patients with end-stage HBV.

Typical Scenario

A 10-year-old boy is diagnosed with acute hepatitis A. How would you treat the parents and siblings who are doing fine? *Think:* IV immunoglobulin.

Hepatitis C

DEFINITION

- Single-stranded RNA virus
- Perinatal transmission described but uncommon except with high-titer HCV

SIGNS AND SYMPTOMS

- Acute infection similar to other hepatitis viruses.
- Mild and insidious onset.
- Fulminant liver failure rare.
- After 20 to 30 years, 25% progress to cirrhosis, liver failure, or primary hepatocellular carcinoma.
- May see cryoglobulinemia, vasculitides, and peripheral neuropathy (extrahepatic).

DIAGNOSIS

- Detection of antibodies to HCV or direct testing for RNA virus
- PCR detection possible
- Increased ALT
- Confirmed by liver biopsy

TREATMENT

- Treat to prevent progression to future complications.
- INF-α-2b for patients with compensated liver disease (response rate long term approximately 25%)
- May use with ribavirin for higher frequency of sustained response

Hepatitis D (Delta Agent)

DEFINITION

- Smallest known animal virus
- Cannot produce infection without HBV infection (co-infective or superinfection)
- Transmission by intimate contact

SIGNS AND SYMPTOMS

- Similar to but more severe than other hepatitis viruses
- In co-infection, acute hepatitis more severe, risk of developing chronic hepatitis low; in superinfection, risk of fulminant hepatitis highest

DIAGNOSIS

Detect IgM antibody to HDV (2–4 weeks after coinfection, 1 week after superinfection).

PREVENTION

No vaccine for hepatitis D, but can minimize against hepatitis B (needs hepatitis B to infect).

Hepatitis E

DEFINITION

- RNA virus with nonenveloped sphere shape with spikes (similar to caliciviruses)
- Non-A, non-B hepatitis

SIGNS AND SYMPTOMS

- Similar to HAV, but more severe
- No chronic illness
- High prevalence of fulminant hepatic failure and death in pregnant women

DIAGNOSIS

- Antibody to HEV exists
- IgM and IgG assays available
- Can detect viral RNA in stool and serum by PCR

PREVENTION

No vaccines available.

Hepatitis G

DEFINITION

- Single-stranded RNA virus of Flaviviridae family.
- Virus not yet isolated.
- Reported in all population groups in approximately 1.5% U.S. blood donors.
- 1% transmission through transfusions but also by organ transplant.
- Vertical transmission occurs.

SIGNS AND SYMPTOMS

- Symptoms associated with hepatic inflammation.
- Co-infection does not worsen course of HBV or HCV.

DIAGNOSIS

Only PCR assays available for testing.

TREATMENT

No method available.

Neonatal Hepatitis

DEFINITION

- Hepatic inflammation of unknown etiology.
- Most result from systemic disease (e.g., sepsis).
- Also caused by CMV, HSV, human immunodeficiency virus (HIV).
- Nonviral causes include congenital syphilis and toxoplasmosis.
- HBV results in asymptomatic infection.

SIGNS AND SYMPTOMS

- Jaundice
- Vomiting
- Poor feeding
- Increased liver enzyme levels
- Fulminant hepatitis

TREATMENT

- Antibiotics for bacteria-associated hepatitis
- Acyclovir for HSV
- Ganciclovir and foscarnet for CMV

Autoimmune (Chronic) Hepatitis

DEFINITION

- Hepatic inflammatory process manifested by increased serum aminotransferase and liver associated autoantibodies
- Variable severity
- 15–20% of cases associated with HBV
- Clinical constellation that suggests immune-mediated disease process responsive to immunosuppressive treatment

SIGNS AND SYMPTOMS

- Variable.
- May mimic acute viral hepatitis.
- Onset insidious.
- May be asymptomatic or may have fatigue, malaise, anorexia, or amenorrhea.
- Extrahepatic signs include arthritis, vasculitis, and nephritis.
- Mild to moderate jaundice.

DIAGNOSIS

- Made clinically.
- Exclude other disease.

TREATMENT

- Corticosteroid
- Azathioprine

REYE'S SYNDROME

DEFINITION

- Acute encephalopathy and fatty degeneration
- Decreased incidence secondary to awareness but relation to acetylsalicylic acid (ASA) ingestion.
- Many other "Reye-like" syndromes exist.

SIGNS AND SYMPTOMS

- Stereotypic, biphasic course
- Usually see prodromal illness, upper respiratory infection (URI), or chickenpox initially, followed by a period of apparent recovery, then see abrupt onset of protracted vomiting 5 to 7 days after illness onset
- May see delirium, combative behavior, and stupor
- Neurologic symptoms including seizures, coma, or death
- Slight to moderate liver enlargement

DIAGNOSIS

- Based on clinical staging.
- Liver biopsy may show yellow to white color because of high triglyceride content.

TREATMENT

- Control intracranial pressure (ICP) secondary to cerebral edema.
- Supportive management depending on clinical stage.

α₁-ANTITRYPSIN DEFICIENCY

The most likely clinical manifestation of α_1-antitrypsin deficiency in the newborn is jaundice (neonatal cholestasis).

DEFINITION

- α_1-Antitrypsin is a major protease inhibitor (PI).
- A small percentage of homozygous patients have neonatal cholestasis, and later in childhood cirrhosis.
- Present in > 20 codominant alleles; only a few associated with defective PI.
- PI ZZ usually predisposes to clinical deficiency (< 20% develop neonatal cholestasis).

SIGNS AND SYMPTOMS

- Variable course
- Jaundice, acholic stools, and hepatomegaly in first week of life; jaundice clears by second to fourth month.
- May have complete resolution, persistent liver disease, or cirrhosis.
- Older children may present with chronic liver disease.

DIAGNOSIS

- Determination of α_1-antitrypsin phenotype
- Confirmed by liver biopsy

TREATMENT

- Liver transplant curative
- No other effective treatment

WILSON'S DISEASE

Consider ordering serum ceruloplasmin for any patient with an unexplained elevation of liver function tests (LFTs).

DEFINITION

- Autosomal recessive disease characterized by excessive copper deposition in brain and liver
- Worldwide incidence: 1/30,000

SIGNS AND SYMPTOMS

- Variable manifestations, including:
  - Asymptomatic in early stages
  - Jaundice, abdominal pain
  - Hepatomegaly, subacute/chronic hepatitis or fulminant liver failure
  - Portal hypertension, ascites, edema, esophageal bleeding
  - Delayed puberty, amenorrhea, or coagulation defect
  - Psychosis
  - Tremors
- Kayser–Fleischer rings are greenish-brown rings of pigment seen at the limbus of the cornea, reflecting deposits of copper in Descemet's membrane. They can be seen with the naked eye in patients with blue eyes. In patients with dark eyes, a slit lamp is often needed to identify them. Ninety percent of patients with Wilson's disease have Kayser–Fleischer rings.

DIAGNOSIS

- Copper indices reveal:
  - Low serum ceruloplasmin
  - High serum copper level
- Liver biopsy for histochemistry and copper quantification
- Genetic testing, including siblings

TREATMENT

- Disease is always fatal if left untreated.
- Zinc: newest Food and Drug Administration (FDA)-approved agent; works by blocking absorption of copper in GI tract.
- Copper-chelating agents to decrease deposition (e.g., penicillamine and trientine).
- Restrict copper intake. Foods high in copper include (Source: Mayo Clinic Diet Manual):
  - Lamb, pork, pheasant, quail, duck, goose, squid, salmon, all organ meats (liver, heart, kidney, brain), all shellfish (oysters, scallops, shrimp, lobster, clams, crab), meat gelatin, soy protein meat substitutes, tofu, all nuts and seeds, dried beans (soybeans, lima beans, baked beans, garbanzo beans, pinto beans), dried peas, and lentils
  - Soy milk, chocolate milk, cocoa, chocolate
  - Nectarines, commercially dried fruits (okay if dried at home)
  - Mushrooms, sweet potatoes, vegetable juice cocktail
  - Barley, bran breads and bran cereals, cereals with more than 0.2 mg of copper per serving (check label), millet, soy flour, soy grits, wheat germ, brewer's yeast
- Patients with hepatic failure require liver transplant.

HEPATIC NEOPLASMS

Hepatoblastoma

DEFINITION

- Rare in children
- Fewer than 65% of malignant tumors are hepatoblastomas.
- Associated with Beckwith–Wiedemann syndrome.
- Usually arises from the right lobe of the liver and is unifocal.
- Two histologic types: epithelial and mixed types.

SIGNS AND SYMPTOMS

- Generally present in first 18 months of life
- Large asymptomatic abdominal mass
- Abdominal distention and increased liver size
- Weight loss, anorexia, vomiting, and abdominal pain (as disease progresses)
- May spread to regional lymph nodes

DIAGNOSIS

- α-Fetoprotein (AFP) level helpful as marker.
- Diagnostic imaging includes ultrasound to detect mass, CT, or magnetic resonance imaging (MRI).

TREATMENT

- Complete resection of tumor
- Cisplatin and doxorubicin adjuvant chemotherapy
- More than 90% survival with multimodal treatment (surgery with chemotherapy)

Echinococcus

DEFINITION

- Most widespread cestode.
- Transmitted from domestic and wild canine animals.
- Two species: *Echinococcus granulosus* and the more malignant *Echinococcus multilocularis*.
- Hosts are dogs, wolves, coyotes, and foxes that eat infected viscera.
- Humans are infected by ingesting contaminated food or water.

SIGNS AND SYMPTOMS

- Majority of cysts in liver; most never symptomatic
- Early, nonspecific symptoms; later on, increased abdominal girth, hepatomegaly, vomiting, or abdominal pain.
- Anaphylaxis secondary to rupture and spillage of contents.
- Second most common site is lungs; symptoms include chest pain and coughing or hemoptysis.

DIAGNOSIS

- Clinical.
- Ultrasound.
- Serologic studies have high false-negative rate.

TREATMENT

- Surgery
- May be CT guided
- If not amenable to surgery, may be treated with albendazole

Avoid spillage during surgery for *Echinococcus*— a major complication.

Amebic Abscess

DEFINITION

A very serious manifestation of disseminated infection.

SIGNS AND SYMPTOMS

Abdominal pain, distention, and liver enlargement with tenderness.

DIAGNOSIS

- May see slight leukocytosis
- Moderate anemia
- Increased ESR
- Nonspecific ALT increase
- Stool exam negative in > 50% of patients
- CT or MRI

TREATMENT

- Metronidazole.
- Chloroquine.
- Aspiration of left lobe abscesses if rupture is imminent.

Respiratory Disease

RESPIRATORY DISTRESS

- Intercostal retractions.
- Nasal flaring.
- Use of accessory muscles for breathing (e.g., abdominals, sternocleido-mastoids).
- Restlessness, agitation.
- Pallor, cyanosis.
- Wheezing may or may not be present.
- See Table 12-1 for normal respiratory rates by age.

COMMON COLD (UPPER RESPIRATORY INFECTION, NASOPHARYNGITIS)

DEFINITION
Multi-etiology illness with a constellation of symptoms including cough, congestion, and rhinorrhea.

ETIOLOGY

- > 200 *viruses*—especially rhinoviruses (one third), parainfluenza, respiratory syncytial virus (RSV), adenovirus
- Risk factors: child care facilities, smoking, passive exposure to smoke, low income, crowding, psychological stress

EPIDEMIOLOGY

- Most frequent illness of childhood (three to eight episodes per year)
- Most common medical reason to miss school
- Occurs in fall and winter especially

SIGNS AND SYMPTOMS

- Nasal and throat irritation.
- Sneezing, nasal congestion, rhinorrhea.
- Sore throat, postnasal drip.
- Low-grade fever, headache, malaise, and myalgia.
- Possible complications include otitis media, sinusitis, and trigger asthma.
- Infants have a variable presentation—feeding and sleeping are difficult due to congestion, vomiting may occur after coughing, may have diarrhea.

Typical Scenario

A 7-year-old girl is well when she leaves for school, but arrives home afterwards with a sore throat and runny nose. *Think:* Rhinovirus.

Typical Scenario

A 17-year-old sexually active adolescent has acute onset of fever, cough, conjunctivitis, and pharyngitis. *Think:* Adenovirus.

Mucopurulent rhinitis may accompany a common cold and doesn't necessarily indicate sinusitis; it is not an indication for antibiotics.

TABLE 12-1. Normal respiratory rates in children.

Age	Birth–6 Weeks	6 Weeks–2 Years	2–6 Years	6–10 Years	Over 10 Years
Respiratory Rate	45–60/min	40/min	30/min	25/min	20/min

The best treatment for the common cold is to increase oral fluids, *not* pharmacologic treatment.

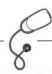

Aspirin is avoided in young children due to theoretical risk of Reye's syndrome.

Influenza is an orthomyxovirus.

Diagnosis of influenza depends on epidemiologic and clinical consideration.

Influenza can be severe in children with congenital heart disease, bronchopulmonary dysplasia (BPD), asthma, cystic fibrosis, and neuromuscular disease.

TREATMENT

- Supportive
- Direct therapy toward specific symptoms

INFLUENZA

DEFINITION

Viral respiratory illness.

ETIOLOGY

- Influenza A and B—epidemic disease
- Influenza C—sporadic

EPIDEMIOLOGY

Common over the winter months.

SIGNS AND SYMPTOMS

- Incubation period: 1 to 3 days.
- Sudden onset of fever, frequently with chills, headache, malaise, diffuse myalgia, and nonproductive cough.
- Conjunctivitis, pharyngitis.
- Typical duration of febrile illness is 2 to 4 days.
- Complications include otitis media, pneumonia, myositis, and myocarditis.

DIAGNOSIS

- Nasal swab
- Atelectasis on chest x-ray (10%)

TREATMENT

- Symptomatic treatment is appropriate for healthy children—fluids, rest, acetaminophen.
- For children at risk, see Table 12-2 for drug options.

VACCINE

- Now recommended for all children over age 6 months, with priority given to high-risk groups.
- High-risk groups include children with chronic diseases such as asthma, renal disease, diabetes, and any other form of immunosuppression.
- Best administered mid-September to mid-November since the peak of the flu season is late December to early March.
- Antibodies take up to 6 weeks to develop in children. Consider prophylaxis in high-risk children during this period.
- Since composition of influenza virus changes, the flu vaccine needs to be administered every year.
- Vaccine is a killed virus and therefore cannot cause the flu.
- Not approved for children under 6 months of age.

TABLE 12-2. Drug treatments for influenza (all pregnancy category C).

	Indications	Age Groups	Rx Dose	Adverse Effects
Amantadine	For type A only Both prophylaxis and treatment	Age > 1 year	200 mg PO bid × 7 days	Central nervous system and gastrointestinal effects
Rimantadine	For type A only Both prophylaxis and treatment	Px: Age > 12 years Tx: Age > 1 year	100 mg PO bid × 7 days	Same as for amantadine, but less frequent and less severe
Zanamivir	For types A and B Treatment only	Age > 12 years	Two inhalations bid × 5 days	Wheezing in patients with asthma, sinusitis, nausea, diarrhea
Oseltamivir	For types A and B Treatment only	Age > 12 years	75 mg PO bid × 5 days	Nausea, vomiting, diarrhea, abdominal pain, bronchitis, dizziness, headache

Tx, treatment; Px, prophylaxis.

PARAINFLUENZA

ETIOLOGY

- Type 1 and 2—seasonal.
- Type 3—endemic.
- See Table 12-3.

SIGNS AND SYMPTOMS

- Incubation period 2 to 6 days
- Causes:
  - Colds
  - Pharyngitis
  - Otitis media
  - Croup
  - Bronchiolitis
- Can be severe in immunocompromised patients

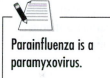

Parainfluenza is a paramyxovirus.

Parainfluenza is a major cause of croup.

TABLE 12-3. Respiratory infections and pathogens.

Respiratory Infection	Most Common Pathogen	Particular Signs and Symptoms
Croup	Parainfluenza virus	Barking cough, steeple sign
Epiglottitis	S. pneumoniae H. influenzae type B	Tripod position, thumb sign
Tracheitis	S. aureus H. influenzae type B	Rapidly progressive
Bronchiolitis	Respiratory syncytial virus	Paroxysmal wheezing
Bronchitis	Viral	Productive cough
Pharyngitis	Viral, group A strep	Sore throat, tonsillar involvement
Bacterial pneumonia	S. pneumoniae	Productive cough, lobar consolidation
Pulmonary abscess	S. aureus	Cavity with air–fluid level

Parainfluenza types 1 and 2 cause croup; type 3 causes bronchiolitis and pneumonia; type 4 is a cause of the common cold.

Croup is the most common cause of stridor in a febrile child.

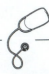

Croup is the most common infectious cause of acute upper airway obstruction.

Typical Scenario

An 18-month-old boy with inspiratory stridor and a barking cough and agitation when lying down is brought at night to the emergency department (ED) by parents. He has steeple sign on x-ray. *Think:* Croup.

Reconsider diagnosis of croup if child is hypoxic.

Minimum observation of child brought in with croup is 3 hours.

TREATMENT

Specific antiviral therapy is not available.

CROUP

Infectious Croup (Acute Laryngotracheobronchitis)

DEFINITION

Viral infection of upper respiratory tract.

ETIOLOGY

Parainfluenza virus types 1 and 2.

EPIDEMIOLOGY

- 3 months to 3 years of age
- Fall and winter months

SIGNS AND SYMPTOMS

- Inspiratory stridor.
- Seal-like, barking cough with retractions and nasal flaring.
- May have coryza and mild fever.
- Can progress to agitation, hypoxemia, hypercapnia, tachypnea, and tachycardia.
- Most cases are mild and last 3 to 7 days.

DIAGNOSIS

- X-ray only if diagnosis is in doubt.
- Steeple sign—narrowing of tracheal air column just below the vocal cords (see Figure 12-1).
- Ballooning—distention of hypopharynx during inspiration.
- Differentiate croup from epiglottitis.

TREATMENT

- Mild—outpatient mist therapy
- Moderate—racemic epinephrine (0.25 mL in 3–5 mL of normal saline [NS]), admit, early corticosteroids

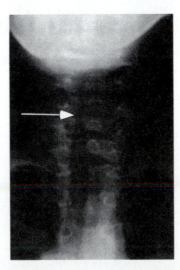

FIGURE 12-1. Radiograph demonstrating steeple sign of croup. Note narrowing of airway (arrow). (Photo courtesy of Dr. Gregory J. Schears.)

- Severe—racemic epinephrine, intensive care unit (ICU), early use of corticosteroids
- Admission criteria include suspected epiglottitis, progressive or severe stridor (i.e., at rest), respiratory distress, hypoxemia, cyanosis, pallor, decreased sensorium, and high fever.

CORTICOSTEROIDS IN RESPIRATORY PROBLEMS

- Dexamethasone (IM or PO 0.6 mg/kg).
- Side effects associated with short-term steroid use are minimal.

Spasmodic Croup (Laryngismus Stridulus, Midnight Croup)

DEFINITION

- Recurrent, sudden onset of barking cough and inspiratory stridor without preceding respiratory tract infection
- Well known to physicians but still defies definition of pathogenesis

ETIOLOGY

- Probable viral etiology
- Other considerations—allergic, psychological, gastroesophageal (GE) reflux

EPIDEMIOLOGY

- Usually at night
- Aggravated by excitement
- Winter months
- 1 to 3 years of age

SIGNS AND SYMPTOMS

- Recurrent episodes of acute-onset barking cough and inspiratory stridor
- No symptoms of infection

DIAGNOSIS

Subglottic, noninflammatory edema.

TREATMENT

- Reassurance and cool mist
- Spontaneous recovery

EPIGLOTTITIS

See Figure 12-2.

DEFINITION

Acute, life-threatening infection of supraglottic tissues.

ETIOLOGY

- Haemophilus influenzae type B
- Other possible pathogens—*Streptococcus pyogenes, Streptococcus pneumoniae, Staphylococcus aureus*

PATHOPHYSIOLOGY

Acute inflammation and edema of epiglottis, aryepiglottic folds, and arytenoids.

EPIDEMIOLOGY

- Decreased incidence due to *H. influenzae* type B vaccine (HiB)
- 2 to 6 years of age, but can occur at any age

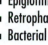

Stridor at rest is an indication for hospital admission.

Give corticosteroids to febrile child with stridor for:
- Croup
- Epiglottitis
- Retropharyngeal abscess
- Bacterial tracheitis

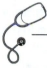

Diagnosis of spasmodic croup can be made only on resolution of the symptoms.

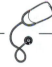

Steroids are not indicated in spasmodic croup.

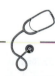

Minutes count in acute epiglottitis.

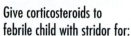

HIGH-YIELD FACTS

Respiratory Disease

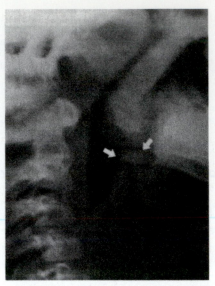

FIGURE 12-2. Radiograph of lateral soft tissue of neck demonstrating epiglottitis. Note the thickening of the epiglottic and ariepiglottic folds (arrows). (Reproduced, with permission, from Schwartz DT, Reisdorff BJ, *Emergency Radiology,* McGraw-Hill, 2002.)

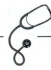

In doubtful cases, radiograph alone should not be used to diagnose epiglottitis.

Epiglottitis is a true medical emergency. If suspected, do not:

- Examine the throat
- Use narcotics or sedatives, including antihistamines
- Attempt venipuncture or other tests
- Place patient supine

SIGNS AND SYMPTOMS

- Sudden onset of inspiratory stridor and respiratory distress.
- "Hot potato" voice.
- High fever.
- Toxic appearing.
- Tripod position—hyperextended neck, leaning forward, mouth open.
- Dysphagia, refusal of food.
- Drooling.
- Not coughing.
- Tachycardia is a constant feature.
- Severe respiratory distress develops within minutes to hours.
- May progress to restlessness, pallor/cyanosis, coma, death.

DIAGNOSIS

- Laryngoscopy—swollen, cherry-red epiglottis
- Lateral neck x-ray to confirm
- Swollen epiglottis (thumbprint sign)
- Thickened aryepiglottic fold
- Obliteration of vallecula

TREATMENT

- **True medical emergency**—potentially lethal airway obstruction
- Comfort
- Anticipate
- Secure airway (Endotracheal intubation in OR)
- Ceftriaxone (100 mg/kg/day) 7 to 10 days
- Rifampin prophylaxis for close contacts

DEFINITION

Rapidly progressive upper airway obstruction due to infection of the trachea and/or larynx.

ETIOLOGY

- *S. aureus* and *H. influenzae* type b
- Also *Moraxella catarrhalis*

SIGNS AND SYMPTOMS

- High fever, toxicity
- Inspiratory stridor

DIAGNOSIS

- X-ray—may be normal or identical to croup.
- Tracheal narrowing.
- Pseudomembrane.
- Endoscopy.
- Copious purulent secretion distal to glottis.
- Secretions should be obtained for Gram stain and culture.

TREATMENT

- Secure an adequate airway.
- Ceftriaxone 100 mg/kg/day.
- Ampicillin–sulbactam 200 mg/kg/day.
- ICU admission.

Bacterial tracheitis has a slower onset than epiglottitis.

DEFINITION

Viral infection of upper and lower respiratory tract (medium and small airways).

ETIOLOGY

- RSV (> 50%)
- Adenovirus, parainfluenza 3, influenza
- *Mycoplasma pneumoniae* (rare)

PATHOPHYSIOLOGY

- Inflammatory obstruction (edema and mucus) of the bronchioles secondary to viral infection.
- Alterations in gas exchange are most frequently the result of mismatching of pulmonary ventilation and perfusion.

EPIDEMIOLOGY

- Occurs in first 2 years of life.
- Ninety percent are aged 1 to 9 months.
- Occurs in winter and early spring.
- Risks: crowded conditions, not breast-fed, mothers who smoke, male gender
- High-risk infants:
  - Cardiac disease
  - Pulmonary disease
  - Neuromuscular disease
  - Premature infants
  - Immunocompromised

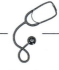

Bronchiolitis is the most common serious respiratory infection of infancy.

More than 50% of cases of bronchiolitis are caused by RSV.

Humans are the only source of RSV infection.

HIGH-YIELD FACTS

Respiratory Disease

SIGNS AND SYMPTOMS

- Starts with mild respiratory illness.
- Respiratory distress gradually develops.
- Paroxysmal wheezing—common but may be absent, cough, dyspnea.
- Apneic spells—young infants should be monitored.
- Frequent complications include bacteremia, pericarditis, cellulitis, empyema, meningitis, and suppurative arthritis.
- Most common complication is hypoxia.
- Dehydration is the most common secondary complication.

DIAGNOSIS

- Viral detection in nasopharyngeal secretions via culture, polymerase chain reaction (PCR), or antigen detection.
- Chest x-ray (rule out pneumonia or foreign body)—hyperinflation of lungs, increased anteroposterior (AP) diameter of rib cage.
- Oxygen saturation is the single best objective predictor.

TREATMENT

- Low threshold for hospitalization for high-risk infants
- Humidified oxygen
- Trial of nebulized albuterol
- Steroids not indicated
- Respiratory isolation
- Ribavirin (aerosol form) if high-risk patient, needs mechanical ventilation, or < 6 weeks old
- RSV intravenous immune globulin (RSV-IVIG) or palivizumab given prior to and during RSV season in high-risk infants < 2 years old

BRONCHIECTASIS

DEFINITION

Abnormal and permanent dilatation of bronchi.

ETIOLOGY

- Viruses: adenovirus, influenza virus
- Bacteria: *S. aureus*, *Klebsiella*, anaerobes
- Primary ciliary dyskinesia
- Kartagener's syndrome
- Cystic fibrosis: *Pseudomonas aeruginosa*
- α_1-antitrypsin deficiency

PATHOPHYSIOLOGY

Consequence of inflammation and destruction of structural components of bronchial wall.

SIGNS AND SYMPTOMS

- Physical exam quite variable
- Persistent or recurrent cough
- Purulent sputum
- Hemoptysis
- Dyspnea
- Wheezing
- Clubbing

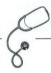

Symptoms of asthma can be identical to bronchiolitis. Suspect asthma if:
- Family history
- Prior episodes
- Response to bronchodilator

Indications for rapid antigen detection in suspected RSV bronchiolitis: cohorting RSV-positive patient or to confirm RSV in high-risk patient.

Typical Scenario

A previously healthy 4-month-old who had rhinorrhea, cough, and a low-grade fever develops tachypnea, mild hypoxemia, and hyperinflation of lungs. *Think:* RSV bronchiolitis.

Typical Scenario

A 7-year-old boy with an upper respiratory infection (URI) occasionally has black, tarry, foul-smelling stools, but is otherwise healthy. X-ray shows two discrete densities located in the right upper lobe of the lungs. *Think:* Bronchiectasis.

DIAGNOSIS

- Chest x-ray
- Bronchography
- Computed tomographic (CT) scan
- Sputum culture

TREATMENT

- Elimination of underlying cause
- Clearance of secretion
- Chest physiotherapy
- Mucolytic agents
- Control of infection—antibiotics
- Reversal of airflow obstruction—bronchodilators

BRONCHITIS

DEFINITION

Infection of conductive airways of lung.

ETIOLOGY

- Viruses: influenza A and B, adenovirus, parainfluenza, rhinovirus, RSV, coxsackievirus
- Bacteria: *Bordetella pertussis*, *M. pneumoniae*, *Chlamydia pneumoniae*, *S. pneumoniae*

SIGNS AND SYMPTOMS

- Acute productive cough (< 1 week)
- Rhinitis
- Myalgia
- Fever
- No evidence of sinusitis, pneumonia, or chronic pulmonary disease
- Normal arterial oxygenation

Cough is the most common symptom of chronic bronchitis.

TREATMENT

- Mostly self-limited.
- Bronchodilators may help.
- Antibiotics (not as a routine).

PHARYNGITIS

DEFINITION

Infection of the tonsils and/or the pharynx.

ETIOLOGY

- Viruses: rhinovirus, adenovirus, coxsackievirus
- Group A beta-hemolytic strep (GABHS)—uncommon in children < 2 years old
- *Mycoplasma*

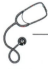

Pharyngitis is the second most common diagnosis in children aged 1 to 15 years in the pediatric clinic.

SIGNS AND SYMPTOMS

- Viral pharyngitis:
  - Gradual onset
  - Fever, malaise, throat pain
  - Conjunctivitis, rhinitis, coryza, viral exanthem, diarrhea

Presence or absence of tonsils does not affect susceptibility to pharyngitis.

163

Acute rheumatic fever occurs more after throat than skin infections and in children who have had acute rheumatic fever before.

- Streptococcal pharyngitis (> 2 years) (see Figure 12-3):
  - Headache, abdominal pain, and vomiting
  - Fever (> 104°F [40°C])
  - Tonsillar enlargement with exudates
  - Fetid odor
  - Cervical adenopathy
  - Palatal petechiae and uvular edema
- It is not possible to distinguish clinically viral from bacterial pharyngitis, though high fever, cervical adenopathy, and absence of URI symptoms suggest bacterial etiology.

DIAGNOSIS

Rapid (DNase) antigen detection test (sensitivity 95–98%):
- Culture if negative.
- Treat if positive.

TREATMENT

- Oral penicillin (25–50 mg/kg/day) for 10 days.
- Erythromycin (50 mg/kg/day) for penicillin-allergic patients for 10 days.
- Alternatively, intramuscular (IM) benzathine and procaine penicillin can be used (single dose, weight based).
- Tetracycline and sulfonamides should not be used to treat GABHS.
- Antibiotics are not indicated for pharyngitis negative for GABHS.

Penicillin remains the drug of choice for GABHS.

COMPLICATIONS SUPPURATIVE

- Suppurative complications of GABHS:
  - Peritonsillar abscess
  - Retropharyngeal abscess
  - Cervical adenitis
  - Otitis media
  - Sinusitis

COMPLICATIONS NONSUPPURATIVE

- Acute glomerulonephritis
- Acute rheumatic fever

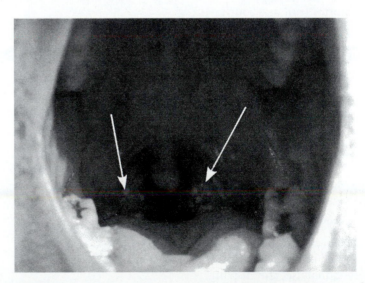

FIGURE 12-3. Streptococcal pharyngitis. Note white exudates (arrows) on top of erythematous swollen tonsils.

DEFINITION

Inflammation of lung parenchyma.

ETIOLOGY

- Viruses: RSV, influenza, parainfluenza, adenovirus
- Bacteria: less common, but more severe—*S. pneumoniae*, *S. pyogenes*, *S. aureus*, *H. influenzae* type b
- *M. pneumoniae*

SIGNS AND SYMPTOMS

- General
  - Tachypnea, dyspnea
  - Fever and feeding difficulty (infant)
  - Productive cough, chest pain (children)
- *Chlamydia trachomatis* (pneumonitis syndrome)
  - 1 to 3 months of age
  - Staccato cough, tachypnea, progressive respiratory distress
  - Lack of fever and other systemic signs
  - Conjunctivitis

DIAGNOSIS

- Chest x-ray (Figure 12-4):
  - Viral (hyperinflation, perihilar infiltrate, hilar adenopathy, and atelectasis)
  - Bacterial (alveolar consolidation)
  - *Mycoplasma* (interstitial infiltrates)
  - Tuberculosis (hilar adenopathy)
  - *Pneumocystis* (reticulonodular infiltrates)
- Blood culture (positive in 10–30% of bacterial cases)

TREATMENT

Inpatient

- 1 to 3 months old: erythromycin (pneumonitis syndrome) or cefuroxime
- 3 months to 5 years old: ampicillin or cefuroxime
- 5 years: erythromycin or cefuroxime

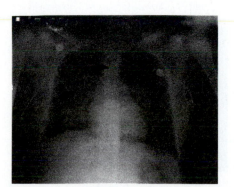

FIGURE 12-4. Chest x-ray demonstrating diffuse bilateral pulmonary infiltrates. Note tip of endotracheal tube (arrow) is in good position.

The more mucous membranes involved, the more likely an infection is viral.

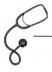
The most reliable sign of pneumonia is tachypnea.

Consider pneumonia in children with neck stiffness or acute abdominal pain.

In young children, auscultation may be normal with impressive x-ray findings.

Pneumonia with hilar adenopathy on chest x-ray. *Think:* Adenovirus.

Round pulmonary infiltrate on chest x-ray. *Think: S. pneumoniae* pneumonia.

HIGH-YIELD FACTS

Respiratory Disease

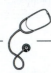

Outpatient

- Patients should have normal O_2 saturation and be able to take oral fluids in order to be outpatients.
- Amoxicillin or erythromycin.

PULMONARY ABSCESS

DEFINITION

Suppurative process resulting in destruction of pulmonary parenchyma and formation of a cavity containing purulent material.

ETIOLOGY

- Aspiration of infected material
- *Bacteroides, Fusobacterium*
- Anaerobic streptococci
- *S. aureus, Klebsiella*
- *Nocardia*, mycobacteria
- Risk factors:
  - Alcohol
  - Drug abuse
  - Tonsillectomy or adenoidectomy
  - Systemic disease
  - Human immunodeficiency virus (HIV) disease

SIGNS AND SYMPTOMS

- Insidious
- Fever, malaise, anorexia, and weight loss

DIAGNOSIS

- Chest x-ray (cavities with air–fluid level) (see Figure 12-5). In infant, consider:
  - Lobar emphysema
  - Cystic adenomatoid malformation
  - Pulmonary sequestration
- Fiberoptic bronchoscopy and/or bronchial alveolar lavage (BAL)

TREATMENT

- Medical—antibiotics (clindamycin)
- Consider surgical if:
  - No radiographic improvement
  - Hemoptysis

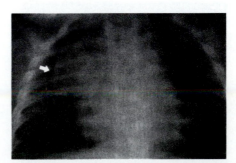

FIGURE 12-5. "Sail sign" (arrow) depicting the enlarged (normal) thymus in a young child. This should not be confused with an infiltrate. (Reproduced, with permission, from Schwartz DT, Reisdorff EJ, *Emergency Radiology*, McGraw-Hill, 2002.)

- Bronchopleural fistula
- Empyema

PERTUSSIS

DEFINITION

- "Whooping cough"
- Highly infectious form of bronchitis

ETIOLOGY

- *Bordetella pertussis* gram-negative coccobacilli.
- Humans are the only known host.
- Whooping cough syndrome also may be caused by:
  - *Bordetella parapertussis*
  - *M. pneumoniae*
  - *C. trachomatis*
  - *C. pneumoniae*
  - Adenoviruses

PATHOPHYSIOLOGY

- Pertussis toxin is a virulence protein that causes lymphocytosis and systemic manifestations.
- Aerosol droplet transmission.

EPIDEMIOLOGY

- Endemic, but epidemic every 3 to 4 years
- 60 million cases/year worldwide
- 500,000 deaths/year worldwide
- July to October
- 1- to 5-year-olds worldwide, 50% < 1-year-olds in United States

SIGNS AND SYMPTOMS

- Incubation period 1 to 2 weeks
- Catarrhal stage: congestion and rhinorrhea
- Paroxysmal stage (2–4 weeks):
  - Paroxysmal cough, with characteristic whoop following (chin forward, tongue out, watery, bulging eyes, purple face)
  - Post-tussive emesis and exhaustion
- Convalescent stage: number and severity of paroxysms plateaus.
- Each stage lasts ~2 weeks; shorter if immunized.
- Complications include apnea, physical sequelae of forceful coughing, brain hypoxia/hemorrhage, secondary infections (bacterial pneumonia is the cause of death).

DIAGNOSIS

- Diagnosis is primarily clinical:
  - Inspiratory whoop
  - Post-tussive emesis
  - Lymphocytosis
- Chest x-ray—perihilar infiltrate or edema (butterfly pattern)
- Positive immunofluorescence test on nasopharyngeal secretions

TREATMENT

- Goal—to decrease number of paroxysms
- Erythromycin for patient and household contacts

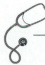

Radiographic resolution of pulmonary abscess cavity may take 2 months.

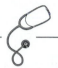

Pertussis means "intense cough."

Despite having "whooping cough," most patients with pertussis do not whoop.

With pertussis, fever may be absent or minimal; cough may be only complaint.

Apnea is common in infants with pertussis.

Suspect pertussis if paroxysmal cough with color change.

- Isolation until cultures become negative after 5 days of therapy
- Admit if:
  - Infant < 3 months
  - Apnea
  - Cyanosis
  - Respiratory distress
- DTP (diphtheria, tetanus, pertussis)/DTaP (diphtheria, tetanus, acellular pertussis) vaccine

No single serologic test is diagnostic for pertussis.

DIPHTHERIA

DEFINITION
Membranous nasopharyngitis or obstructive laryngotracheitis.

ETIOLOGY

- *Corynebacterium diphtheriae.*
- Humans are the only reservoir.

There is a risk of hypertrophic pyloric stenosis in infants younger than 6 weeks treated with oral erythromycin.

SIGNS AND SYMPTOMS

- Incubation period 2 to 7 days
- Erosive rhinitis with membrane formation
- Tonsillopharyngeal—sore throat, membranous exudate
- Cardiac symptoms
- Tachycardia out of proportion to fever

DIAGNOSIS

- Culture (nose, throat, mucosal, or cutaneous lesion).
- Material should be obtained from beneath the membrane or a portion of membrane.
- All C. *diphtheriae* isolates should be sent to diphtheria laboratory.

For treatment of diphtheria, antibiotics are not a substitute for antitoxin.

TREATMENT

- Antitoxin—dose depends on:
  - Site of membrane
  - Degree of toxic effects
  - Duration of illness
- Antibiotics:
  - Erythromycin for 14 days or
  - Penicillin G for 14 days
- Elimination of organism should be documented by two consecutive cultures.

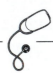

Most tuberculosis infections in children are asymptomatic with positive PPD.

TUBERCULOSIS (TB)

DEFINITION

- Signs and symptoms and/or radiographic manifestations caused by M. *tuberculosis* are apparent.
- May be pulmonary, extrapulmonary, or both.

ETIOLOGY
Mycobacterium tuberculosis.

PATHOPHYSIOLOGY
Primary portal of entry into children is lung.

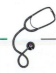

A patient may develop TB despite prior bacillus Calmette–Guérin (BCG) vaccination.

EPIDEMIOLOGY

- Children are never the primary source (look for adult contacts).
- Risk factors:
  - Urban living
  - Low income
  - Recent immigrants
  - HIV

SIGNS AND SYMPTOMS

- Chronic cough (nonproductive)
- Hemoptysis
- Fever
- Night sweats
- Weight loss
- Anorexia
- Lymphadenopathy
- Present to ED with:
  - Primary pneumonia
  - Miliary TB (may mimic sepsis)

DIAGNOSIS

- When to suspect TB:
  - Hilar adenopathy
  - Pulmonary calcification
  - Pneumonia with infiltrate and adenopathy
  - Pneumonia with pleural effusion
  - Painless unilateral cervical adenopathy
  - Meningitis of insidious onset
  - Bone or joint disease
  - When any of the above are unresponsive to antibiotics
- PPD test (Mantoux test):
- Induration > 5 mm
  - Children in close contact with known or suspected cases of active TB
  - Children suspected to have TB based on a consistent chest x-ray or clinical findings
  - Immunosuppressed children
- Induration > 10 mm
  - Children < 4 years
  - Children with chronic illness (lymphoma, diabetes mellitus, renal failure
- Induration > 15 mm
  - Children ≥ 4 years of age without any risk factors
- Chest x-ray.
- Culture (gastric aspirates, sputum, pleural fluid, cerebrospinal fluid, urine, or other body fluids).
- Look for the adult source.

TREATMENT

Two to four or more drugs (isoniazid, rifampin, pyrazinamide, ethambutol, streptomycin) for a minimum of 6 months.

A positive PPD skin test results from infection, not from exposure.

Asymptomatic children with a positive PPD should be considered infected and get treatment.

All cases of active TB should be referred to public health department.

Persons with TB should be tested for HIV.

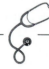

TB in children < 4 years of age is much more likely to disseminate; prompt and vigorous treatment should be started when the diagnosis is suspected.

CYSTIC FIBROSIS (CF)

Cystic fibrosis is the most common lethal inherited disease of Caucasians.

The gene for cystic fibrosis is CFTR; the mutation is delta F508.

A patient with severe CF breathing room air can have an arterial blood gas (ABG) showing decreased chloride and increased bicarbonate.

Typical Scenario

A 3-year-old has had six episodes of pneumonia, with *Pseudomonas* being isolated from sputum; loose stools; and is at the 20th percentile for growth. *Think:* CF.

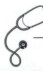

False-positive sweat test (not CF):
- Nephrogenic diabetes insipidus
- Myxedema
- Mucopolysaccharidosis
- Adrenal insufficiency
- Ectodermal dysplasia

DEFINITION

Disease of exocrine glands that causes viscous secretions:
- Chronic respiratory infection
- Pancreatic insufficiency
- Increased electrolytes in sweat

ETIOLOGY

- Defect of cyclic adenosine monophosphate (cAMP)-activated chloride channel of epithelial cells in pancreas, sweat glands, salivary glands, intestines, respiratory tract, and reproductive system
- Autosomal recessive

PATHOPHYSIOLOGY

- Chloride does not exit from cells.
- Increased osmotic pressure inside cells attracts water and leads to thick secretions.

EPIDEMIOLOGY

Most common cause of severe, chronic lung disease in children.

SIGNS AND SYMPTOMS

- Respiratory:
  - *Cough*—most common pulmonary symptom
  - Wheezing, dyspnea, exercise intolerance
  - Bronchiectasis, recurrent pneumonia
  - Sinusitis, *nasal polyps*
  - Reactive airway disease, hemoptysis
  - Increased AP chest diameter
  - Hyperresonant lungs
  - Clubbing of nails
- Gastrointestinal (GI):
  - *Failure to thrive*
  - *Meconium ileus* (10%)
  - Constipation, rectal prolapse
  - Intestinal obstruction
  - Pancreatic insufficiency:
    - *Malabsorption*
    - Fat-soluble vitamin deficiencies
    - Glucose intolerance
  - Biliary cirrhosis (uncommon): jaundice, ascites, hematemesis from esophageal varices
- Reproductive tract: decreased/absent fertility—female, thick cervical secretions; male azoospermic
- Sweat glands:
  - Salty skin
  - Hypochloremic alkalosis in severe cases
- Complications may include pneumothorax, chronic pulmonary hypertension, cor pulmonale, atelectasis, allergic bronchopulmonary aspergillosis, respiratory failure, GE reflux.

DIAGNOSIS

- Sweat test—chloride concentration > 60 mEq/L.
- Hypoelectrolytemia with metabolic alkalosis.
- Chest x-ray—blebs.

- Pulmonary function tests (PFTs)—obstructive and restrictive abnormalities.
- Prenatal diagnosis via gene proves CF mutations or linkage analysis.

TREATMENT

- Multidisciplinary team approach—pediatrician, physiotherapist, dietitian, nursing staff, teacher, child, and parents
- Respiratory:
  - Chest physical therapy
  - Exercise
  - Coughing to move secretions and mucous plugs
  - Bronchodilators
  - Normal saline aerosol
  - Anti-inflammatory medications
  - Dornase-alpha nebulizer (breaks down DNA in mucus)
- Pancreatic/digestive:
  - Enteric coated pancreatic enzyme supplements (add to all meals)
  - Fat-soluble vitamin supplements
  - High-calorie, high-protein diet
- Antibiotics—tobramycin with cephalosporin or penicillin for bacterial infections. Pseudomonal infections are especially common.
- Lung transplant
- Gene therapy being aggressively studied

PROGNOSIS

- Advances in therapy have increased life expectancy into adulthood.

TONSILS/ADENOIDS

Tonsillitis/Adenoiditis

DEFINITION

Inflammation of:
- Tonsils—two faucial tonsils
- Adenoids—nasopharyngeal tonsils

SIGNS AND SYMPTOMS

- Sore throat
- Pain with swallowing
- May have whitish exudate on tonsils
- Chronic tonsillitis:
  - Seven in past year
  - Five in each of the past 2 years
  - Three in each of the past 3 years

TREATMENT

- Less than 2 to 3 years old: Tonsillectomy is performed for obstructive sleep symptoms.
- Large size alone is not an indication to remove tonsils.

Enlarged Adenoids

DEFINITION

Nasopharyngeal lymphoid tissue.

SIGNS AND SYMPTOMS

- Mouth breathing
- Persistent rhinitis
- Snoring

Features of CF: **CF PANCREAS**
- **Chronic cough**
- **Failure to thrive**
- **Pancreatic insufficiency**
- **Alkalosis**
- **Nasal polyps**
- **Clubbing**
- **Rectal prolapse**
- **Electrolytes increased in sweat**
- **Absence of vas**
- **Sputum mucoid**

Ninety-nine percent of cases of meconium ileus are due to CF.

Fat-soluble vitamin deficiencies:
A—night blindness
D—decreased bone density
E—neurologic dysfunction
K—bleeding

DIAGNOSIS

- Digital palpation
- Indirect laryngoscopy

TREATMENT

- Adenoidectomy:
  - Persistent mouth breathing
  - Hyponasal speech
  - Adenoid facies
  - Recurrent otitis media or nasopharyngitis
- Tonsillectomy should not be performed routinely unless separate indication exists.

Peritonsillar Abscess

DEFINITION

Walled-off infection occurring in the space between the superior pharyngeal constrictor muscle and tonsils.

ETIOLOGY

- GABHS
- Anaerobes

EPIDEMIOLOGY

Usually preadolescent.

SIGNS AND SYMPTOMS

- Preceded by acute tonsillopharyngitis
- Severe throat pain
- Trismus
- Refusal to swallow or speak
- "Hot potato voice"
- Markedly swollen and inflamed tonsils
- Uvula displaced to opposite side

TREATMENT

- Antibiotics (penicillin)
- Incision and drainage

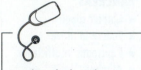

Tonsils and adenoids are part of Waldeyer's ring that circles the pharynx.

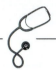

It can be normal for tonsils to be relatively large during childhood.

Trismus is limited opening of the mouth.

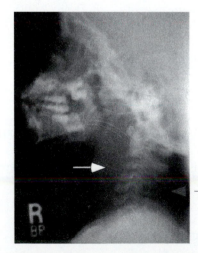

FIGURE 12-6. Lateral radiograph of the soft tissue of the neck. Note the large amount of prevertebral edema (solid arrow) and the collection of air (dashed arrow). Findings are consistent with retropharyngeal abscess. (Photo courtesy of Dr. Gregory J. Schears.)

RETROPHARYNGEAL ABSCESS

DEFINITION

Potential space between the posterior pharyngeal wall and the prevertebral fascia.

ETIOLOGY

Usually a complication of pharyngitis:
- GABHS
- Oral anaerobes
- *S. aureus*

SIGNS AND SYMPTOMS

- Sudden onset of high fever with difficulty in swallowing
- Refusal of feeding
- Throat pain
- Hyperextension of the head
- Toxicity is common
- May cause meningismus

DIAGNOSIS

Lateral neck x-ray: normal retropharyngeal space should be less than one half of width of adjacent vertebra (see Figure 12–6).

TREATMENT

- Clindamycin or Ampicillin–sulbactam

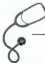

Usually lymph nodes in the retropharyngeal space disappear by third to fourth year of life.

ASTHMA

DEFINITION

Reversible airway obstruction characterized by airway narrowing.

ETIOLOGY

Hyperresponsiveness to a variety of stimuli:
- Respiratory infection
- Air pollutants
- Allergens
- Foods
- Exercise
- Emotions

PATHOPHYSIOLOGY

- Bronchospasm (acute)
- Mucus production (acute)
- Inflammation and edema of the airway mucosa (chronic)
- Two types:
  - Extrinsic
    - Immunologically mediated
    - Develop in childhood
  - Intrinsic
    - No identifiable cause
    - Late onset
    - Worsen with age
- Underlying abnormalities in asthma include increased pulmonary vascular pressure, diffuse narrowing of airways, increased residual volume

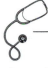

Asthma is the most common chronic lung disease in children.

Asthma is the most common cause of cough in school-age children.

The most important risk factor for development of asthma is the combination of RSV-related bronchiolitis and a genetic predisposition for atopic disease.

and functional residual capacity, and increased total ventilation maintaining normal or reduced P_{CO_2} despite increased dead space.

SIGNS AND SYMPTOMS

- Cough, wheezing, dyspnea.
- Increased work of breathing (retractions, use of accessory muscles, nasal flaring, abdominal breathing).
- Decreased breath sounds.
- Prolongation of expiratory phase.
- Acidosis and hypoxia may result from airway obstruction.
- See Table 12-4 for classification of severity.

DIAGNOSIS

- Clinical diagnosis, usually.
- Peak expiratory flow rate (PEFR):
  - Maximal rate of airflow during forced exhalation after a maximal inhalation
  - Normal values depend on age and height:
    - Mild (80% of predicted)
    - Moderate (50–80% of predicted)
    - Severe (< 50% of predicted)
- Chest x-ray will demonstrate hyperinflation and can be useful to look for pneumonia.
- Pulse oximetry may demonstrate hypoxia.
- Fever and focal lung exam—think pneumonia.
- Unresponsive to usual URI therapy.
- Complete blood count (CBC)—eosinophilia > 250 to 400 cells/mm³.
- ABG—hypoxia
- Bloodwork should not be routinely ordered in the evaluation of asthma.

Classic trilogy of asthma:
- Bronchospasm
- Mucus production
- Inflammation and edema of the airway mucosa

Respiratory drive is not inhibited in asthma.

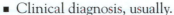

All wheezing is not caused by asthma; all asthmatics do not wheeze.

TABLE 12-4. Asthma severity classification.

Step	Symptoms	Pulmonary Function Tests (PFTs)
1—Mild intermittent	■ Up to 2×/week ■ Asymptomatic, normal PFTs between exacerbations	■ PEFR variability not more than 20% ■ PEFR or FEV_1 at least 80% predicted
2—Mild persistent	■ > 2×/week, but < 1×/day ■ Exacerbations may affect activity	■ PEFR variability 20–30% ■ PEFR or FEV_1 at least 80% predicted
3—Moderate persistent	■ Daily symptoms ■ Daily use of inhaled short acting β_2 agonist ■ Exacerbations affect activity ■ Exacerbations may last days and occur ≥ 2×/week	■ PEFR variability > 30% ■ PEFR or FEV_1 60–80% predicted
4—Severe persistent	■ Continual symptoms ■ Limited physical activity ■ Frequent exacerbations	■ PEFR or FEV_1 < 60% predicted ■ PEFR variability > 30%

PEFR, peak expiratory flow rate; FEV_1, forced expiratory volume in one second.

Reproduced from NHLBI guidelines, publication 97-4051, 1997.

TREATMENT

Goals: Improve bronchodilation, avoid allergens, decrease inflammation, educate patient.

First-Line Agents

1. Oxygen
2. Inhaled β_2 agonist
   - Albuterol (2.5 mg) (nebulized)
   - Short-acting/rescue medication—treats only symptoms, not underlying process
   - Bronchial smooth muscle relaxant
   - Side effects: tachycardia, tremors, hypokalemia
3. Corticosteroids (sooner is better)
   - For treatment of chronic inflammation
   - Oral prednisone (2 mg/kg, max 60 mg) or
   - IV methylprednisolone 2 mg/kg max 125 mg)
   - Contraindication: active varicella or herpes infection
4. Anticholinergic agents
   - Ipratropium bromide (nebulized)
   - Act synergistically with albuterol
   - Bind to cholinergic receptors in the medium and large airways

Second-Line Agents

1. Magnesium sulfate—bronchodilation via direct effect on smooth muscle
2. Epinephrine or terbutaline
3. No role in acute asthma for theophylline; not recommended

Others

1. Heliox—mixture of 60–70% helium and 30–40% oxygen
   - Decreases work of breathing by improving laminar gas flow (nonintubated patient)
   - Improves oxygenation and decreases peak airway pressure (intubated patients)
2. Mechanical ventilation indications:
   - Failure of maximal pharmacologic therapy
   - Hypoxemia
   - Hypercarbia
   - Change in mental status
   - Respiratory fatigue
   - Respiratory failure
3. Leukotriene modifiers
   - Inflammatory mediators
   - Improve lung function
   - No role in acute asthma
4. Cromolyn and nedocromil
   - Effective in maintenance therapy
   - Exercise-induced asthma
   - May reduce dosage requirements of inhaled steroid

Admit if:
- Respiratory failure requiring intubation
- Status asthmaticus
- Return ED visit in 24 hours
- Complete lobar atelectasis

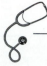

Asthmatic patient in severe respiratory distress may not wheeze.

Spirometry is the most important study in asthma.

Typical Scenario

A 5-year-old boy with a history of sleeping problems presents with a nonproductive nocturnal cough and shortness of breath and cough during exercise. *Think:* Asthma, and start on a trial of a bronchodilator.

O_2 is indicated for all asthmatics to keep O_2 saturation > 95%.

Long-acting β_2 agonist (salmeterol) should not be used for acute asthma exacerbation.

Asthmatic child's ability to use inhaler correctly should be regularly assessed.

Nedocromil is not Food and Drug Administration (FDA) approved for children under 12 years of age.

Most important risk factor for morbidity is failure to diagnose asthma from recurrent wheezing.

Typical Scenario

A young patient being treated as an inpatient for asthma exacerbation is anxious, has a flushed face, and is vomiting repeatedly. *Think:* Aminophylline toxicity.

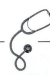

Increased white blood cell (WBC) count does not always signify infection in status asthmaticus.

- Pneumothorax/pneumomediastinum
- Underlying cardiopulmonary disease

Status Asthmaticus

DEFINITION

- Life-threatening form of asthma
- Condition in which a progressively worsening attack is unresponsive to usual therapy

SIGNS AND SYMPTOMS

Look for:

- Pulsus paradoxus > 20 mm Hg
- Hypotension, tachycardia
- Cyanosis
- One- to two-word dyspnea
- Lethargy
- Agitation
- Retractions
- Silent chest (no wheezes—poor air exchange)

FOREIGN BODY ASPIRATION

PATHOPHYSIOLOGY

Cough reflex usually protects against aspiration.

EPIDEMIOLOGY

Twice as likely to occur in males, particularly 6-month-olds to 3-year-olds.

SIGNS AND SYMPTOMS

- Determined by nature of object, location, and degree of obstruction.
- Initial respiratory symptoms may disappear for hours to weeks after incident.
- Vegetal/arachidic bronchitis due to vegetable (usually peanut) aspiration causes cough, high fever, and dyspnea.
- Complications if object is not removed include pneumonitis/pneumonia, abscess, bronchiectasis, pulmonary hemorrhage, erosion, and perforation.

DIAGNOSIS/TREATMENT

Larynx

- Croupy cough, may have wheezing, aphonia, hemoptysis, cyanosis
- Lateral x-ray
- Direct laryngoscopy—confirm diagnosis and remove object

Trachea

- Wheezing, audible slap and palpable thud due to expiratory impaction
- Chest x-ray (see Figure 12-7), bronchoscopy

Bronchi

- Initial choking, gagging, wheezing, coughing
- Latent period with some coughing, wheezing, possible hemoptysis, recurrent lobar pneumonia, or intractable asthma
- Tracheal shift, decreased breath sounds
- Midline obstruction can cause severe dyspnea or asphyxia
- Leads to chronic bronchopulmonary disease if not treated

- Direct bronchoscopic visualization (Figure 12-8)
- Lobectomy if vegetal foreign body for extended period of time
- Antibiotics for secondary infection
- Emergency treatment of local upper airway obstruction if necessary

TRACHEOESOPHAGEAL FISTULA (TEF)

DEFINITION

Connection between the trachea and esophagus (see Figure 12-9).

ETIOLOGY

- Congenital
- Acquired

SIGNS AND SYMPTOMS

- Suspect esophageal atresia
- Maternal polyhydramnios
- Inability to pass catheter into stomach
- Increased oral secretions—drooling
- Choking, cyanosis, or coughing with an attempt to feed
- Tachypnea

DIAGNOSIS

- X-ray: Radiopaque feeding tube passes no further than proximal esophagus.
- Barium swallow: Aspiration of barium into the tracheobronchial tree.

TREATMENT

Esophageal atresia is a surgical emergency.

TRACHEOMALACIA/LARYNGOMALACIA

DEFINITION

- Floppy epiglottis and supraglottic aperture
- Disproportionately small and soft larynx

SIGNS AND SYMPTOMS

- Usually begins within first month
- Noisy breathing
- Stridor

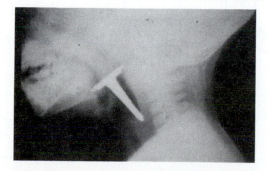

FIGURE 12-7. Radiograph of lateral soft tissue of the neck demonstrates a foreign body (nail) in the pharynx. (Photo courtesy of Dr. Gregory J. Schears.)

Dehydration may be present in status asthmaticus, but overhydration should be avoided (risk for syndrome of inappropriate antidiuretic hormone secretion [SIADH]).

Prevention is key! Keep small food and objects away from young children.

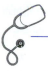

Foreign Body Aspiration
- Toddlers: R = L mainstem
- Adults: R mainstem predominates

Percussion of lung fields:
- Hyperresonant = overinflation
- Dull = atelectasis

Typical Scenario

A 2-year-old boy is brought to the ED with the acute onset of audible wheezing. His respiratory rate is 24, and he has mild intercostal retractions. His babysitter found him playing in his room. *Think:* Foreign body aspiration.

177

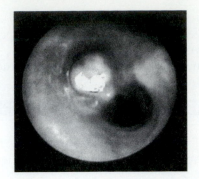

FIGURE 12-8. Foreign body (peanut) in the right mainstem bronchus visualized by bronchoscopy. Foreign bodies tend to lodge most commonly in the right mainstem bronchus due to the larger anatomic angle that makes traveling down right mainstem easier. (Photo courtesy of Dr. Gregory J. Schears.)

There is an association of tracheoesophageal fistulae with esophageal atresia.

H-type tracheoesophageal fistula is the least common but the most likely to be seen in ED.

- Hoarseness or aphonia (laryngeal crow)
- Feeding difficulty
- Symptoms worse when crying or lying on back

DIAGNOSIS

- Direct laryngoscopy
- Collapse of laryngeal structures during inspiration especially arytenoid cartilages

TREATMENT

- Reassurance
- No specific therapy required
- Usually resolves spontaneously by 18 months

CONGENITAL LOBAR EMPHYSEMA (INFANTILE LOBAR EMPHYSEMA)

DEFINITION

Overexpansion of the airspaces of a segment or lobe of the lung.

PATHOPHYSIOLOGY

No significant parenchymal destruction.

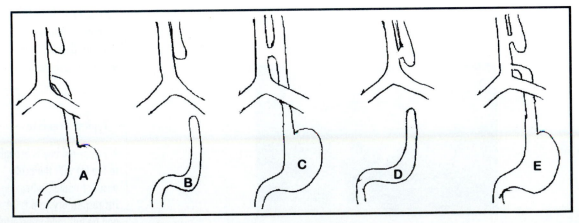

FIGURE 12-9. Types of tracheoesophageal fistulas (TEFs). Type A, esophageal atresia (EA) with distal TEF (87%). Type B, isolated EA. Type C, isolated TEF. Type D, EA with proximal TEF. Type E, EA with double TEF.

SIGNS AND SYMPTOMS

- Normal at birth
- Cough, wheezing, dyspnea, and cyanosis within a few days

DIAGNOSIS

- Chest x-ray
- Radiolucency
- Mediastinal shift to opposite side
- Flattened diaphragm

TREATMENT

- Remove bronchial obstruction (foreign bodies, mucous plug)
- Lobectomy

CYSTIC ADENOMATOID MALFORMATION

DEFINITION

- Excessive overgrowth of bronchioles
- Increase in terminal respiratory structure

SIGNS AND SYMPTOMS

- Neonatal respiratory distress
- Recurrent respiratory infection
- Pneumothorax

DIAGNOSIS

- Chest x-ray (posteroanterior [PA], lateral, and decubitus)
- Cystic mass (multiple grape-like sacs) and mediastinal shift
- Air–fluid level
- CT scan

TREATMENT

Surgical excision of affected lobe.

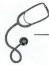

Laryngomalacia is the most frequent cause of stridor in infants.

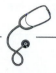

Symptoms of laryngomalacia can be intermittent.

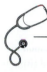

Congenital lobar emphysema is the most common congenital lung lesion.

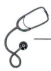

Cystic adenomatoid malformation is the second most common congenital lung lesion.

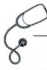

Cystic adenomatoid malformation may be confused with diaphragmatic hernia in neonatal period.

In patients with cystic
adenomatoid malformation,
avoid attempted aspiration
or chest tube placement, as
there is the risk of
spreading infection.

Cystic adenomatoid
malformation increases the
risk for pulmonary
neoplasia.

Cardiovascular Disease

MURMURS

NORMAL HEART SOUNDS

- S1 may split.
- S2 normally splits with respiration.
- S3 can represent normal, rapid ventricular refilling.
- P2 should be soft.

EPIDEMIOLOGY

- Fifty percent or more of children have a murmur.
- Two to seven percent of murmurs in children represent pathology.

DESCRIPTION AND GRADING

Murmurs are graded for intensity on a six-point system:

- **Grade I:** Very soft murmur detected only after very careful auscultation.
- **Grade II:** Soft murmur that is readily heard but faint.
- **Grade III:** Moderately intense murmur not associated with a palpable precordial thrill.
- **Grade IV:** Loud murmur; a palpable precordial thrill is not present or is intermittent.
- **Grade V:** Loud murmur associated with a palpable precordial thrill; the murmur is not audible when the stethoscope is lifted from the chest.
- **Grade VI:** Loud murmur associated with a palpable precordial thrill. It can be heard even when the stethoscope is lifted slightly from the chest.

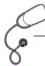

The difference between grade I and II murmur: a grade I can be heard only in a quiet room with a quiet child.

SITES OF AUSCULTATION

See Figure 13-1 to correlate the following points:

1. This site corresponds to the location of the **carotid arteries.** Common murmurs heard here: carotid bruit, aortic stenosis (AS). AS is usually louder at the right upper sternal border (RUSB) and often has an associated ejection click.
2. **Aortic valve.** Right upper sternal border. Common murmurs: aortic valve stenosis (supravalvar, valvar, and subvalvar). Valvar stenosis will often have an ejection click, whereas the others will not.
3. **Pulmonic valve.** Left upper sternal border. Common murmurs: pulmonary valve stenosis, atrial septal defect (ASD), pulmonary flow murmur, pulmonary artery stenosis, aortic stenosis, coarctation of the aorta, patent ductus arteriosus (PDA), total anomalous pulmonary venous return (TAPVR).

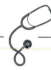

Murmur grading is usually written as "Grade [#]/6."

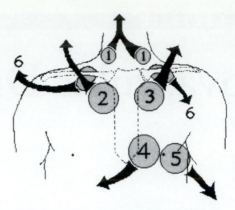

FIGURE 13-1. Sites of auscultation. (Artwork by Dr. John Brienholt.)

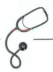

Reminders for a systematic cardiac exam:

1. Assess the child's appearance, color, etc.
2. Palpate the precordium.
3. Listen in a quiet room, during systole and diastole.
4. Listen first for heart sounds, then repeat your "sweep" of the chest for murmurs.
5. Don't forget to listen to the back and in the axillae.
6. Move the patient in different positions.
7. Feel the pulses and assess capillary refill.
8. Palpate the liver.

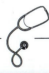

Any murmur > grade III is likely pathologic.

4. **Tricuspid valve.** Left lower sternal border. Common murmurs: ventricular septal defect (VSD), Still's murmur, hypertrophic obstructive cardiomyopathy (HOCM), tricuspid regurgitation, endocardial cushion defect.
5. **Mitral valve.** Apex. Common murmurs: mitral regurgitation, mitral valve prolapse, Still's murmur, aortic stenosis, HOCM.
6. This site correlates with areas of venous confluence. Common murmurs: venous hum.

Accentuation Maneuvers

Various positions and activities can diminish and intensify a murmur (see Table 13-1). The following section also reiterates the positions that aid in diagnosing innocent murmurs.

INNOCENT MURMURS

- **Pulmonary flow murmurs, physiologic pulmonary branch stenosis,** and **Still's murmurs** can all be heard best when the patient is supine versus upright.
- A Still's murmur may disappear with the Valsalva maneuver.
- Pulmonary flow murmurs are augmented by full exhalation, diminished by inhalation.
- **Venous hum** can be extinguished or accentuated with head and neck movement. It disappears in the supine position, and can also be eliminated with digital compression of the jugular vein.

PATHOLOGIC MURMURS

See Table 13-1.

Innocent Murmurs

- Common to all innocent murmurs are:
  - Absence of structural heart defects
  - Normal heart sounds (S1, S2)
  - Normal peripheral pulses
  - Normal chest radiographs and electrocardiogram (ECG)
  - Asymptomatic
- Usually systolic and graded less than III
- See Table 13-2.

TABLE 13-1. **Accentuation maneuvers for pathologic murmurs.**

Murmur	Increased with	Decreased with
Patent ductus arteriosus	Supination	
Atrial septal defect	(Valsalva can cause a temporary middiastolic murmur)	(Occasional crescendo–decrescendo systolic ejection murmur heard with ASD will not decrease in intensity with the Valsalva maneuver like the pulmonary murmur)
Aortic stenosis	Valsalva release, sudden squatting, passive leg raising	Valsalva maneuver, handgrip, standing
Subaortic stenosis	Valsalva maneuver, standing	
Hypertrophic obstructive cardiomyopathy	Valsalva maneuver, standing	Handgrip, squatting, leg elevation
Mitral valve prolapse	(Click and murmur occur earlier and the murmur is longer [not louder] with inspiration, when upright, and during the Valsalva maneuver)	
Mitral regurgitation	Sudden squatting, isometric handgrip	Valsalva maneuver, standing
Pulmonic stenosis	Valsalva release	Valsalva maneuver, expiration
Tricuspid regurgitation	Inspiration, passive leg raising	Expiration
Aortic regurgitation	Sudden squatting, isometric handgrip	
Mitral stenosis	Exercise, left lateral position, isometric handgrip, coughing	
Tricuspid stenosis	Inspiration, passive leg raising	Expiration

INTERPRETATION OF PEDIATRIC ECGs

Always approach an ECG systematically:

1. Measure atrial and ventricular rates.
2. Define the rhythm (sinus, or other).
3. Measure the P-R interval, QRS duration, and Q-T interval.
4. Measure the axes of the P waves, QRS complexes, and T waves.
5. Look for abnormalities of wave patterns and voltages.

Cardiology consultation is indicated with any "non-innocent" murmur.

Rate

Age-dependent—see Table 13-3.

ECG Paper

- Speed = 25 mm/s
- Small box = 0.04 sec = 1 mm
- Large box = 0.20 sec = 5 mm

Atrial Rate

- Look for P wave count that exceeds QRS complex count.
- If P wave number is greater than QRS complex number, an atrial dysrhythmia may be present.

	TABLE 13-2. Innocent murmurs.				
Murmur	**Cause**	**Epidemiology**	**Location**	**Sound**	**Characteristics**
Pulmonary flow murmur	Turbulent flow through a normal pulmonary valve	Most common between 8 and 14 years	Mid to upper left sternal border	Midfrequency, crescendo–decrescendo, systolic	Louder when patient is supine than upright
Still's (vibratory) murmur	Possibly turbulent flow in the left ventricular outflow tract region	Most common between 3 and 6 years; uncommon < 2 years	Lower left sternal border	Musical or vibratory with midsystolic accentuation	Louder supine, may disappear with Valsalva, softer during inspiration
Venous hum	Turbulent flow of systemic venous return in the jugular veins and superior vena cava	Most common between 3 and 6 years	Infra- and supraclavicular, base of neck	High frequency, best heard with diaphragm, during systole and diastole	More prominent on right than left, can be accentuated or eliminated with head position, disappears supine or digital compression of jugular vein
Carotid bruit	Turbulent flow from abrupt transition from large-bore aorta to smaller carotid and brachiocephalic arteries	Any age	Over carotid arteries with radiation to head	Systolic	Rarely, a faint thrill is palpable over the artery
Physiologic pulmonary branch stenosis	Turbulent flow as blood enters right and left pulmonary arteries that are relatively hypoplastic at birth due to patent ductus arteriosus predominance	Newborns, especially low birth weight (usually disappears by 3–6 months)	Upper left sternal border, axillae, and back	Crescendo–decrescendo, systolic	Louder supine
Patent ductus arteriosus	Turbulent flow as blood is shunted left to right from the aorta to the pulmonary artery	Can be innocent in newborns, abnormal if persists	Upper left sternal border	Continuous, machinery-like, louder in systole	

VENTRICULAR RATE

- Count number of small boxes between 2 R waves, then divide into 1,500.
- Count R-R cycles in six large divisions, then multiply by 50 (use with irregular or fast rate).

BRADYCARDIA

Found in sleep, sedation, vagal stimulation (stooling or cough), hypothyroid, hyperkalemia, hypothermia, hypoxia, athletic heart, second- or third-degree atrioventricular (AV) block, junctional rhythm, increased intracranial pressure, medicine (i.e., digitalis, β blockers).

TABLE 13-3. Heart rate by age.

Age	Normal Range (Average)
< 1 day	93–154 bpm (123)
1–2 days	91–159 bpm (123)
3–6 days	91–166 bpm (129)
1–3 weeks	107–182 bpm (148)
1–2 months	121–179 bpm (149)
3–5 months	106–186 bpm (141)
6–11 months	109–169 bpm (134)
1–2 years	89–151 bpm (119)
3–4 years	73–137 bpm (108)
5–7 years	65–133 bpm (100)
8–11 years	62–130 bpm (91)
12–15 years	80–119 bpm (85)
> 16 years	60–100 bpm

TACHYCARDIA

Found in fever, anxiety, hypovolemia, sepsis, congestive heart failure (CHF), hyperthyroidism, supraventricular tachycardia (SVT), ventricular tachycardia, atrial flutter and fibrillation, medicine (i.e., theophylline).

SINUS ARRHYTHMIA

Normal variation in heart rate, due to inspiration and expiration.

Rhythm

Check for sinus rhythm:
- Verify a P wave before every QRS complex.
- Verify a QRS complex after every P wave.
- All P waves should look the same.
- Normal P wave axis (0° to +90°).
- Upright P waves in leads I and aVF.

P-R INTERVAL

- Beginning of P to beginning of QRS.
- Prolonged P-R (first-degree AV block): found in myocarditis, digitalis, hyperkalemia, ischemia, increased vagal tone, hyperthyroidism.
- Short P-R: found in ectopic atrial pacemaker, preexcitation syndromes (Wolff–Parkinson–White syndrome [WPW], Lown–Ganong–Levine syndrome), and glycogen storage disease. It may show patient is at risk for SVT.

QRS DURATION

Prolonged: found in right bundle branch block (RBBB), left bundle branch block (LBBB), WPW, premature ventricular contractions (PVCs), mechanical pacemaker rhythms.

QT and QTc

- QTc—corrected QT
- Normal—< 0.45 (< 6 months), < 0.44 (> 6 months).
- Beginning of Q to end of T.
- QTc = QT interval (sec) divided by the square root of the R-R interval (sec).
- Causes of prolonged QT: long QT syndrome, hypokalemia, hypomagnesemia, hypocalcemia, neurologic injury.
- Long QT predisposes to ventricular tachycardia and is associated with sudden death.

Abnormal Rhythms

Premature Atrial Contraction (PAC)

- Preceded by a P wave, followed by a normal QRS.
- The length of two cycles (R-R) including a PAC is usually shorter than the length of two normal cycles.
- No hemodynamic significance.

Premature Ventricular Contraction (PVC)

- Premature and wide QRS, no P wave, T wave opposite to QRS
  - *Multifocal PVCs:* different-shaped PVCs in same strip
  - *Bigeminy:* coupled beat (sinus, PVC, sinus, PVC)
  - *Trigeminy* (sinus, sinus, PVC, sinus, sinus, PVC)
  - *Couplets* (sinus, sinus, PVC, PVC, sinus, sinus)
- May be normal if they are uniform and decrease with exercise

Atrial Flutter

- A rapid atrial rate (~300 bpm) with a varying ventricular rate, depending on degree of block (i.e., 2:1, 3:1)
- Sawtooth pattern (II, III, aVF, V1)
- Normal QRS
- Usually suggests significant pathology

Atrial Fibrillation

- Very fast atrial rate (350–600 bpm)
- Irregularly irregular ventricular response
- No P waves; normal QRS
- Usually suggests significant pathology

Ventricular Tachycardia

- Series of 3++ PVCs with a heart rate between 120 and 200 bpm
- Wide, unusually shaped QRS complexes
- T waves in opposite direction of QRS complex
- Usually suggests significant pathology

Ventricular Fibrillation

- Very irregular QRS complexes.
- The rate is rapid and irregular.
- This is a terminal arrhythmia because the heart cannot maintain effective circulation.

Axis

QRS Axis

- Examine leads I and aVF.
    - In lead I, count all forces above the baseline by the number of boxes (mm) and subtract all forces below baseline. If the total is +[+], the axis range is between ++90° and −90°.
    - Do the same in aVF. If the total is +[+], the QRS is also between 0° and ++180°.
    - Superimpose the ranges. Region of overlap is quadrant QRS lies in.
- Find lead with isoelectric QRS complex. The axis points perpendicular to that lead.
- If all leads are equiphasic, the axis is perpendicular to all leads and perpendicular to that plane. It is directed anterior or posterior and called indeterminate.

Abnormal Axes

- Right axis deviation (RAD): caused by severe pulmonary stenosis with right ventricular hypertrophy (RVH), pulmonary hypertension (HTN), conduction disturbances (RBBB).
- Left axis deviation (LAD) with RVH is highly suggestive of AV canal. Consider especially with Down's syndrome.
- Mild LAD with left ventricular hypertrophy (LVH) in a cyanotic infant suggests tricuspid atresia.

Quick Way to QRS Axis

Normal = [+] in lead I, [+] in aVF
- I−, aVF− = Extreme axis deviation (direction based on Q-wave)
- I +, aVF− = LAD
- I, aVF+ = RAD

P Axis

- Normal defines sinus rhythm and normally related atria (atrial situs solitus).
- A P axis between 0 and −90° may result from an ectopic low right atrial pacemaker (in absence of sinus node dysfunction, it is not significant).
- A P axis > +90° suggests atrial inversion or misplaced leads.

T Axis

- If differs by > 60 to 90° from QRS axis in presence of ventricular hypertrophy, it is called a "strain pattern" and may be a sign of ischemia.
- If strain is present, examine left precordial leads (V5, V6) for abnormal repolarization (indicated by T-wave inversion).
- LVH with strain in patients with aortic stenosis or hypertrophic cardiomyopathy is an ominous finding indicating severe disease.

Abnormal Wave Patterns and Voltages

Abnormal Q waves

- If no narrow Q waves in inferior (II, III, aVF) and leftward leads (I, V5, V6), suspect CHD with ventricular inversion.
- Q waves of new onset or of increased duration of previous Q waves, with or without notching of Q, may represent myocardial infarction (MI).
- ST elevation or prolonged QTc is also supportive of MI.
- Causes of ischemia and infarction: anomalous origin of left coronary artery from pulmonary artery, coronary artery aneurysm and thrombosis

187

in Kawasaki's disease, asphyxia, cardiomyopathy, severe aortic stenosis, myocarditis, cocaine use.

- A deep, wide Q wave in aVL is a marker for LV infarction. Suspect anomalous origin of left coronary artery, particularly in a child < 2 months old.

ST-T Segment

- End of S to beginning of T.
- Causes of ST displacement: pericarditis, cor pulmonale, pneumopericardium, head injury, pneumothorax, early ventricular repolarization, and normal atrial repolarization.
- Elevation may result from ischemia or pericarditis; depression is consistent with subendocardial ischemia or effects of digoxin.

T Wave

- Peaked, pointed T waves occur with hyperkalemia, LVH, and head injury.
- Flattened T waves are seen in hypokalemia and hypothyroidism.

Right Atrial Enlargement

- Peaked P waves (leads II and V1): P = > 2.5 mm (> 6 months) or > 3 mm (< 6 months)
- Causes include cor pulmonale (pulmonary hypertension, RVH), anomalous pulmonary venous connection, large ASD (uncommon)

Left Atrial Enlargement

- Wide P wave (notched in II, deep terminal inversion in V1): P = > 0.08 sec (< 12 months old) or > 0.10 sec (> 12 months old).
- Causes include VSD, PDA, mitral stenosis.
- The wider and deeper the terminal component, the more severe the enlargement.

Right Ventricular Hypertrophy (RVH)

- R wave > 98% in V1 or S wave > 98% in I or V6.
- Increased R/S ratio in V1 or decreased R/S in V6.
- RSR′ in V1 or V3R in the absence of complete RBBB. RSR′ with R > 15 mm (> 1 year) is characteristic of RVH secondary to right ventricular overload.
- In newborns, a pure R wave in V1 > 10 mm = pressure-type RVH.
- Upright T wave in V1 (> 3 days).
- Presence of a Q wave in V1, V3R, V4R.
- Adult pattern may occur as early as 6 years.
- A qR pattern of Q wave in V1 suggests severe RVH.
- Causes include ASD, TAPVR, pulmonary stenosis, tetralogy of Fallot (TOF), large VSD with pulmonary HTN, coarctation in the newborn.

Left Ventricular Hypertrophy (LVH)

- R > 98% in V6, S > 98% in V1.
- Increased R/S ratio in V6 or decreased R/S in V1.
- Q > 5 mm in V6 with peaked T (occurs with LV diastolic overload and denotes septal hypertrophy)
- Flat or inverted T waves in lead I or V6, in presence of LVH, suggests severe LVH.
- Excessive LAD supports LVH but is not sufficient to make the diagnosis.
- Causes include VSD, PDA, anemia, complete AV block, aortic stenosis,

systemic HTN, obstructive and nonobstructive hypertrophic cardiomy-opathies.

COMBINED VENTRICULAR HYPERTROPHY (CVH)

- If criteria for RVH exist and left ventricular forces exceed normal mean values for age, the patient has CVH.
- If LVH present, similar reasoning may apply to the diagnosis of RVH.
- In the presence of RVH, dominant RV forces diminish apparent LV forces, causing lower LV voltages (small R in V6 and small S in V1).
- Large equiphasic voltages in limb leads and midprecordial leads are called Katz–Wachtel phenomenon and suggest biventricular hypertrophy.
- Causes include left-to-right shunts with pulmonary HTN (large VSD) and complex structural heart disease.
- Cannot diagnose ventricular hypertrophy in the absence of normal conduction (RBBB).

DECREASED QRS VOLTAGE

- < 5 mm in limb leads.
- Causes include pericardial effusion, pericarditis, hypothyroidism.
- Sometimes normal newborns have decreased voltages—not a concern.

BASICS OF ECHOCARDIOGRAPHY

There are four basic cross-sectional views taken of the heart with **transthoracic echocardiography:**

- The parasternal (long and short axis) view
- The apical view
- The subcostal view (taken in the midline below the xiphoid process)
- The suprasternal view

Transesophageal echocardiography employs a transducer introduced down the esophagus for enhanced imaging during cardiac surgery or catheterization.

2-D Echocardiography

- Cross-sectional images of the heart are seen via this method.
- *Parasternal views:*
    - Long axis: left ventricular inflow and outflow tracts
    - Short axis: aortic valve, pulmonary valve, pulmonary artery and branches, right ventricular outflow tract, atrioventricular valves, right side of heart
- *Apical views:* atrial and ventricular septa, atria and ventricles, atrioventricular valves, pulmonary veins
- *Subcostal views:* atrial and ventricular septa, atrioventricular valves, atria and ventricles, and pulmonary venous drainage
- *Suprasternal views:* ascending and descending aorta, pulmonary artery size, systemic and pulmonary veins

Color-Flow Doppler Echocardiography

- Blood flow and direction can be seen via this method.
- Red indicates blood moving toward the transducer.
- Blue indicates blood flowing away from the transducer.
- When blood flow velocity exceeds a certain limit (called the Nyquist limit), the color signal is often yellow. This is indicative of high veloci-

ties that may be seen in VSDs, ASDs, and valvar regurgitation and stenosis.

M MODE ECHOCARDIOGRAPHY
- In this mode, the information from one scan point is measured over time.
- Motion creates a graph of depth of structures (i.e., valves, ventricular wall, etc.) versus time.
- This modality is used to determine cardiac chamber dimension, valve annuli size, fractional shortening and ejection fraction, left ventricular mass.

INTERPRETATION OF PEDIATRIC CHEST X-RAYS

Heart Size

Cardiothoracic ratio:
- Measure largest width of the heart and divide by the largest diameter of the chest. A normal ratio is < 0.5.
- The chest x-ray (CXR) must have a good inspiratory effort. For this reason, newborns and infants are difficult to evaluate by this method.
- Cardiomegaly on CXR is most suggestive of volume overload; ECG better reflects increased pressure.

Cardiac Chamber Enlargement

Left Atrial Enlargement (LAE)
- May produce a "double density" on the PA CXR.
- More severe LAE can elevate the left mainstem bronchus.

Right Atrial Enlargement (RAE)
RAE is noted most at the right lower cardiac border; however, it is difficult to diagnose by CXR alone.

Left Ventricular Enlargement
- The apex is seen further to the left and downward.
- On lateral CXR, the posterior cardiac border is further displaced posteriorly.

Right Ventricular Enlargement
- RVH is not seen well on PA CXR because it does not make up the cardiac silhouette.
- On lateral CXR, it is noted by filling the retrosternal space.

Pulmonary Vascular Markings

Increased Pulmonary Vascular Markings
- Noted by the visualization of pulmonary vasculature in the lateral one third of the lung field.
- In an **acyanotic** child this could be ASD, VSD, PDA, endocardial cushion defect, or partial anomalous pulmonary venous return.
- In a **cyanotic** child this could be transposition of the great arteries, TAPVR, hypoplastic left heart syndrome, persistent truncus arteriosus, or single ventricle.

In newborns and small infants, the upper aspects of the heart are obscured by a large "boat sail–shaped" opacity — the thymus. This organ will involute after puberty. It is often not seen in premature newborns.

Decreased Pulmonary Vascular Markings
- The lung fields are dark, with small vessels.
- Seen in pulmonary stenosis and atresia, tricuspid stenosis and atresia, tetralogy of Fallot.

Pulmonary Venous Congestion
- Manifested as hazy lung fields.
- Kerley B lines are often present.
- Caused by LV failure or obstruction of the pulmonary veins.
- Seen in mitral stenosis, TAPVR, cor triatriatum, hypoplastic left heart syndrome, or any left-sided obstructive lesion with heart failure.

Abnormal Cardiac Silhouettes

Tetralogy of Fallot
- A "boot-shaped" heart with decreased pulmonary vascular markings is sometimes seen. The boot is due to the hypoplastic main pulmonary artery.
- RVH is noted.
- About 25% will have a right aortic arch.

Transposition of the Great Arteries
- An "egg-shaped" heart is sometimes seen.
- The narrow superior aspect of the cardiac silhouette is due to the absence of the thymus and the irregular relationship of the great arteries.

Total Anomalous Pulmonary Venous Return
- A "snowman" shape is sometimes seen.
- The left vertical vein, left innominate vein, and dilated superior vena cava create the "snowman's" head.

RHEUMATIC FEVER

DEFINITION
- Rheumatic fever is the immunologic sequela of a previous group A streptococcal infection of the pharynx (not of the skin).
- Affects the brain, heart, joints, and skin.

EPIDEMIOLOGY
- Although an uncommon disease in the United States, small outbreaks occur in various regions.
  - Peak age range: 6 to 15 years.
  - A positive family history of rheumatic fever increases risk.
- Incidence: 0.3–3% in developed countries
  - Risk of RF after untreated strep pharyngitis is 1–3%.
  - Patients with the infection < 3 weeks have a 0.3% risk.
- Follows pharyngitis by 1 to 5 weeks (average: 3 weeks).
- Rate of recurrent RF with subsequent strep infection may approach 65%.
- Recurrence rate decreases to < 10% over 10 years.

DIAGNOSIS
- To diagnose acute rheumatic fever you must fulfill the following combination of the Jones Criteria:
  - 2 major manifestations *or*

- 1 major and 2 minor manifestations
- In addition to the major and minor manifestations, patients may appear pale and complain of abdominal pain and epistaxis.
- Aschoff bodies (found in atrial myocardium) are diagnostic.

Jones Criteria (Modified)
2 major or 1 major + 2 minor
Major—J ♥ NES:
- Joints — polyarthritis
- ♥ — carditis
- Nodules, subcutaneous
- Erythema marginatum
- Sydenham's chorea

Minor
- Arthralgia
- Fever
- Elevated erythrocyte sedimentation rate (ESR) or C-reactive protein (CRP)
- Prolonged P-R interval

Plus
- Laboratory evidence of antecedent group A strep infection (ASO titer)

CARDITIS

- Incidence: 50% of patients
- Clinical presentation:
  - Tachycardia is common.
  - Heart murmur, most commonly due to valvulitis of the following (in order of decreasing frequency):
    - Mitral valve regurgitation
    - Aortic valve regurgitation
    - Tricuspid valve regurgitation—less common
- Pericarditis (a friction rub may be heard).
- Cardiomegaly.
- CHF (a gallop may be heard).

ARTHRITIS

- Most common manifestation, affecting 70%.
- Usually affects the large joints, but can affect the spine and cranial joints.
- Migratory in nature, affecting a new joint as other affected joints resolve (can affect more than one joint at a time).
- Joints are red, warm, swollen, and very tender, particularly if moved.
- Responds well to aspirin therapy (give once diagnosis is confirmed).
- Duration is usually < 1 month, even without treatment.

CHOREA

- Incidence: 15% of patients; most commonly prepubertal girls.
- Movements last on average 7 months before slowly diminishing (can last up to 17 months).
- Characteristics:
  - Initial emotional lability: Behaviors characteristic of attention deficit/hyperactivity disorder (ADHD) and obsessive–compulsive disorder (OCD) have been noted to precede the movement disorder.
  - Loss of motor coordination.
  - Spontaneous, purposeless movement.
  - Motor weakness.

Absence of tachycardia or murmur usually excludes the diagnosis of myocarditis.

ERYTHEMA MARGINATUM

- Incidence: < 10% of patients
- Pink, erythematous macular rash
- Often has a clear center and serpiginous outline
- Nonpruritic
- Evanescent and migratory
  - Disappears when cold
  - Reappears when warm
- Found primarily on the trunk and proximal extremities

Rheumatic fever can cause long-term valvular disease, both stenosis and insufficiency.

SUBCUTANEOUS NODULES

- Incidence: 2–10% of patients
- Hard, painless, small (0.5–1 cm) swellings over bony prominences, primarily the extensor tendons of the hand
- Can also be found on the scalp and along the spine
- Not transient, lasting for weeks

DIAGNOSIS

- Streptococcal antibody tests are the most reliable evidence of preceding group A strep infection leading to acute rheumatic fever.
  - Antistreptolysin O (ASO) titer is the most commonly used. It is elevated in 80% of patients with acute rheumatic fever (ARF) and 20% of normal individuals.
  - Other antibody tests exist (antihyaluronidase, antistreptokinase, antideoxyribonuclease B) wherein at least one will be positive in 95% of patients with ARF.
- Positive throat cultures and "rapid strep tests" are less reliable because they do not differentiate acute infection versus chronic carrier state.

TREATMENT

- Upon diagnosis, the patient should receive benzathine penicillin G 1.2 million units IM to eradicate the streptococci (if < 27 kg = 600,000 U).
  - Patients allergic to penicillin can receive 4 days of erythromycin 40 mg/kg/day.
- Prophylaxis should be initiated:
  - Benzathine penicillin G 1.2 million units IM every 3 weeks *or*
  - Penicillin 200,000 units PO three times per day *or*
  - Sulfadiazine 1 g PO once per day
- Length of prophylaxis is undetermined, but often advocated at least throughout adolescence if not indefinitely. Obviously, compliance becomes a difficult issue.
- Seventy-five percent of patients recover within 6 weeks, and less than 5% are symptomatic beyond 6 months. Seventy percent of those with carditis recover without permanent cardiac damage.

ENDOCARDITIS

ETIOLOGY

- **α-Hemolytic streptococci** are most common.
  - *Streptococcus viridans* is the organism in 67% of cases.
- ***Staphylococcus aureus*** is also common, accounting for 20% of cases.
- If felt to be secondary to cardiac surgery complications, *Staphylococcus epidermidis,* gram-negative bacilli, and fungi should be considered.
- Most endocarditis is left-sided.
- Right-sided endocarditis is associated with IV drug use.

PATHOPHYSIOLOGY

Most likely to occur on congenitally abnormal valves, valves damaged by rheumatic fever, acquired valvular lesions, prosthetic replacement valves, and any cardiac defect leading to turbulent blood flow.

SIGNS AND SYMPTOMS

- Fever is most common.
- New or changing heart murmur.
- Chest pain, dyspnea, arthralgia, myalgia, headache.
- Embolic phenomena:
  - Hematuria with red cell casts
  - Transient ischemic attacks
  - Roth spots, splinter hemorrhages, Osler nodes, Janeway lesions (less common in children)

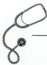

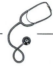

If a patient's arthritis doesn't improve within 48 hours of therapeutic aspirin therapy, he or she probably does not have rheumatic fever.

The chorea of rheumatic fever is known as Syndenham's chorea or St. Vitus' dance.

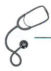

Erythema marginatum is never found on the face.

Subcutaneous nodules are also found in connective tissue diseases such as systemic lupus erythematosus (SLE) and rheumatoid arthritis.

Subcutaneous nodules in rheumatic fever have a significant association with carditis.

Cardiovascular Disease

A history of sore throat or scarlet fever is insufficient evidence for rheumatic fever without a positive strep test.

Carditis is the only manifestation of rheumatic fever that can cause permanent cardiac damage. Therefore, once definitively diagnosed, anti-inflammatory therapy (with prednisone in extreme cases, or aspirin) should be started.

Janeway lesions — painless
Osler's nodes — painful

Risk factors for endocarditis:
- Previous endocarditis
- Dental procedures
- Gastrointestinal and genitourinary procedures
- IV drug use (usually affects the tricuspid valve)
- Indwelling central venous catheters
- Prior cardiac surgery

PREDISPOSING CONDITIONS
- High risk:
    - Prosthetic cardiac valves
    - Previous bacterial endocarditis (due to scar formation on valve)
    - Congenital heart disease—complex cyanotic types
    - Surgical pulmonary–systemic shunts
- Moderate risk:
    - Congenital cardiac diseases not in high and low risk
    - Acquired valvular dysfunction
        - Rheumatic heart disease, Libman–Sacks valve, antiphospholipid syndrome–associated valve disease
        - Hypertrophic cardiomyopathy
    - Complicated mitral valve prolapse (valvular regurgitation, thickened valve leaflets)
- Low risk:
    - Isolated ASD, secundum type
    - Surgically repaired cardiac defects > 6 months postoperative (ASD, VSD, PDA)
    - Heart murmurs with normal echocardiogram (physiologic or functional, flow murmurs)
    - Systemic diseases without cardiac valve involvement:
        - Kawasaki disease: normal echo only
        - Rheumatic heart disease: normal echo only
    - Cardiac pacemakers and implantable defibrillators

DIAGNOSIS
- Four sets of blood cultures over 48 hours from different sites.
- Most common findings:
    - Positive blood cultures
    - Elevated ESR
    - Hematuria
    - Anemia
- Echocardiographic evidence of vegetations or thrombi is diagnostic.

TREATMENT
- Four to eight weeks of organism-specific antibiotic therapy.
- Surgery is necessary when endocarditis is refractory to medical treatment. Also considered in cases of prosthetic valves, fungal endocarditis, and hemodynamic compromise.
- Antibiotic prophylaxis is necessary for children with structural heart disease and other predisposing conditions.

PROPHYLAXIS RECOMMENDATIONS
Prophylaxis is recommended with:
- Most dental and periodontal procedures
- Tonsillectomy or adenoidectomy
- Rigid bronchoscopy or surgery involving gastrointestinal (GI) or upper respiratory mucosa
- Gallbladder surgery
- Catheterization in setting of urinary tract infection, cystoscopy, urethral dilation
- Urinary tract surgery including prostate surgery
- Incision and drainage of infected tissues
    - Vaginal hysterectomy in high-risk patients only or vaginal delivery with infection present
Prophylaxis is *not* usually recommended with:
- Intraoral injection of local anesthetic

- Shedding of primary teeth
- Tympanostomy tube insertion
- Endotracheal tube insertion
- Bronchoscopy with flexible bronchoscope
- Transesophageal echo
- Cardiac catheterization
- Cesarean section (only when no infection present)
- GI endoscopy, with or without biopsy (prophylaxis for high-risk patients)
- Genitourinary (GU) procedures with no infection present (except those above)
- Circumcision

Typical Scenario

A 6-year-old girl with PDA develops fever and anorexia. Hgb is 9, she has hematuria, increased ESR, positive rheumatoid factor (RF), and immune complexes are present. *Think:* Bacterial endocarditis.

MYOCARDITIS

ETIOLOGY

- Most often caused by viruses. Coxsackieviruses and echoviruses are most common. Recent evidence suggests adenovirus as a common etiology.
- Immune-mediated diseases (e.g., acute rheumatic fever, Kawasaki's disease).
- Collagen vascular diseases.
- Toxic ingestions.

EPIDEMIOLOGY

Clinically recognizable myocarditis is rare in the United States.

SIGNS AND SYMPTOMS

- Presentation depends on the degree of myocardial injury.
- Ranges from asymptomatic to fulminant CHF.
- Common symptoms are fever, dyspnea, upper respiratory symptoms, vomiting, and lethargy.
- CHF should be considered if patient is tachycardic and tachypneic and has a gallop on auscultation.

DIAGNOSIS

- ECG findings: low voltages, S-T changes, prolonged QT interval, premature beats.
- Radiology: Chest radiographs will show cardiomegaly.
- Echocardiography: Chamber enlargement is present with impaired ventricular function.

TREATMENT

- First, treat the underlying cause (i.e., antibiotics if bacterial).
- Since it is most often viral, treatment is largely supportive. Rest and activity limitation is important.
- Treatment of CHF may be necessary (i.e., diurectics, inotropic agents if severely ill). Gamma globulin also has been effective.

PERICARDITIS

ETIOLOGY

- Viral (most common)
- Bacterial infection (also common): acute rheumatic fever, *S. aureus, Haemophilus influenzae, Neisseria meningitides,* streptococci, tuberculosis
- Complications from heart surgery

- Collagen vascular diseases
- Uremia
- Medications (i.e., dantrolene, oncology agents)

SIGNS AND SYMPTOMS

- Precordial pain with radiation to the shoulder and neck (often relieved by standing)
- **Pericardial friction rub** on auscultation
- Signs of cardiac tamponade:
    - Distant heart sounds
    - Tachycardia
    - Pulsus paradoxus
    - Hepatomegaly and venous distention

DIAGNOSIS

- CXR: A pear- or water bottle–shaped heart indicates a large effusion.
- Echocardiography is diagnostic (can also detect tamponade).

TREATMENT

- Treat the underlying disease process.
- Supportive treatment for viral etiologies.
- Pericardiocentesis is indicated if effusion is present.
- Urgent drainage is indicated when symptoms of tamponade are present.

Digitalis is typically not given in pericarditis, as this blocks the compensatory tachycardia the heart utilizes to overcome decreased venous return.

CONGESTIVE HEART FAILURE (CHF)

ETIOLOGY

- Caused from either congenital heart disease (CHD) or acquired heart disease.
- CHD: Most common cause is from volume or pressure overload.
- VSD, PDA, and endocardial cushion defects are the most common causes of CHF in the first 6 months of life.
- ASD can cause CHF in adulthood if unrepaired.
- Acquired heart disease: Potential causes of CHF are metabolic abnormalities (i.e., hypoxia, acidosis, hypoglycemia, hypocalcemia), myocarditis, rheumatic fever with carditis, cardiomyopathy, and drug toxicity.

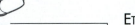

Onset of CHF is dependent on the fall of pulmonary vascular resistance and the subsequent increased left-to-right shunting.

SIGNS AND SYMPTOMS

- Often similar symptoms to those found in respiratory illnesses: tachycardia, tachypnea, shortness of breath, rales and rhonchi, intercostal retractions.
- Poor weight gain/poor feeding.
- Cold sweat on forehead.
- Older children develop peripheral edema.
- Gallop on auscultation.
- Hepatomegaly, jugular venous distention (JVD).

A left-to-right shunt usually takes about 6 weeks to become significant enough to stress the left ventricle.

DIAGNOSIS

- CXR: cardiomegaly, evidence of pulmonary edema
- Echo: Enlarged ventricular chamber, impaired ventricular function

TREATMENT

- Treat the underlying cause (i.e., surgical correction of CHD, correction of metabolic defects).

- Oxygen can be used if patient is hypoxic or in respiratory distress.
- Medication:
  - *Digitalis* is used to improve ventricular function. Contraindicated in complete heart block and hypertrophic cardiomyopathy.
  - *Diurectics* are used to decrease volume overload and pulmonary edema. Most common are the "loop diurectics" (i.e., furosemide).
  - *Afterload-reducing agents* (i.e., angiotensin-converting enzyme [ACE] inhibitors, calcium channel blockers, nitroglycerin) are used to dilate peripheral vasculature and thus decrease the work on the heart.

VASCULITIDES

Henoch–Schönlein Purpura

- Immune-mediated vasculitis that affects the GI tract, joints, and kidneys and causes a characteristic rash (see dermatology chapter).
- Most often occurs in winter months, following a group A streptococcal upper respiratory infection (URI).
- GI involvement is most significant, leading to vomiting and upper and lower GI bleeding.
- Renal involvement, in the form of glomerulonephritis, can progress to acute renal failure.
- Treatment is supportive, with full recovery within 4 to 6 weeks.

Kawasaki's disease

DEFINITION

Also known as mucocutaneous lymph node syndrome.

ETIOLOGY

Unknown etiology, but believed to have an infectious cause.

EPIDEMIOLOGY

- Affects children (> 80% under age 4 years)
- More common in Asians than other racial groups
- More common in males than females (ratio 1.5:1)
- Most common in winter/spring months
- Associated with carpet cleaning and living near body of water

SIGNS AND SYMPTOMS

- Sterile pyuria
- Aseptic meningitis
- Thrombocytosis
- Desquamation of fingers and toes
- Elevated ESR or CRP
- Most significant sequelae:
  - Coronary aneurysms (usually resolve within 12 months of adequate therapy)
  - Pericardial effusion
  - CHF

DIAGNOSIS

- Diagnostic criteria (need 5+):
  1. Fever (to 104°F [40°C]), for > 5 days
  2. Bilateral conjunctivitis (without exudate)
  3. Mucocutaneous lesions ("strawberry" tongue; dry, red, cracked lips; diffuse erythema of oral cavity)

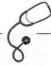

Use of diurectics in CHF is preferred to salt and fluid restriction.

Watch out for hypokalemia, as increased potassium is lost with some diuretic use.

Hypokalemia can precipitate digitalis toxicity.

4. Changes in upper and lower extremities (erythema and/or edema of hands/feet)
5. Polymorphic rash (usually truncal)
6. Cervical lymphadenopathy (> 1.5 cm in diameter), usually unilateral
- Echocardiogram: initial study at diagnosis to establish baseline and to evaluate for early coronary aneurysms; follow-up echo to establish presence or absence

TREATMENT

- Intravenous gamma globulin (IVIG): usually one dose.
- High-dose aspirin (80–100 mg/kg/day).
- Aspirin is reduced after 2 weeks of therapy or until the patient is afebrile for 48 hours.
- Use of steroids is controversial and under investigation.

Polyarteritis Nodosa

DEFINITION

A necrotizing inflammation of the small and medium-sized muscular arteries.

SIGNS AND SYMPTOMS

- Prolonged fever, weight loss, malaise, subcutaneous nodules on extremities.
- Various rashes can be associated with this condition.
- Respiratory symptoms: rhinorrhea, congestion.
- Often waxes and wanes.
- Gangrene of distal extremities is found in severe disease.

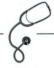

Hypertension and abdominal pain can be important clues in polyarteritis nodosa.

DIAGNOSIS

- No diagnostic tests.
- Associated with abnormal cell counts (thrombocytosis, leukocytosis), abnormal urinalysis, elevated acute-phase reactants, p-ANCA.
- Conclusive with findings of medium-sized artery aneurysms.
- Echocardiographic evidence of coronary artery aneurysms is diagnostic if other clinical evidence is present.

TREATMENT

- Corticosteroids suppress the clinical manifestations.
- Cyclophosphamide or azathioprine may be required to induce remission.

Takayasu's Arteritis

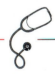

Takayasu's arteritis is also known as "pulseless disease."

DEFINITION

- Also known as aortoarteritis
- Chronic inflammatory disease involving:
  - Aorta
  - Arterial branches from the aorta
  - Pulmonary vasculature

PATHOPHYSIOLOGY

- Lesions are segmental and often obliterative.
- Aneurysmal and saccular dilation also occur.
- Thoracoabdominal aorta is the predominantly affected site in the pediatric population.

Essentially, Takayasu's arteritis is giant cell arteritis of the aorta (and large branches).

EPIDEMIOLOGY

Most patients are female, ages 4 to 45 years.

SIGNS AND SYMPTOMS

- A significant number of patients experience LV dysfunction and CHF (even in the absence of coronary artery involvement, hypertension, or valvar abnormalities).
- A lymphocytic infiltration consistent with myocarditis is present in about 50% of patients.
- Other symptoms include fever, polyarthralgias, polyarthritis, and loss of radial pulsations.

TREATMENT

Corticosteroids may induce remission.

Wegener's Granulomatosis

DEFINITION

A rare vasculitis of both arteries and veins leading to widespread necrotizing granumolas.

EPIDEMIOLOGY

Most common in adults, although occurrence in children has been described.

SIGNS AND SYMPTOMS

- Rhinorrhea, nasal mucosa ulcers, sinusitis
- Hematuria
- Cough, hemoptysis, pleuritis
- Heart involvement: granulamatous inflammation of cardiac muscle causing arrhythmias

DIAGNOSIS

- Antineutrophil cytoplasmic antibodies (c-ANCA) are present.
- ESR is greatly elevated.
- Organ biopsy (kidney and/or lung) may be essential to establish early diagnosis.

TREATMENT

- Corticosteroids alone may be unsuccessful.
- Cyclophosphamide or azathioprine is recommended (have changed a once uniformly fatal disease into an excellent prognosis).

Children with cyanotic heart disease are at increased risk for strokes and scoliosis.

CYANOTIC HEART DEFECTS

See Figure 13-2.

Tetralogy of Fallot (TOF)

DEFINITION

Four anomalies constitute the tetralogy:
1. Right ventricular outflow tract obstruction (RVOTO)
2. VSD
3. Aortic override
4. RVH

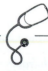

Cyanotic Heart Defects
T's
Tetralogy of Fallot
Transposition of the great vessels
Truncus arteriosus
Total anomalous pulmonary venous return (obstructive)

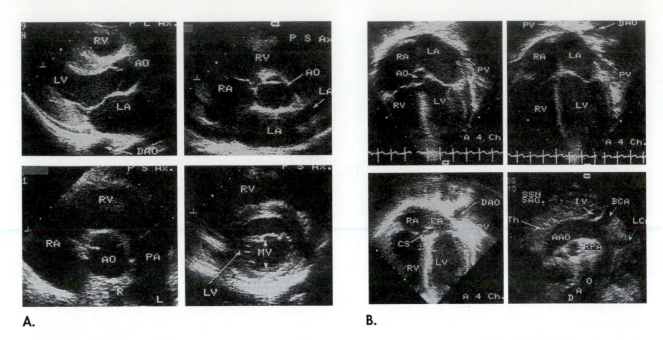

A.

B.

FIGURE 13-2. Basic Echocardiography Views. **A.** *Top left:* this frame, taken from a normal subject, is a parasternal long-axis (P L Ax) view taken slicing the heart from a parasternal location at the fourth left interspace, subtending a sector with the right ventricle (RV) anteriorly. The sound beams then pass through the ventricular septum and the aorta (AO), the left ventricular cavity (LV), and the left ventricular posterior wall. Behind the ascending aortic root is the left atrium (LA). Posterior to the heart behind the pericardium, the descending aorta (DAO) can be seen running in its cross-section, indicating how far from the sagittal body plane this image is as the descending aorta runs on the left of the spine. *Bottom left:* from the same normal subject in the parasternal short-axis (P S Ax) view from the third intercostal space. The sector subtends the right side of the heart as it winds around the aortic root (AO) in the center of image. The right atrium (RA) is separated from the right ventricle (RV) by the tricuspid valve. The pulmonary artery (PA) is separated from the right ventricle by the pulmonary valve. The cusps of the aortic valve can also be identified in this figure. The pulmonary artery bifurcates into its left (L) and right branches. *Top right, bottom right:* these parasternal short-axis (P S Ax) views taken from the same normal subject are sequential scans through the heart from the top to the bottom (from the cranial-to-caudal direction). The *top frame* represents a short-axis view of the entire right heart. In the center, the aortic valve (AO) cusps are seen in their open position, demonstrating a trileaflet aortic valve. Posteriorly, the left atrium (LA), with the left atrial appendage (LAA) extending to the left side of the heart, are observed. The interatrial septum separates the left atrium from the right atrium (RA). The tricuspid valve separates the right atrium from the right ventricle (RV). In the *bottom frame* with the caudal scan, the right (RV) and left (LV) ventricles are seen. The ventricular septum is seen between the two ventricles. The mitral valve (MV) is seen in its open position with the anterior cusp (arrow) at the top and the posterior cusp (arrow) at the bottom. **B.** This is a series of apical four-chamber views (A 4 Ch) from a normal subject, demonstrating the scan from the anterior to the posterior aspect of the heart (from the apex to base). The electrocardiogram shown on the bottom indicates the timing within the cardiac cycle. The *top frame* is taken in systole. A left pulmonary vein (PV) can be seen entering the left atrium (LA). The right atrium (RA) is separated from the left atrium (LA) by the faint echo of the interatrial septum. The aortic root (AO) can be seen to be arising out of the heart, and the left and right ventricles (LV, RV) can be seen separated from their respective atria by the tricuspid and mitral valves in the closed position, and from each other by the ventricular septum. The *second frame,* taken with more caudal scanning, demonstrates the descending aorta in cross-section, the pulmonary veins (PV) from the left and the right (arrows), the atria, and the ventricles. This is an end-systolic frame, as seen from the electrocardiogram. The *third frame,* taken with most caudal scanning, demonstrates the descending aorta (DAO) posteriorly, and a small portion of the left atrium (LA) with a coronary sinus (CS) running inferiorly at the crux of the heart. The other labels are as for the previous panels. The *fourth frame* shows the aortic arch from the suprasternal notch sagittal view (SSN, SAG) in a normal infant. The scan comes from the suprasternal notch area, and the sector subtends the innominate vein (IV) superiorly, as it crosses in front of the ascending aorta (AAO). The whole arch is seen from the ascending aorta to the descending aorta (DAO). The brachiocephalic artery (BCA) and left carotid artery (LCA) can be seen arising from the aortic arch. The circular right pulmonary artery can be seen running under the arch (RPA). The label obscures the area of the right bronchus, lying between the aortic arch and the right pulmonary artery. Anteriorly, the thymus (Th) is identified.

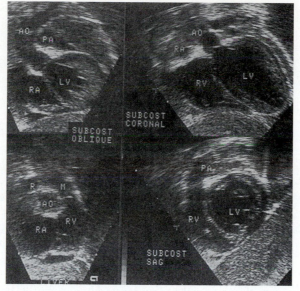

C.

FIGURE 13-2. Basic Echocardiography Views *(continued).* **C.** These images from a normal subject are taken with the subcostal transducer position in coronal and sagittal (SAG) planes. The scans pass from the subcostal region through the liver and diaphragm, and into the heart. *Right panels:* in the *top right panel* with posterior angulation, the left ventricle (LV) and right ventricle (RV) are identified. The aorta (AO) arises from the left ventricle, separated from it by the aortic valve; the right atrium (RA) and right ventricle (RV) can be identified. The *bottom right panel,* taken in an orthogonal cut in the sagittal plane, demonstrates the left ventricle (LV) cut in cross-section with its papillary muscles; the right ventricle (RV) and pulmonary artery (PA) can be seen wrapping around the left ventricle. *Left panels:* these subcostal oblique cuts demonstrate the exit of the aorta (AO) and the pulmonary artery (PA) from their respective ventricles, the left ventricle (LV) and the right ventricle (RV). In the *upper left panel,* the aorta (AO) can be seen arising from the left ventricle (LV) and arching toward the left side over the main pulmonary artery (PA). In the *bottom left panel,* taken with an orthogonal view and more anterior angulation, the right-sided structures, right atrium (RA), right ventricle (RV), main (M) pulmonary artery, and right (R) pulmonary artery can be seen as they surround the aortic valve (AO). (Reproduced, with permission, from *Rudolph's Pediatrics,* 20th ed. Appleton & Lange, 1996.)

ETIOLOGY

Prenatal factors associated include maternal rubella or viral illness.

PATHOPHYSIOLOGY

RVOTO dictates degree of shunting:

- *Minimal obstruction:* Leads to increased pulmonary blood flow as pulmonary vascular resistance (PVR) decreases, leading to CHF.
- *Mild obstruction:* Hemodynamic balance pressure between right and left ventricles is equal, thus no net shunting ("pink tet").
- *Severe obstruction:* Decreased pulmonary blood flow, leading to cyanosis.

EPIDEMIOLOGY

Most common cyanotic heart defect in children who survive infancy.

SIGNS AND SYMPTOMS

- Failure to thrive (FTT) (if diagnosed late)
- "Conotruncal facies"
- Variable cyanosis (clubbing later if unrepaired)
- Right ventricular impulse; occasional thrill; single S2, systolic ejection murmur at the upper left sternal border with or without ejection click
- Squatting is a common posture in older, unoperated children with TOF:
  - Often occurs after exercise

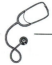

Two key features are required for diagnosis of TOF:

- **VSD** (typically large enough to equalize pressures in right and left ventricles).
- **RVOTO** (e.g., pulmonary stenosis).
- **Aortic override** is variable.
- **RVH** is secondary to the RVOTO.

- Causes trapping of desaturated blood in the lower extremities and increases systemic vascular resistance (SVR) while the RVOTO remains fixed. Thus, it:
  - Decreases right-to-left shunting
  - Increases pulmonary blood flow
  - Increases arterial saturation

"TET SPELLS"

- Most common: 2 to 6 months of age
- Occur in the morning or after a nap when SVR is low
- Precipitating factors:
  - Stress
  - Drugs that decrease SVR
  - Hot baths
  - Fever
  - Exercise
- Mechanism: Unknown, but likely due to increased cardiac output with fixed RVOT, leading to increased right-to-left shunting, which increases cyanosis
- If prolonged or severe: syncope, seizures, cardiac arrest

DIAGNOSIS

- CXR (Figure 13-3)
- "Boot-shaped heart"
- Decreased pulmonary vascular markings
- Right aortic arch (25%)

TREATMENT

- Patient's clinical status may prevent definitive repair initially.
- Shunting (i.e., Blalock–Taussig shunt) is often used when pulmonary stenosis is severe and an alternative route for blood to reach the lungs is necessary.
- Complete repair entails:
  - VSD closure
  - Relief of RVOTO
  - Ligation of shunts
  - ASD/patent foramen ovale (PFO) closure

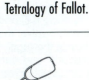

CXR with the boot shape, decreased pulmonary vascular markings, and a right aortic arch. *Think:* Tetralogy of Fallot.

Without repair of TOF, mortality is:
- 50% by 3 years
- 90% by 20 years
- 95% by 30 years

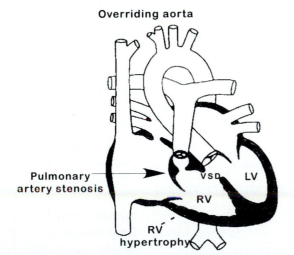

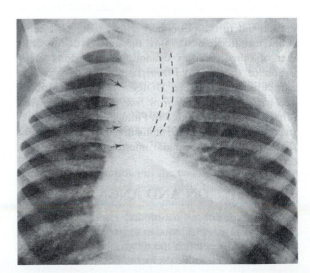

FIGURE 13-3. Chest x-ray in tetralogy of Fallot. Arrows indicate right-sided aortic arch and upper thoracic aorta. Dashed lines indicate right-sided aortic indentation on the air bronchogram. (Reproduced, with permission, from *Rudolph's Pediatrics*, 20th ed. Appleton & Lange, 1996.)

Transposition of the Great Vessels

PATHOPHYSIOLOGY

- This lesion occurs when, in the development of the heart, the primitive heart loops to the left instead of the right and the following result (see Figure 13-4):
    - Aorta originates from the RV.
    - Pulmonary artery originates from LV.
        - Aorta is anterior; pulmonary trunk is posterior.
    - Right and left hearts are in parallel:
        - Pulmonary venous return is via the pulmonary artery.
        - Systemic venous return is via the aorta.
- An ASD and/or VSD is essential to allow mixing.
- A PDA alone is usually not sufficient to allow adequate mixing.

EPIDEMIOLOGY

Most common cyanotic congenital heart defect presenting in the neonatal period.

TYPES

I: Short common pulmonary trunk arising from right side of common trunk, just above truncal valve.

II: Pulmonary arteries (PAs) arise directly from ascending aorta, from posterior surface.

III: Similar to type II, with PAs arising more laterally and more distant from semilunar valves.

Intact Ventricular Septum (with no valve abnormality)

SIGNS AND SYMPTOMS

- Early cyanosis, a single S2, and no murmur.
- An intact atrial septum or very restrictive PFO is a medical emergency.

DIAGNOSIS

- ECG will be normal initially, but will demonstrate right ventricular hypertrophy by 1 month.
- CXR: "Egg on a string."

With VSD (a large VSD allows adequate mixing)

- Symptoms are related to increased pulmonary blood flow, with CHF sometimes occurring early.
- May have little cyanosis.

- ECG: Right or biventricular hypertrophy.

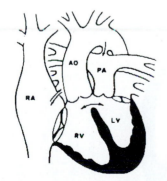 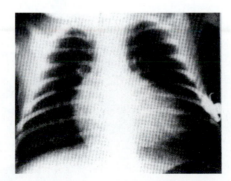

FIGURE 13-4. Transposition of the great vessels. "Egg on a string"—spinal column serving as the string and the globular presentation of the heart as the egg. (Reproduced, with permission, from Moller JH, Neal WA. *Fetal, Neonatal, and Infant Cardiac Disease*, 2nd ed. Appleton & Lange, 1992: 532.)

TREATMENT

- Patient is "ductal dependent" and will require prostaglandin E_1 (PGE_1) to keep the PDA patent.
- Early **balloon atrial septostomy** (BAS) is necessary to allow mixing of oxygenated and deoxygenated blood.
- Arterial switch procedure is definitive.
- BAS if VSD does not allow adequate mixing.
- PA band to control increased pulmonary blood flow.
- Arterial switch with VSD closure is definitive.

Truncus Arteriosus

DEFINITION

A persistent truncus is a single arterial trunk that emerges from the ventricles, supplying the coronary, pulmonary, and systemic circulations (see Figure 13-5).

PATHOPHYSIOLOGY

- The valve has 2, 3, or 4 leaflets and is usually poorly functioning.
- The truncus overrides a VSD.

SIGNS AND SYMPTOMS

Symptoms usually occur within the first few weeks of life:

- Initial left-to-right shunt symptoms:
  - Dyspnea
  - Frequent respiratory infections
  - Failure to thrive
- If pulmonary vascular resistance increases, cyanosis increases.
- Second heart sound is prominent and single due to the single semilunar valve.
- Peripheral pulses are strong, often bounding.
- Often, a systolic ejection click can be appreciated.

DIAGNOSIS

CXR shows cardiomegaly and increased pulmonary vascular markings.

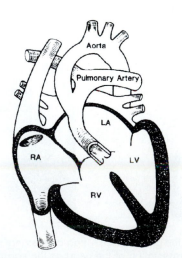

FIGURE 13-5. Truncus arteriosus. (Artwork by Dr. John Brienholt.)

- Surgery must occur before patient develops significant pulmonary vascular disease (usually 3–4 months of age).
- VSD is surgically closed, leaving the valve on the left ventricular side.
- The pulmonary arteries are freed from the truncus and are connected to a valved conduit (Rastelli procedure), which will serve as the new pulmonary trunk.

Hypoplastic Left Heart Syndrome (HLHS)

DEFINITION

The syndrome consists of the following (see Figure 13-6):

- Aortic valve hypoplasia, stenosis, or atresia.
- Hypoplasia of the ascending aorta.
- LV hypoplasia or agenesis.
- Mitral valve stenosis or atresia.
- The result is a single (right) ventricle that provides blood to the pulmonary system, the systemic circulation via the PDA, and coronary system via retrograde flow after crossing the PDA.
- Ductal dependent requiring patency until intervention undertaken.

EPIDEMIOLOGY

The second most common congenital heart defect presenting in the first week of life (and the most common cause of death from CHD in the first month).

HLHS accounts for 25% of all cardiac deaths in the first year of life.

SIGNS AND SYMPTOMS

- Pulses range from normal to absent (depending on ductal patency).
- Hyperdynamic RV impulse.
- Single S2 of increased intensity.
- Gallop at apex due if there is heart failure.
- Nonspecific systolic murmur at left sternal border (LSB).
- Skin may have a characteristic grayish pallor.

DIAGNOSIS

- CXR: cardiomegaly with globular shaped heart; increased pulmonary vascular markings, pulmonary edema.
- Echocardiogram is diagnostic.

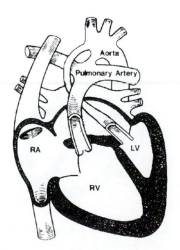

FIGURE 13-6. Hypoplastic left heart syndrome. Note small size of left ventricle. (Artwork by Dr. John Brienholt.)

- No intervention: Due to the high mortality and complicated surgical course of this disease, ethical dilemmas are frequent as to how far physicians should intervene.
- Three-stage surgery
  - *Norwood procedure:* The pulmonary trunk is used to reconstruct the hypoplastic aorta, and the right ventricle subsequently becomes the functional left ventricle. This leaves the pulmonary arteries connected but separated from the heart. The pulmonary blood flow is then reestablished via systemic to pulmonary conduits from the subclavian arteries to the pulmonary arteries.
  - *Glenn procedure:* The superior vena cava is connected to the right PA, restoring partial venous return to the lungs.
  - *Fontan procedure:* The inferior vena cava is anastamosed to the PAs, resulting in complete venous diversion from the systemic circulation to the lungs.
- Heart transplant: This alternative occurs either as a primary intervention (if an organ is available) or after any of the previous palliative surgeries have provided maximal but ultimately insufficient benefit.

ACYANOTIC HEART DEFECTS

Left-to-right shunt (see Figure 13-7).

Subendocardial Cushion Defect

PATHOPHYSIOLOGY

- Related to the ostium primum ASD, this defect results from abnormal development of the AV canal (endocardial cushions) resulting in:
  - A VSD
  - An ostium primum ASD
- Clefts in the mitral and tricuspid valves

EPIDEMIOLOGY

- Thirty percent of patients with this defect have trisomy 21.
- Also frequently found with asplenia and polysplenia syndromes.

> Subendocardial cushion defects are associated with Down's syndrome.

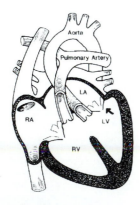 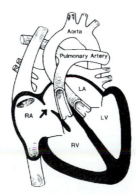 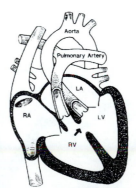 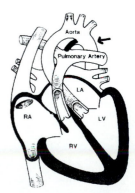

Subendocardial cushion defect   Atrial septal defect   Ventricular septal defect   Patent ductus arteriosus

FIGURE 13-7. Acyanotic heart defects. (Artwork by Dr. John Brienholt.)

SIGNS AND SYMPTOMS

- Often the result of the specific components of the accumulated defects:
  - Holosystolic murmur from the VSD, if restrictive
  - Systolic murmur from mitral and tricuspid valve insufficiency
- High risk of developing Eisenmenger's syndrome

TREATMENT

- Surgical correction is sometimes the only option (despite high risk) when patient has an unbalanced AV canal.
- Some benefit from PA banding if shunting is predominantly at the ventricular level (rare).

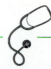

Children with trisomy 21 often have more favorable anatomy for surgical intervention.

Atrial Septal Defect (ASD)

DEFINITION

- Three types:
  - *Secundum defect* (most common—50–70%)
    - Located in the central portion of the atrial septum
  - *Primum defect* (about 30% of ASDs)
    - Located at the atrial lower margin
    - Associated with abnormalities of the mitral and tricuspid valves
  - *Sinus venosus defect* (about 10% of ASDs)
- Located at the upper portion of the atrial septum, and often extends into the superior vena cava

ASD is the most common congenital heart lesion recognized in adults.

EPIDEMIOLOGY

- A common "co-conspirator" in CHD.
- As many as 50% of patients with congenital heart defects have an ASD as one of the defects.
- More common in females (male-to-female ratio 1:2).

SIGNS AND SYMPTOMS

- Children with ASDs are typically asymptomatic.
- Widely split and fixed S2. Murmurs are uncommon, but may occur as patient gets older.
- Symptoms of CHF and pulmonary HTN occur in adults (second and third decades).

DIAGNOSIS

ECG: The left-to-right shunt may produce right atrial enlargement and RVH.

TREATMENT

- Nearly 90% will close spontaneously.
  - 100% close if < 3 mm.
  - ASDs > 8 mm are unlikely to close spontaneously.
- Surgical or catheter closure (via a "clamshell" or "umbrella" device) are used when indicated.

Patent Foramen Ovale (PFO)

- The foramen ovale is used prenatally to provide oxygenated blood from the placenta to the left atrium.
- It normally functionally closes when increased left atrial pressure causes the septa to press against each other (many remain "probe-patent" into adulthood).

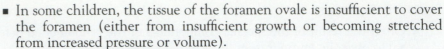

- In some children, the tissue of the foramen ovale is insufficient to cover the foramen (either from insufficient growth or becoming stretched from increased pressure or volume).
- Some CHDs require a PFO for patient survival after birth (e.g., tricuspid and mitral atresia, TAPVR).

Ventricular Septal Defect (VSD)

EPIDEMIOLOGY

- The most common form of congenital heart disease (30–60% of all patients with CHDs)
- Usually membranous, as opposed to in the muscular septum

SIGNS AND SYMPTOMS

Dependent on defect size:
- Small VSDs
  - Usually asymptomatic
  - Normal growth and development
  - High-pitched, holosystolic murmur
  - No ECG or CXR changes
- Large VSDs
  - Can lead to CHF and pulmonary HTN
  - May have failure to thrive
  - Lower-pitched murmur; intensity dependent on the degree of shunting

DIAGNOSIS

- ECG: LVH
- CXR: cardiomegaly

TREATMENT

- Spontaneous closure:
  - Muscular defects are most likely to close (up to 50%), with closure occurring during the first year of life.
  - Inlet and infundibular defects do not reduce in size or close.
- Intervention is based on the development of CHF, pulmonary HTN, and growth failure.
- Initial management with diuretics and digitalis.
- Surgical closure is indicated when therapy fails.
- Catheter-induced closure devices are less commonly used with VSDs than ASDs.

Patent Ductus Arteriosus (PDA)

PATHOPHYSIOLOGY

- Most often a problem in premature neonates:
  - Left-to-right shunts are handled poorly by premature infants.
  - Many develop idiopathic respiratory distress syndrome.
  - Some progress to develop left ventricular failure.
- Failure of spontaneous closure:
  - Premature infants: due to ineffective response to oxygen tension
  - Mature infants: due to structural abnormality of ductal smooth muscle

EPIDEMIOLOGY

- PDA is more common in females (male-to-female ratio 1:3).
- Incidence is higher at higher altitudes due to higher atmospheric oxygen tension.
- Maternal rubella in the first trimester has also been implicated in PDA.

VSD is the most common congenital heart disorder.

Typical Scenario

A 2-month-old male born at term appeared well until 3 weeks ago when he became dyspneic and had difficulty feeding. A loud pansystolic murmur is heard at the left lower sternal border, and ECG shows LVH and RVH. *Think:* VSD.

Spontaneous closure occurs in 30–50% of VSDs.

A PDA murmur is common (and normal) in newborn infants. It will usually disappear within the first 12 hours of life.

In the normal neonate, the ductus arteriosus closes primarily in response to a ductal $PO_2 > 50$ mm Hg.

SIGNS AND SYMPTOMS

- Small PDAs usually are asymptomatic.
- Large PDAs increase incidence of lower respiratory tract infections and CHF.
- Machinery-like murmur.
- Bounding peripheral pulses and wide pulse pressure.
- If Eisenmenger's syndrome results, patient may have cyanosis restricted to the lower extremities.

TREATMENT

- Indomethacin: used in premature infants. Inhibits prostaglandin synthesis, leading to closure.
- Catheter closure via devices such as double-umbrella devices and coils in older children.
- Surgical ligation and division via a left lateral thoracotomy:
  - An occasional complication is recurrent laryngeal nerve injury leading to hoarseness.
  - Eisenmenger's syndrome is a contraindication to surgery.

Subacute bacterial endocarditis (SBE) is more common in small PDAs than large ones.

Eisenmenger's Syndrome

- Can occur in unrepaired left-to-right shunts (i.e., VSD) that cause an increased pressure load on the pulmonary vasculature.
- Pressure overload on the pulmonary vasculature can result in irreversible changes in the arterioles.
- This develops into pulmonary vascular obstructive disease, usually over several years.
- The pulmonary HTN reduces the left-to-right shunt and previous LVH often resolves.
- Persistent HTN maintains an enlarged right ventricle and can dilate the main pulmonary segment (this becomes evident on CXR).
- Avoidance of this condition via surgical correction of CHD is essential, as it causes irreversible changes.

Infective endocarditis is the most common complication of PDA in late childhood.

CONGENITAL VALVAR DEFECTS

See Figure 13-8.

Tricuspid Atresia

DEFINITION

RV inlet is absent or nearly absent:

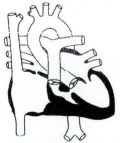

Tricuspid atresia

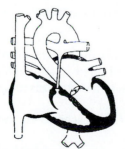

Pulmonary atresia

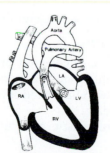

Aortic insufficiency

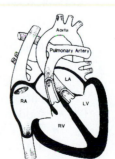

Mitral stenosis

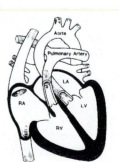

Mitral valve prolapse

FIGURE 13-8. Congenital valvular defects. (Artwork by Dr. John Brienholt.)

- Eighty-nine percent have no evidence of tricuspid valve tissue, only dimple.
- Seven percent have a membranous septum forming part of the right atrial floor.
- Three percent are Ebstein's.
- One percent have a tiny, imperforate valve-like structure.

EPIDEMIOLOGY

- ASD and/or VSD is usually present.
- Seventy-five percent will present with cyanosis within the first week.

SIGNS AND SYMPTOMS

LV impulse displaced laterally.

DIAGNOSIS

ECG: LVH, prominent LV forces (due to decreased RV voltages).

TREATMENT

- PGE_1 to maintain ductal patency
- Surgical intervention
- Modified Blalock–Taussig (BT) shunt
- Glenn procedure, followed by Fontan procedure

Pulmonary Atresia (with Intact Ventricular Septum)

SIGNS AND SYMPTOMS

- Cyanosis within hours of birth (PDA closing)
- Hypotension, tachypnea, acidosis
- Single S2, with a holosystolic murmur (tricuspid regurgitation)

DIAGNOSIS

- ECG: decreased RV forces and occasionally RVH
- CXR: normal to enlarged RV with decreased pulmonary vascular markings

TREATMENT

- PGE_1 to maintain ductal patency
- Balloon atrial septostomy (sometimes)
- Reconstruction of RVOT with transannular patch or pulmonary valvotomy
- ASD left open to prevent systemic venous HTN

Aortic Stenosis

EPIDEMIOLOGY

Eighty-five percent of congenitally stenotic aortic valves are bicuspid.

SIGNS AND SYMPTOMS

- Severe stenosis generally presents shortly after birth.
- Older children may complain of chest or stomach pain (epigastric).
- Patients with untreated severe aortic stenosis are at risk for syncope and sudden death.
- The characteristic murmur is a **crescendo–decrescendo systolic murmur.**
- A **systolic ejection click** is also common (particularly if bicuspid aortic valve).

Typical Scenario

A 4-year-old boy with recurrent episodes of syncope while playing has a harsh systolic murmur radiating to the carotids, diminished cardiac pulses, and severe LVH. *Think:* Congenital aortic stenosis.

Supravalvular aortic stenosis is associated with idiopathic hypercalcemia.

- In severe disease, paradoxical splitting of S2 occurs (split narrows with inspiration).

DIAGNOSIS

- Clinical findings, including ECG findings, and symptoms can be deceiving.
- Echo or catheterization to evaluate pressure differences between the aorta and left ventricle is essential.

TREATMENT

- Surgical or interventional balloon.
- Valvotomy is most common intervention:
  - Indication is usually if the measured catheterization gradient is > 50 mm Hg.
  - High incidence of recurrent stenosis.
- Valve replacement: deferred, when possible, until patient completes growth.

Aortic Insufficiency

EPIDEMIOLOGY

Uncommon and usually associated with mitral valve disease, or aortic stenosis.

SIGNS AND SYMPTOMS

- A diastolic, decrescendo murmur is present at the left upper sternal border.
- Presentation with symptoms indicates advanced disease.
- Chest pain and CHF are ominous signs.

DIAGNOSIS

CXR: LV enlargement, dilated ascending aorta.

TREATMENT

- Surgery or balloon valvuloplasty to treat aortic stenosis may worsen the insufficiency.
- Aortic valve replacement is the only definitive therapy.

Mitral Stenosis

EPIDEMIOLOGY

- Rare in children; usually a sequela of acute rheumatic fever.
- Congenital forms are generally severe.

SIGNS AND SYMPTOMS

- When symptomatic, dyspnea is the most common symptom.
- Weak peripheral pulses with narrow pulse pressure.
- An **opening snap** is heard on auscultation; also, a **presystolic murmur** may be heard.
- Pulmonary venous congestion occurs, leading to:
  - CXR evidence of interstitial edema
  - Hemoptysis from small bronchial vessel rupture

TREATMENT

- Balloon valvuloplasty
- Surgical:
  - Commissurotomy
  - Valve replacement

People with Marfan's disease frequently have aortic insufficiency as well.

Mitral Valve Prolapse

PATHOPHYSIOLOGY

Caused by thick and redundant valve leaflets that bulge into the mitral annulus.

EPIDEMIOLOGY

- Usually occurs in older children and adolescents.
- Has a familial component (autosomal dominant).
- Nearly all patients with Marfan's syndrome have it.

SIGNS AND SYMPTOMS

- Auscultation: midsystolic click and late systolic murmur
- Often asymptomatic with some history of palpitations and chest pain

TREATMENT

Management is symptomatic (e.g., β blocker for chest pain).

OTHER CONGENITAL CARDIOVASCULAR DEFECTS

Coarctation of the Aorta

PATHOPHYSIOLOGY

- Most commonly found in the juxtaductal position (where the ductus arteriosus joins the aorta).
- Development of symptoms may correspond to the closure of the ductus arteriosus (the patent ductus provides additional room for blood to reach the postductal aorta).

EPIDEMIOLOGY

- More common in males than females (male-to-female ratio 2:1)
- Seen in one third of patients with Turner's syndrome

Coarctation of the aorta is associated with Turner's syndrome.

SIGNS AND SYMPTOMS

Clinical Presentation of Symptomatic Infants
- Failure to thrive, respiratory distress, and CHF develop in the first 2 to 3 months of life.
- Lower extremity changes: decreased pulses in the lower extremities.
- Acidosis may develop as the lower body receives insufficient blood.
- Usually, a murmur is heard over the left back.

Clinical Presentation of Asymptomatic Infants or Children
- Normal growth and development
- Occasional complaint of leg weakness or pain after exertion
- Decreased pulses in the lower extremities
- Upper extremity HTN (or at least greater than in the lower extremities)

DIAGNOSIS

CXR: "3 sign," dilated ascending aorta that displaces the superior vena cava to the right (see Figure 13-9).

TREATMENT

- Resection of the coarctation segment with end-to-end anastomosis is the intervention of choice for initial treatment.
- Allograft patch augmentation can also be used.

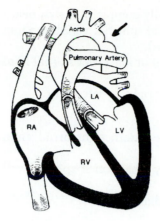

FIGURE 13-9. Coarctation of the aorta. (Artwork by Dr. John Brienholt.)

- Catheter balloon dilation can be used:
  - Has a higher restenosis rate than surgery.
  - Has an increased risk of producing aortic aneurysms.
  - Balloon dilation is more frequently used when stenosis occurs at the surgical site of a primary reanastamosis.

Ebstein's Anomaly

DEFINITION

Components of the defect (see Figure 13-10):
- The tricuspid valve is displaced apically in the right ventricle.
- The valve leaflets are redundant and plastered against the ventricular wall, often causing functional pulmonary atresia.
- Right atrium is frequently the largest structure.

EPIDEMIOLOGY

Without intervention:
- CHF in first 6 months
- Nearly 50% mortality

SIGNS AND SYMPTOMS

- Growth and development can be normal depending on severity of the lesion.

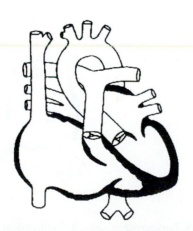

FIGURE 13-10. Ebstein's anomaly. (Artwork by Dr. John Brienholt.)

- Older patients usually complain of dyspnea, cyanosis, and palpitations.
- Widely split S1, fixed split S2, variable S3 and S4 (characteristic triple or quadruple rhythm).
- Holosystolic murmur at left lower sternal border.
- Opening snap.
- Cyanosis from atrial right-to-left shunt.

DIAGNOSIS

- ECG: right axis deviation, right atrial enlargement, RBBB; WPW is present in 20%.
- CXR: Cardiomegaly ("balloon-shaped") "wall-to-wall heart" in severely affected infants.
- Echocardiogram is diagnostic.

TREATMENT

Intervention (87% do well):
- Glenn procedure to increase pulmonary blood flow.
- Severely affected infants may require aortopulmonary shunt.
- Tricuspid valve replacement or reconstruction.
- Right atrial reduction surgery.
- Ablation of accessory conduction pathways.

Total Anomalous Pulmonary Venous Return (TAPVR)

PATHOPHYSIOLOGY

- See Figure 13-11A and B.
- No communication exists between the pulmonary veins and the left atrium.
  - All pulmonary veins drain to a common vein.
  - The common vein drains into the:
    - Right superior vena cava (50%)
    - Coronary sinus or right atrium (20%)
    - Portal vein or inferior vena cava (20%)
    - Combination of the above types (10%)
- An ASD is needed for survival.

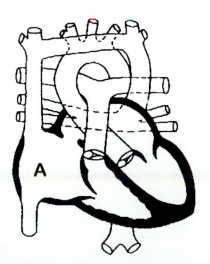 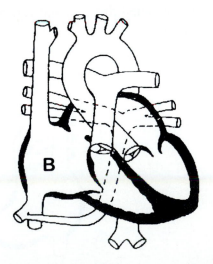

FIGURE 13-11. Total anomalous pulmonary venous return. **A.** Supracardiac view. **B.** Infracardiac view. (Artwork by Dr. John Brienholt.)

Dramatically more common in males (male-to-female ratio 4:1).

SIGNS AND SYMPTOMS/ DIAGNOSIS/TREATMENT

- Presence or absence of obstruction of pulmonary venous return changes the clinical presentation.
- TAPVR with obstruction.

TAPVR WITH OBSTRUCTION

- Obstruction leads to increased pulmonary artery pressure (and subsequent pulmonary edema) that increases pulmonary then right atrial and ventricular pressures. This causes a right-to-left shunt and resultant cyanosis.
- Presents with early, severe respiratory distress and cyanosis, no murmur, and hepatomegaly.
- CXR: normal-size heart, pulmonary edema.
- Echocardiogram is diagnostic.
- Management: BAS or immediate corrective surgery.

TAPVR WITHOUT OBSTRUCTION

- Free communication between RA and LA
- Large right-to-left shunt ("large ASD")
- Presents later during first year of life, with mild FTT, recurrent pulmonary infections, tachypnea, right heart failure, and rarely cyanosis
- CXR: cardiomegaly, large PAs; increased pulmonary vascular markings ("snowman" or "figure eight" sign)
- Management: surgical movement of pulmonary veins to the left atrium

Renal, Gynecologic, and Urinary Disease

ACID–BASE DISORDERS

Normal Acid–Base Balance

pH, 7.4; P_{CO_2}, 40; O_2 sat, 98

DIAGNOSIS

- Diagnose acid–base disorders by obtaining an arterial blood gas (pH and P_{CO_2}) and a electrolyte panel (HCO_3).
- Assess the acid–base disorder step by step:
    - Is the primary disorder an acidosis (pH < 7.4) or alkalosis (pH > 7.4)?
    - Is the disorder respiratory (pH and P_{CO_2} move in opposite directions)?
    - Is the disorder metabolic (pH and P_{CO_2} move in the same direction)?
    - Is the disorder a simple or mixed disorder?

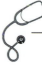

The notation for arterial blood gases is: pH/P_{CO_2}/P_{O_2}/calculated HCO_3/calculated Sa_{O_2}— bicarbonate may also be included.

Metabolic Acidosis

- Decreased serum pH caused by a decrease in plasma HCO_3 from diarrhea or increase in H+ from exogenous sources (MUDPILES), increased endogenous production (lactic acidosis/sepsis), or decreased elimination of H+.
- Treat metabolic acidosis by correcting the underlying disorder. Treat patients with pH < 7.15 with HCO_3.

To interpret metabolic acid–base disturbances, you need a measured HCO_3 from a serum chemistry panel.

Respiratory Acidosis

- Decreased serum pH due to pulmonary retention of CO_2 secondary to sedative overdose, hypoxemia, pneumonia, brain stem injury, airway obstruction, bronchospasm, or pulmonary edema.
- Treat respiratory acidosis by stimulating the ventilation independently or mechanically.

Anion Gap is:
$Na - (Cl + HCO_3) = 12 \pm 2$

Metabolic Alkalosis

- Increased pH due to increased HCO_3. Alkalosis is caused by excessive loss of H+ (vomiting), excessive parenteral HCO_3 administration (licorice, Cushing's syndrome, hyperaldosteronism), or contraction of the extracellular fluid volume.
- Treat metabolic alkalosis with volume repletion.

Respiratory Alkalosis

- Increased pH due to decreased CO_2.
- Caused by hyperventilation seen in asthma and pulmonary embolism, for example.
- Alkalosis causes decrease in serum K and ionized Ca, resulting in paresthesia, carpopedal spasm, and tetany.
- Treat respiratory alkalosis by treating the underlying disorder. Breathing into a paper bag can be useful in cases of psychogenic hyperventilation.

Causes of anion gap metabolic acidosis:
MUDPILES
Methanol
Uremia
Diabetic ketoacidosis (DKA)
Paraldehyde
Isoniazid
Lactate
Ethylene glycol
Salicylate

Typical Scenario

A 6-week-old child has a 2-week history of projectile vomiting that is not bile-stained. He is dehydrated and slightly jaundiced. *Think:* Hypochloremic metabolic alkalosis. Most likely lab findings: Na 138, K 3.0, Cl 88, HCO_3 35, pH 7.52.

If an asthmatic in respiratory distress has a normal pH and normal P_{CO_2}, beware of impending respiratory failure.

The primary defect in distal renal tubular acidosis is a defect in secretion of hydrogen ions.

RENAL TUBULAR ACIDOSIS (RTA)

DEFINITION

Systemic hyperchloremic acidosis due to impaired urinary acidification.

ETIOLOGY

- Three types:
  - **Type 1: Distal RTA.** Distal RTA is caused by increased hydrogen ion secretion by the distal tubule and collecting duct. Distal RTA is associated with hypercalciuria, which may lead to nephrocalcinosis, nephrolithiasis, and renal parenchymal destruction.
  - **Type 2: Proximal RTA.** Proximal RTA is caused by decreased proximal tubular reabsorption of bicarbonate. Proximal RTA may occur as an isolated disorder or as part of a generalized defect in proximal tubular transport, such as Fanconi's syndrome. Proximal RTA can be complicated by rickets, secondary to phosphate wasting.
  - **Type 3: Mineralcorticoid deficiency RTA.** Mineralcorticoid deficiency RTA results from inadequate production or reduced distal tubular responsiveness to aldosterone. This can be due to decreased aldosterone production by the adrenal gland (Addison's disease, congenital adrenal hyperplasia, primary hypoaldosteronism) or a decreased production of renin by the juxtaglomerular apparatus (interstitial damage).

SIGNS AND SYMPTOMS

Polyuria, dehydration, anorexia, vomiting, constipation, and hypotonia. Children often present with growth failure.

TREATMENT

- Correct acidosis.
- Correct electrolyte abnormalities to maintain bicarbonate and potassium levels.

PROGNOSIS

Distal RTA can be a lifelong disease and may lead to renal failure. Proximal RTA and mineralocorticoid RTA usually resolves within 12 months.

DEFINITION

- Acute renal failure develops when renal function is diminished to the point where body fluid homeostasis can no longer be maintained.
- There are three main causes of ARF: prerenal, renal, and postrenal.

PATHOPHYSIOLOGY

- **Prerenal:** Prerenal ARF is caused by hypoperfusion of the kidneys secondary to hemorrhage, sepsis, heart failure, or salt/protein wasting disease.
- **Renal:** ARF is caused by renal parenchyma damage, usually from glomerulonephritis, acute tubular necrosis, interstitial nephritis, or small-vessel thrombosis such as HUS or renal vein thrombosis.
- **Postrenal:** ARF is caused by an obstruction of the urine collection system by tumors or renal stones.

SIGNS AND SYMPTOMS

- Oliguria
- Edema (salt and water overload)
- Hypertension (HTN)
- Congestive heart failure (CHF)
- Seizures
- Mental status change (uremic encephalopathy)

DIAGNOSIS

- Obtain a careful history to determine the cause of renal failure.
- In children with postrenal ARF, a renal ultrasound will show dilation of the renal pelvis and collecting system.

TREATMENT

- Catheterize the patient to monitor urine output and relieve obstruction.
- Treat patients with hypovolemia with volume replacement.
- Treat patients who fail to produce adequate urine output with fluid restriction.

COMPLICATIONS OF UNTREATED ACUTE RENAL FAILURE

- **Hyperkalemia** can develop secondary to impaired renal tubule function. A potassium > 7 mEq/L must be treated emergently with calcium gluconate to stabilize the myocardium, bicarbonate, glucose and insulin, and Kayexalate.
- **Hypocalcemia** and **hyperphospatemia** can lead to tetany. Hypocalcemia is treated by lowering phosphate and replacing active vitamin D.
- **Anemia** is often caused by lowered erythropoietin levels.
- **Hyponatremia** secondary to excessive administration of hypotonic fluids to oliguric patients. Patients with a serum sodium < 120 are at risk for developing cerebral edema and central nervous system (CNS) hemorrhage. Treat patients with water restriction.
- **Metabolic acidosis** is due to decreased excretion of hydrogen and ammonia.

Typical Scenario

A 1-year-old child is brought into the emergency department (ED) with vomiting, constipation, and decreased urine production. The child is found to be acidotic. A renal ultrasound reveals medullary nephrocalcinosis. *Think:* Distal renal tubular acidosis.

The most common cause of ARF in toddlers is hemolytic–uremic syndrome (HUS).

Typical Scenario

A 2-year-old boy develops bloody diarrhea a few days after eating in a fast food restaurant. A few days later, he develops facial edema, pallor, lethargy, and decreased urine output. Bloodwork shows a low hematocrit and platelet count. A urinalysis (UA) reveals blood and protein in the urine. *Think:* HUS secondary to *Escherichia coli* 0157:H7 infection.

Oliguria is < 1–2 mL/kg/hr urine production.

HIGH-YIELD FACTS

Renal, Gynecologic, and Urinary Disease

In patients with prerenal ARF, serum BUN/Cr is > 20.

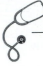

Patients with ARF could be either volume overloaded or volume depleted. Always assess a patient's hydration status. A low pressure, tachycardia, poor skin turgor, flattened fontanels, and sunken eyes indicate severe dehydration. Treat these patients with a bolus of normal saline (NS). A patient with CHF can be treated with diuretics and nitrates.

CHRONIC RENAL FAILURE (CRF)

DEFINITION

Chronic renal failure is a result of kidney damage leading to end-stage renal failure.

ETIOLOGY

- CRF in children under the age of 5 is most often due to anatomic abnormalities, such as renal hypoplasia, dysplasia, or malformations.
- After the age of 5, CRF usually results from glomerular diseases such as HUS or glomerulonephritis, hereditary diseases such as Alport syndrome, or cystic diseases.

SIGNS AND SYMPTOMS

- The development of chronic renal disease is usually insidious and non-specific.
- Patients may present with headache, fatigue, lethargy, anorexia, vomiting, polydipsia, polyuria, and growth failure.
- Most patients with CRF are weak and have HTN.
- See Table 14-1 for a listing of symptoms of uremia.

DIAGNOSIS

Glomerular filtration rate (GFR) < 20% of normal.

TREATMENT

- Dialysis and renal transplant is indicated for patients when serum Cr is > 10 mL/dL.
- **Diet:** Children with CRF are growth retarded. Children should be given adequate caloric intake. Nasogastric (NG) tube feeds and recombinant human growth hormone therapy has been shown to improve linear growth. Water-soluble vitamins, zinc, and iron should be supplemented.

TABLE 14-1. Symptoms of uremia.

Azotemia (accumulation of nitrogen products)
Acidosis
Sodium wasting
Sodium retention
Urinary concentrating defect
Hyperkalemia
Renal osteodystrophy
Growth retardation
Anemia
Bleeding tendency
Infection
Neurologic (fatigue, poor concentration, headache, drowsiness, muscle weakness, seizures, coma)
Gastrointestinal ulceration
Hypertension
Hypertriglyceridemia
Pericarditis and cardiomyopathy
Glucose intolerance

- **Renal osteodystrophy:** Children with CRF are unable to excrete phosphate. The resulting hyperphosphatemia and hypocalcemia stimulate parathyroid hormone (PTH). Excessive PTH leads to fibrosis of the bone marrow space (osteitis fibrosis cystica). Symptoms of renal osteodystrophy include muscle weakness, bone pain, and growth retardation. Treatment includes normalization of the serum calcium and phosphorus levels.
- **Anemia:** Anemia results from inadequate erythropoietin production by the kidneys. Children with Hgb < 6 should be transfused with packed red blood cells (RBCs). Erythropoietin can also be administered subcutaneously.
- **Hypertensive emergencies:** HTN should be treated with salt restriction and a combination of angiotensin-converting enzyme (ACE) inhibitors and β blockers.

END-STAGE RENAL DISEASE (ESRD)

DEFINITION

End-stage renal disease (ESRD) occurs when the serum Cr rises above 10 mg/dL.

TREATMENT

- **Dialysis:** Peritoneal dialysis is the standard technique for infants and children. However, dialysis patients remain uremic, which restricts normal growth and development.
- **Renal transplant:** Renal transplantation is the preferred mode of treatment of most children with ESRD. Preparation for transplantation from living donors or listing for cadaver donor transplant should begin in all children with ESRD. The contraindications for transplant include children with human immunodeficiency virus (HIV) and children with metastatic malignancy.

WILMS' TUMOR

DEFINITION

Most common renal tumor in children < 15 years old.

ETIOLOGY

Wilms' tumors are associated with mutations of the p53 tumor suppressor gene chromosome 11.

PATHOLOGY

- Stage 1: Tumor limited to kidneys and can be removed with an intact capsule
- Stage 2: Grows beyond the kidney but can be completely removed
- Stage 3: Nonhematogenous extension into the abdomen
- Stage 4: Hematogenous metastases
- Stage 5: Bilateral renal metastasis

HISTORY

- Age < 3 years
- Abdominal/flank mass
- Vomiting
- HTN due to obstruction of renal artery

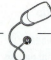

Indications for emergent dialysis: **AEIOU**
Acidosis
Electrolyte abnormalities
Toxic **I**ngestion
Fluid **O**verload
Uremia

Typical Scenario

On a routine exam, a 10-year-old girl has HTN that is confirmed by repeated measurements. Her blood pressure is 160/90 in the right arm and similar in the left arm and right leg. *Think:* Renal disease. The most appropriate next diagnostic test is UA.

The most common causes of HTN in children are secondary causes—renal (75%), infection, glomerulonephritis, HUS, obstructive uropathy.

Patients will often present with bleeding due to defective platelets secondary to uremia. Uncontrolled bleeding can be treated with dialysis and desmopressin.

DIAGNOSIS

Renal ultrasound (US) and computed tomography (CT).

TREATMENT

- Stage 1–3 tumors are treated with nephrectomy and chemotherapy with or without radiation.
- Stage 4 tumors are treated with pulmonary irradiation and three-drug combination chemotherapy in addition to above.

POLYCYSTIC KIDNEY DISEASE (PKD)

DEFINITION

Congenital malformation of the urinary tract resulting in cysts within the kidneys.

PATHOPHYSIOLOGY

- **Autosomal recessive PKD** ("infantile polycystic disease"): Cysts are a dilation of the collecting ducts. Many patients also have cysts in the liver, cirrhosis, and portal HTN.
- **Autosomal dominant PKD** ("adult polycystic disease"): Cortical and medullary cysts that are primarily dilated tubules.

SIGNS AND SYMPTOMS

Autosomal Recessive PKD (ARPKD)

- Decreased urine formation by the fetus leads to oligohydraminos, Potter's syndrome (flat nose, recessed chin, epicanthal folds, low-set abnormal ears, limb abnormalities), and pulmonary hypoplasia.
- At birth, infants may present with renal insufficiency or hypertension. Children will also present with bilateral flank masses at birth.

Autosomal Dominant PKD (ADPKD)

- Commonly presents in the fourth or fifth decade of life with hematuria, bilateral flank pain or masses, and HTN. ADPKD is also associated with hepatic cysts and aneurysms of the cerebral circulation.

DIAGNOSIS

US of the kidneys reveals enlarged and hyperechogenic kidneys.

TREATMENT

Treatment is supportive. PKD results in ESRD. Treat patients with ESRD with dialysis and kidney transplant.

RENAL DYSPLASIA

DEFINITION

Abnormal metanephric differentiation resulting in nonrenal components affecting all or part of the kidney. A dysplastic kidney can contain nonrenal elements such as cartilage.

RENAL HYPOPLASIA

DEFINITION

- Nondysplastic small kidney that has decreased calyces and nephrons.
- Children with bilateral hypoplasia usually present with chronic renal failure.
- This is the leading cause of ESRD during the first decade of life.

HORSESHOE KIDNEY

DEFINITION

Midline fusion of the lower kidney poles.

EPIDEMIOLOGY

- Seven percent of horseshoe kidneys are associated with Turner's syndrome and are four times more common in children with Wilms' tumor.
- Horseshoe kidneys occur in 1:500 births.

NEPHROTIC SYNDROME

DEFINITION

Nephrotic syndrome is characterized by proteinuria, hypoproteinemia, edema, and hyperlipidemia.

ETIOLOGY

- Eighty-five percent of nephrotic syndrome in children is caused by minimal change disease.
- Other causes of nephrotic syndrome include mesangial proliferation and focal sclerosis.

PATHOPHYSIOLOGY

A loss of negatively charged glycoproteins in the capillary walls causes an increase in basement membrane permeability.

EPIDEMIOLOGY

More common in boys than girls (2:1).

SIGNS AND SYMPTOMS

- Proteinuria > 3.5 g/24 hr
- Pitting edema
- Hyperlipidemia
- Periorbital edema
- Oliguria
- Anasarca

DIAGNOSIS

- The diagnosis of is usually made clinically.
- A confirmatory renal biopsy shows fusion of the epithelial foot process by electron microscopy.

TREATMENT

- Most children will respond to steroids, and repeated relapses can be treated with steroids until the disease resolves spontaneously toward the end of the second decade.
- Salt restriction to decrease edema.

Horseshoe kidneys are "caught" by the inferior mesenteric artery during development.

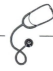

The major pathologic finding in congenital nephrotic syndrome is dilation of the proximal tubules.

Patients can develop a hypercoagulable state due to nephrotic loss of antithrombin III.

Typical Scenario

A 2-year-old boy has a 1-week history of edema. On examination his BP is 100/60 and he has generalized edema and ascites. Lab values show Cr 0.4, albumin 1.4 g/dL, and cholesterol 569 mg/dL. A UA shows 4+ protein and no blood. *Think:* Minimal change disease (nephrotic syndrome).

Typical Scenario

A 4-year-old girl presents with malaise, periorbital edema, and smoky-colored urine. She had a strep throat infection 2 weeks prior. A serum complement level is decreased, and an antistreptolysin O (ASO) titer is increased. *Think:* PSGN.

POSTSTREPTOCOCCAL GLOMERULONEPHRITIS (PSGN)

DEFINITION

Immune complex disease caused by group A β-hemolytic streptococcus types 12 and 49. Typically occurs 10 to 14 days following a strep infection.

DIAGNOSIS

- **Light microscopy:** Enlarged glomeruli with mesangial proliferation and exudation of neutrophils.
- **Immunofluorescent microscopy:** Granular pattern of immunoglobulin deposition.
- **Electron microscopy:** Electron microscopy reveals electron-dense humps (immune complexes) on the epithelial side of the glomerular basement membrane (GBM).

TREATMENT

- Treat with penicillin for 10 days to prevent spread of nephrogenic strain.
- Treat renal and cardiac failure with peritoneal dialysis.
- Microscopic hematuria may take up to 1 year to resolve.

RAPIDLY PROGRESSIVE GLOMERULONEPHRITIS (RPGN)

DEFINITION

- Rapidly progressive describes the clinical course of several forms of glomerulonephritis.
- The underlying abnormality is the presence of crescents in the majority of the glomeruli.

SYMPTOMS

RPGN presents with nephritic or nephrotic episodes and rapidly progresses to ARF within weeks to months after onset.

DIAGNOSIS

Light, immunofluorescent, and electron microscopy show crescents on the inside of Bowman's capsule. The crescents are composed of the proliferative epithelial cells of the capsule, fibrin, and macrophages.

TREATMENT

The prognosis is poor for patients with RPGN, although some patients respond to steroids or cyclophosphamide.

MEMBRANOPROLIFERATIVE GLOMERULONEPHRITIS

DEFINITION

Most common cause of chronic glomerulonephritis in older children.

DIAGNOSIS

- **Light microscopy:** Glomeruli arranged in a lobular pattern, often appearing duplicated or "split"
- **Immunofluorescent microscopy:** Lobular deposits of C3 and immunoglobulins
- **Electron microscopy:** Immune complex deposits in mesangial and subendothelial regions

SIGNS AND SYMPTOMS

- Nephrotic syndrome
- Hematuria
- HTN

TREATMENT AND PROGNOSIS

- Poor prognosis. Most cases progress to ESRD.
- There is no definitive therapy, although some patients respond to prednisone.

MEMBRANOUS GLOMERULONEPHRITIS

DEFINITION

Membranous glomerulonephritis is an immune complex disease of the kidney.

EPIDEMIOLOGY

It is the most common cause of nephrotic syndrome in adults and is uncommon in children.

SIGNS AND SYMPTOMS

- Presents as a nephrotic syndrome.
- Some patients have microscopic hematuria.

DIAGNOSIS

- **Light microscopy:** Diffuse thickening of the GBM without proliferative changes
- **Immunofluorescent microscopy:** Granular deposits of immunoglobulin G (IgG) and C3
- **Electron microscopy:** Deposits of IgG and C3 located on the epithelial side of the membrane

TREATMENT

Most cases resolve spontaneously in children, although some children will have persistent proteinuria. Nephrotic syndrome is best controlled with salt restriction and diuretics.

FEVER/EXERCISE/POSTURAL PROTEINURIA

DEFINITION

- Proteinuria up to 150 mg/day may be normal.
- Proteinuria consists of plasma, albumin, and Tamm–Horsfall proteins.
- **Postural proteinuria:** Proteinuria is increased from laying in supine to upright position due to unknown cause.
- **Febrile proteinuria:** Proteinuria caused by fever > 101°F (41.1°C). Febrile proteinuria will normalize after fever resolves.
- **Exercise proteinuria:** Proteinuria following vigorous exercise. Usually resolves after 48 hours of rest.

INTERSTITIAL NEPHRITIS: ACUTE AND CHRONIC

DEFINITION

Inflammation in the interstitium between the glomeruli in the areas surrounding the tubules.

Typical Scenario

A patient presents with hemoptysis, sinusitis, and glomerulonephritis. *Think:* Wegener's granulomatosis.

A patient presents with dyspnea, hemoptysis, and ARF. *Think:* Goodpasture's syndrome.

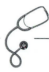

The most common cause of gross hematuria in children is IgA nephropathy.

Electron microscopy of membranous glomerulonephritis shows a "spike and dome" on the epithelial side of the GBM.

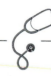

Degrees of Proteinuria
1+: 30 mg/dL
2+: 100 mg/dL
3+: 300 mg/dL
4+: > 2,000 mg/dL

HIGH-YIELD FACTS

Renal, Gynecologic, and Urinary Disease

RISK FACTORS

- **Acute:** Drugs (penicillin, cephalosporins, sulfonamides, rifampin, phenytoin, thiazides, furosemide, allopurinol, amphotericin B, non-steroidal anti-inflammatory drugs [NSAIDs]), infections, sarcoid, glomerulonephritis, transplant rejection
- **Chronic:** Drugs (analgesics, lithium), infections, vesicoureteral reflux

PATHOPHYSIOLOGY

Interstitial nephritis is often associated with tubular damage, edema, and necrosis between tubules.

SIGNS AND SYMPTOMS

- **Acute:** Most patients present with ARF of generalized tubular dysfunction.
- **Chronic:** Children usually present with symptoms of CRF such as nausea and vomiting, headache, fatigue, HTN, and growth failure.

DIAGNOSIS

- **Acute:** A renal biopsy demonstrates an interstitial infiltrate of lymphocytes, plasma cells, eosinophils, and neutrophils. Edema is present, and the glomeruli are typically normal.
- **Chronic:** In chronic interstitial nephritis, the inflammatory cells consist of lymphocytes and plasma cells. Fibrosis is present, and the glomeruli are sclerosed, secondary to ischemia.

TREATMENT

- Treat renal failure.
- Children with acute interstitial nephritis may recover completely after withdrawal of the inciting agents. Children with chronic interstitial nephritis progress to ESRD.

SYSTEMIC LUPUS ERYTHEMATOSUS (SLE)

DEFINITION

- A systemic autoimmune disease characterized by fever, weight loss, rash, hematologic abnormalities, and arthritis.
- Lupus nephritis is the most common manifestation of SLE in childhood.

PATHOPHYSIOLOGY

Immune complexes deposit into the glomeruli, causing characteristic kidney diseases. See Table 14-2 for classification.

EPIDEMIOLOGY

Most common in adolescent females.

SIGNS AND SYMPTOMS

See Table 14-2.

DIAGNOSIS

SLE is suggested by detecting circulating antinuclear antibodies that cross-react with native DNA (anti-DNA antibodies).

TREATMENT

Immunosuppressive therapy (e.g., prednisone, azathioprine).

TABLE 14-2. SLE Nephritis—World Health Organization (WHO) classification and symptoms.

Classification	Histopathology	Symptoms
WHO Class I	No histologic abnormalities detected.	No symptoms
Class II	Mesangial lupus nephritis. Glomeruli have mesangial deposits containing immunoglobulin and complement.	Hematuria Normal renal function Proteinuria of < 1 g/24 hr
Class III	Focal segmental lupus glomerulonephritis. Mesangial deposits in all glomeruli and subendothelial deposits in some.	Hematuria ± Proteinuria ± Reduced renal function ± Nephrotic syndrome
Class IV	Diffuse proliferative lupus nephritis. All glomeruli contain massive mesangial and subendothelial deposits of immunoglobulin and complement.	Hematuria ± Proteinuria ± Reduced renal function ± Nephrotic syndrome
Class V	Membranous lupus nephritis. Resembles idiopathic membranous glomerulopathy.	Nephrotic syndrome

RENAL VEIN THROMBOSIS (RVT) IN INFANCY

DEFINITION

- Thrombus formation in the renal vein.
- In infants, RVT is associated with dehydration, shock, and sepsis.
- In older children, RVT is associated with nephrotic syndrome (membranous nephropathy), cyanotic heart disease, hypercoagulable states, and contrast agents.

SIGNS AND SYMPTOMS

- Acute gross hematuria
- Flank masses
- Flank pain

DIAGNOSIS

- US shows enlarged kidneys.
- Doppler flow studies show little renal function.

TREATMENT

- Correct fluid and electrolyte abnormalities.
- Prophylactic anticoagulation with heparin.

NEUROGENIC BLADDER

DEFINITION

Abnormal innervation to the bladder and sphincter muscles, associated with spinal abnormalities such as CNS tumors, teratomas, and myelodysplasia.

SIGNS AND SYMPTOMS

- Urinary incontinence
- Urinary tract infections (UTIs)
- Upper tract deteriorations

UROLITHIASIS

DEFINITION

Accumulation of crystals in the calyx that aggregate to form a calculus.

EPIDEMIOLOGY

More common in boys girls (2:1), children with metabolic abnormalities, neuropathic bladder, enterocystoplasty.

ETIOLOGY

- Most stones are made of calcium, struvite, uric acid, or cystine that accumulates in the calyx or bladder.
- **Calcium stones:** Radiopaque stones due to increased intestinal calcium absorption or decreased renal absorption.
- **Struvite stones:** Radiopaque stones composed of magnesium, ammonium, and phosphate. Most commonly secondary to chronic UTIs by urea-splitting bacteria such as *Proteus*.
- **Uric acid stones:** Radiolucent stones associated with high serum uric acid levels, such as hyperuricosuria, Lesch–Nyhan syndrome, after chemotherapy, myeloproliferative disorders, and inflammatory bowel disease.
- **Cystine stones:** Radiopaque stones associated with cystinuria, an autosomal recessive disorder causing decreased absorption of dibasic amino acids (cystine, lysine, arginine, and ornithine) by the renal epithelial cells.

SIGNS AND SYMPTOMS

- Microscopic or gross hematuria
- Urinary tract obstruction
- Abdominal/flank pain radiating to the genitalia (renal colic)

DIAGNOSIS

- Plain abdominal x-ray will show radiopaque stones (calcium and struvite). Ninety percent of stones are radiopaque.
- Abdominal CT can be better at detecting stones and will also yield information on the presence of hydronephrosis.

TREATMENT

- Pain management. NSAIDs are mainstay; opiates occasionally needed.
- Remove calculi if they are > 5 to 6 mm via urethral stent or lithotripsy, especially if they are associated with obstruction and hydronephrosis.
- **Calcium stones:** Treat with thiazide diuretic to reduce renal calcium excretion or potassium citrate, an inhibitor of calcium stones.
- **Struvite stones:** Treat with antibiotics to prevent recurrence of bacterial infections.
- **Uric acid stones:** Treat with allopurinol and urine alkalization.
- **Cystine stones:** Treat with D-penicillamine to chelate cystine.

> **Typical Scenario**
>
> An 8-year-old boy presents with left flank pain radiating to his left testicle. The pain does not change with movement or positioning and is colicky in nature. Urine dip is positive for blood. *Think:* Urolithiasis.

> Consider nosocomial UTIs with *Pseudomonas* and methicillin-resistant *Staphylococcus aureus* in institutionalized or recently hospitalized patients.

URINARY TRACT INFECTION (UTI)

DEFINITION

- Infection of the urinary system by bacterial pathogens. UTIs are often ascending infections from fecal flora.

- The most common bacteria are *E. coli*, followed by *Klebsiella*, *Proteus*, enteroccci, and *Staphylococcus saprophyticus*.

PREDISPOSING FACTORS

- Female
- Uncircumcised male
- Vesicoureteral reflux
- Toilet training (wiping from back to front)
- Tight clothing
- Bubble baths
- Nylon panties, bathing suit

CLASSIFICATION OF UTIs

- **Pyelonephritis:** Infection of the kidney characterized by abdominal or flank pain, fever, malaise, nausea, vomiting, and diarrhea.
- **Cystitis:** Infection of the bladder. Common symptoms include dysuria, urgency, frequency, suprapubic pain, incontinence, and malodorous urine. Cystitis does not cause fever.
- **Asymptomatic bacteriuria:** Presence of > 100,000/mL of a single bacteria on two successive urine cultures in a patient without any UTI-like symptoms.

SIGNS AND SYMPTOMS

Symptoms vary with age:
- Neonates: failure to thrive, feeding irregularities, diarrhea, vomiting, fever, hyperbilirubinemia
- 1 months–2 years: colic, irritability, gastrointestinal (GI) complaints
- > 2 years: urgency, frequency, dysuria, abdominal and flank pain

DIAGNOSIS

- Presence of > 100,000 colonies of a single bacteria or > 10,000 colonies in a symptomatic child or any bacterial growth from a properly obtained specimen
- Leukocytes > 5
- Hematuria
- White cell casts

TREATMENT

- Treatment varies depending on the age of the child:
  - 2 months–2 years: UTIs are often associated with bacteremia in this age group and 10 to 14 days of parenteral antibiotics is the treatment of choice. Trimethoprim–sulfamethoxazole, fluoroquinolones, and aminopenicillins are effective.
  - Older children: 5 to 7 days of oral antibiotics.
  - Pyelonephritis: 14-day therapy of IV β-lactam/cephalosporin.
- Further investigations:
  - All children under the age of 5 and all male children should have a renal US to identify anatomic abnormalities including hydronephrosis, dilation of distal ureters, or bladder hypertrophy and to rule out pyelonephritis.
  - Voiding cytourethrogram (VCUG) is indicated in children < 5 years to uncover reflux. VCUG is performed by placing a catheter through the urethra into the bladder and instilling a radionuclide testing agent until the bladder is full and the child voids. Images are taken to record reflux disease.

DEFINITIONS

- Retrograde flow of urine from the bladder to the ureter and renal pelvis.
- Reflux predisposes to renal infections by facilitating the transport of bacterial from the bladder to the upper urinary tract.
- The repeated infections can result in renal scarring and ESRD.
- See Table 14-3 for grading of vesicoureteral reflux.

EPIDEMIOLOGY

- Eighty percent of children with reflux are female.
- Average age of diagnosis is 2 to 3 years.

SIGNS AND SYMPTOMS

Most reflux is diagnosed during a workup for a UTI.

DIAGNOSIS

VCUG or radionuclide cystogram.

TREATMENT

- The goal of treatment is to prevent pyelonephritis and renal injury.
- Children with low-grade reflux are managed medically with low-dose antibiotic prophylaxis and UA and cultures every 3 to 4 months.
- Surgical therapy is performed in children with breakthrough UTI on antibiotic prophylaxis, unresolving reflux, and grade IV or V reflux.

OVARIAN/TESTICULAR TORSION

DEFINITION

Twisting of the ovary or testicle on its vascular pedicle.

EPIDEMIOLOGY

Testicular torsion is the most common cause of testicular pain in boys > 12 years and is most often due to poor fixation of the testis inside the scrotum (bell clapper deformity).

SIGNS AND SYMPTOMS

- **Ovarian torsion:** acute unilateral intermittent sharp lower abdominal pain
- **Testicular torsion:** acute pain and swelling of the scrotum

---

> **Typical Scenario**
>
> A 15-year-old boy presents with severe pain in his right testicle. This occurred suddenly while playing basketball. A physical exam reveals a tender, swollen, firm testicle with a transverse lie. There is no cremasteric reflex on the right. *Think:* Testicular torsion.

> **Typical Scenario**
>
> A 16-year-old previously healthy boy experiences a sudden onset of abdominal and scrotal pain. A physical exam shows severe tenderness in the inguinal canal on the right, and the right side of scrotum is empty. A UA is within normal limits. *Think:* Testicular torsion of an undescended testicle. The most effective management is an immediate operation.

Grade	Associated Symptom
I	Reflux into a nondilated ureter
II	Reflux into the upper collecting system without dilation
III	Reflux into dilated ureter and blunting of calyces
IV	Reflux into a grossly dilated ureter
V	Massive reflux, with significant ureteral dilation and tortuosity and loss of the papillary impression

TABLE 14-3. Grading of vesicoureteral reflux.

DIAGNOSIS

Doppler US shows low blood flow.

TREATMENT

- Manual detorsion, followed by surgical fixation.
- Time is of the essence. The longer the ovary or testis remains torsed, the lesser the chance of salvageability.

POLYCYSTIC OVARIAN (PCO) SYNDROME/OVARIAN CYSTS

DEFINITION

- PCO syndrome is the most commonly diagnosed ovarian cause of hirsutism.
- Other causes of ovarian cysts include ovarian hyperthecosis.

SIGNS AND SYMPTOMS

PCO: hirsutism, amenorrhea, infertility, obesity, insulin resistance.

DIAGNOSIS

- Hyperandrogenism.
- US shows multicystic ovaries resembling a "pearl necklace."

TREATMENT

- Ovarian suppression with estrogen or progestins.
- Hirsutism can be treated with spironolactone and electrolysis.

UNDESCENDED TESTES

DEFINITION

- Failure of one or both testes to descend into the scrotum. The undescended testes are usually found in the inguinal canal.
- Cryptorchidism is the failure of the testes to descend by 6 months of age.

SIGNS AND SYMPTOMS

- Cryptorchidism is associated with infertility, seminomas, hernias, and testicular torsion.
- The risk of seminomas is increased even if the testis is surgically placed into the scrotum; however, repositioning the testes makes them accessible for periodic examinations.
- Orchiopexy also helps to decrease the risk of testicular torsion by decreasing the mobility of the testis.

TREATMENT

- **If testes are not palpated in the inguinal canal:** Orchiopexy after age 12 months.
- **If testes are palpated in the inguinal canal:** Hormonal therapy with luteinizing hormone–releasing hormone (LHRH) is controversial.

CHORIOCARCINOMA

- Malignant tumor of syncytiotrophoblasts and cytotrophoblasts.
- Choriocarcinomas are associated with a high human chorionic gonadotropin (hCG) level.
- Treated with surgery followed by chemotherapy and irradiation.

SEMINOMA/DYSGERMINOMA

- Seminomas are the most common germ cell tumor. β-hCG is elevated. Treated with radiation good prognosis.
- Dysgerminomas are associated with XY gonadal dysgenesis. Y-DNA probes are important in diagnosis.

YOLK SAC CARCINOMA

- Malignant germ cell tumor.
- Yolk sac tumors are associated with an increase in serum α-fetoprotein.
- The peak incidence is during infancy and childhood.

GONADOBLASTOMA

Malignant germ cell tumor, with a 100% 10-year survival rate in girls < 10 years old.

SERTOLI CELL TUMORS

DEFINITION

- Malignant sex chord stroma tumors.
- Sertoli cell tumors produce estrogens and cause feminization and precocious puberty.
- Sertoli cell tumors are diagnosed with CT and hormone measurements.
- Treated with surgery and chemotherapy.

SEXUALLY TRANSMITTED DISEASES (STDS)

See Table 14-4.

EPIDEMIOLOGY

- Sexually transmitted diseases affect ~25% of adolescents.
- In infants and children, detection of an STD is an important clue to sexual abuse.

RISK FACTORS

- Sexual contact with person(s) with a history of STD
- Multiple sexual partners
- Street involvement (e.g., homelessness)
- Intercourse with new partner during last 2 months
- More than two sexual partners during previous 12 months
- No contraception or use of nonbarrier methods
- Injection drug use
- Men who have sex with men
- "Survival sex" (e.g., exchanging sex for money, drugs, shelter, or food)

SCREENING AND PREVENTION

- All sexually active adolescent women should receive a Papanicolaou smear annually to screen for cervical dysplasia. In additional, screen all asymptomatic sexually active patients annually for HIV, herpes simplex virus (HSV), hepatitis B, and chlamydia.

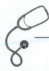

PainFUL ulcers:
Chancroid
Herpes
PainLESS ulcers:
Lymphogranuloma venereum (LGV)
Syphilis
Urethral discharge:
Gonorrhea
Chlamydia
Trichomonas

"Whiff test": Two drops of KOH mixed with the discharge and heated onto a slide produces a fishy smell. This is characteristic of both *Trichomonas* and bacterial vaginosis.

— **Typical Scenario** —

A 16-year-old boy presents with lower left abdominal pain and left testicular pain for 2 weeks. Palpation of the testes is normal except for isolated tenderness of the epididymis. Cremasteric reflex is normal. *Think:* Epididymitis.

TABLE 14-4. Sexually transmitted diseases in children.

	Urethritis and Cervicitis	Epididymitis	Vulvovaginitis	Pelvic Inflammatory Disease	Condyloma acuminata	Genital Ulcers
Definition	Inflammation of the urethra or cervix with mucopurulent discharge	Inflammation of the epididymis with mucopurulent discharge	Infectious causes of vaginal discharge, vulvar itching, and irritation	Inflammation of the upper female genital tract	Anogenital warts caused by human papillomavirus (HPV)	Ulcerative lesions on vagina, vulva, or penis
Symptoms	Urethral discharge Dysuria Possible proctitis or pharyngitis Women are symptomatic half as often as men Complications can include PID in women and Reiter's syndrome in men, disseminated infection in both	Scrotal swelling Tenderness of the epididymis	Pruritus Vaginal discharge	Abdominal pain Fever Vomiting Cervical motion tenderness Adnexal tenderness Peritonitis Long-term complications result from scarring of the fallopian tubes, including infertility, ectopic pregnancy, and perihepatitis (Fitz-Hugh–Curtis syndrome)	Large, fleshy warts around anus	Lesion can be painful or painless, depending on etiology Inguinal lymphe-denopathy Urethritis
Pathogens	*Chlamydia trachomatis* *Neisseria gonorrhoeae*	*C. trachomatis* *N. gonorrhoeae*	*Trichomonas vaginalis* *Gardnerella vaginalis* (causes bacterial vaginosis [BV]) *Candida albicans*	*C. trachomatis* *N. gonorrhea*	**HPV:** Types 6 and 11 are most frequently in genital warts, and types 16 and 18 are most common in cervical dysplasia	PAINFUL: Herpes simplex virus (HSV) *Haemophilus ducreyi* *Treponema pallidum* PAINLESS: *T. pallidum* Lympho-granuloma venereum (LGV)

(continues)

TABLE 14-4. Sexually transmitted diseases in children (continued).

HIGH-YIELD FACTS

Renal, Gynecologic, and Urinary Disease

	Urethritis and Cervicitis	Epidymitis	Vulvovaginitis	Pelvic Inflammatory Disease	Condyloma Acuminata	Genital Ulcers
Diagnosis	Gram stain of urethral/vaginal discharge Polymerase chain reaction (PCR)/enzyme-linked immunosorbent assay (ELISA) Culture (gonorrhea on Thayer–Martin agar)	UA shows pyuria (> 10 WBC/high-power field)	**Trichomoniasis:** Flagellated protozoan on wet preparation **BV:** Fishy odor of vaginal discharge; "clue cells" and pH > 4.5 on wet prep *Candida:* Cottage cheese discharge without odor; yeast or pseudohyphae with KOH stain present	Diagnosis is made clinically. A positive culture for *N. gonorrhoeae* or *C. trachomatis* seen ~ 75% of the time	Acetic acid whitening is used to indicate the extent of infection (colposcopy) Pap smears detect cervical abnormalities	**HSV:** Tzanck smear **Syphilis:** *T. pallidum* on dark-field microscopy **Chancroid:** Gram stain reveals gram-positive cocci arranged in boxcar formation. **LGV:** Elevated Ab titers on complement fixation and microimmuno-fluorescence tests.
Treatment	**Chlamydia:** Single-dose oral azithromycin or doxycycline, erythromycin, levofloxacin, or ofloxacin for 7 days **Gonorrhea:** IM ceftriaxone or oral cefixime, ciprofloxacin, or ofloxacin (Treat for both bugs and treat both partners)	Scrotal supporter for comfort Trimethoprim–sulfamethoxazole	**Trichomoniasis and BV:** Metronidazole *Candida:* Topical azoles	Doxycycline for 2 weeks	Posodilox Cryotherapy Surgical removal	**HSV:** Acyclovir **T. Pallidum:** Penicillin **Chancroid + LGV:** Azithromycin

- Educate all children how to limit STDs, such as limiting number of sexual partners, using condoms, having regular check-ups, and engaging in open discussions about STDs.
- If sexual abuse is suspected, social services and law enforcement agencies must be contacted to ensure the child's protection.

PHIMOSIS/PARAPHIMOSIS

DEFINITION

- **Phimosis:** Inability to retract the prepuce (foreskin). Phimosis is normal in boys younger than 3 years. In older males, phimosis may be due to the inflammation at the tip of the foreskin.
- **Paraphimosis:** Inability to reduce to foreskin due to venous congestion of the foreskin. Paraphimosis can progress to arterial compromise and gangrene.

SIGNS AND SYMPTOMS

Phimosis may cause urinary retention secondary to pain or obstruction of the urethra.

TREATMENT

- **Phimosis:** Steroid cream applied to the foreskin to loosen the phimotic ring. Circumcision is recommended for chronic phimosis in children older than 10 years.
- **Paraphimosis:** Lubrication and compression of the foreskin and glans. Superficial vertical incision of the ligating band may be needed in refractory cases.

HYPOSPADIAS

DEFINITION

- Ventral opening of the urethra on the penile shaft due to incomplete development of the foreskin "dorsal hood."
- Hypospadias is sometimes associated with in vivo exposure to estrogens or antiandrogens.

TREATMENT

Surgical repair at 6 to 12 months.

Typical Scenario

A 15-year-old female presents to the ED with a fever for 1 day, dyspareunia, and vaginal discharge. She had unprotected sexual intercourse with a new male partner 2 weeks ago. Physical exam reveals adnexal tenderness, cervical motion tenderness, and a friable cervix. *Think:* Pelvic inflammatory disease.

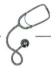

Due to the high rate of concurrent gonorrhea infection with chlamydia infection (60%), treatment for gonorrhea should always be included with that for chlamydia (and vice versa).

Typical Scenario

A 3-year-old girl presents with malodorous bloody vaginal discharge. *Think:* Foreign body.

Do not force retraction of the foreskin in phimosis. This may lead to paraphimosis.

It is important to not circumcise children with hypospadias, as the foreskin is used in the repair.

Hematologic Disease

Normal values of hemoglobin and red cell parameters vary with age (see Table 15-1).

ANEMIA

DEFINITION
Reduced circulating red blood cell (RBC) mass.

CLASSIFICATION
- Size and hemoglobin content (mean corpuscular volume [MCV], mean corpuscular hemoglobin concentration [MCHC]) (see Table 15-2)
- Mechanism—loss/sequestration, increased destruction, decreased production

TABLE 15-1. Normal hemoglobin and mean corpuscular volume (MCV) by age.

Age	Hgb (g/dL)	MCV (fl)
Birth	13.5–24.0	95–121
< 1 month	10.0–20.0	
1–2 months	10.0–18.0	
2–6 months	9.5–14.0	
6 months–2 years	10.5–13.5	70–86
2–6 years	11.5–13.5	
6–12 years	11.5–15.5	
12–18 years (female)	12.0–16.0	78–102
12–18 years (male)	13.0–16.0	78–98
> 18 years (female)	12.1–15.1	78–98
> 18 years (male)	13.7–17.7	78–98

TABLE 15-2. Anemias.

MCV	MCHC	Anemia	RDW	Smear	Labs
Microcytic < 80 (decreased Hgb production)	Hypochromic	Iron deficiency	↑	Elliptocytes Anisocytosis	↓ ferritin, ↓ TIBC ↑ platelets ↑ Red cell count
		Thalassemia	Nl		
		Lead toxicity		Stippled RBCs	
	Normochromic	Neoplastic			
Normocytic 80–100	Normochromic	Acute blood loss			
		Hemolytic (microangiopathic)	Nl	Schistocytes	Bilirubin/LDH
		Anemia of chronic disease	Nl		↓ TIBC
		Hemoglobinopathy	Nl	Target cell	
		Renal disease		Acanthocyte	BUN/creatinine
Macrocytic > 100 (defective DNA synthesis)	Normochromic	Hemolytic (autoimmune)	↑	Spherocytes	Bilirubin/LDH Direct Coombs' test
		Alcohol	Nl	Round	
		Liver disease	Nl	Round, target, echinocyte, acanthocyte	
		Reticulocytosis			
		Aplastic anemia	Nl		
		Hypothyroidism		Round	T_4/TSH
		Drug effect (e.g., hydroxyurea)		Oval	
		Myelodysplasia	↑	Oval, dacrocyte	
Megaloblastic > 110 (defective DNA synthesis)		Folate deficiency	↑	Oval PMN segmented	↓ reticulocytes ↓ serum folate ↑ homocysteine
		B_{12} deficiency/pernicious anemia	↑	Oval PMN segmented	↓ serum cobalamin Schilling test ↓ reticulocytes ↑ serum methylmalonic acid and homocysteine

MCV, mean corpuscular volume; MCHC, mean corpuscular hemoglobin concentration; RDW, red cell distribution width; RBC, red blood cell; PMN, polymorphonuclear neutrophil; TIBC, total iron-binding capacity; BUN, blood urea nitrogen; LDH, lactic dehydrogenase; T_4, thyroxine; TSH, thyroid-stimulating hormone.

PATHOPHYSIOLOGY

- Less oxygen transport
- Decreased blood volume
- Increased cardiac output

SIGNS AND SYMPTOMS

- Somnolence, light-headedness, headache
- Angina, dyspnea, palpitations, flow murmur
- Fatigue, claudication, edema
- Pallor—conjunctiva, palmar creases
- Hepatosplenomegaly in some cases
- Irritability
- Pica: desire to eat unusual things (e.g., clay)

DIAGNOSIS

- Family history
- Exposure history
- Past medical history, including medications
- Physical exam
- Complete blood count (CBC):
    - Decreased hematocrit (Hct)—volume of packed cells
    - Decreased hemoglobin (Hgb)
- MCV
    - Normal 80 to 100 (age-dependent)
    - Microcytic—abnormal Hgb synthesis
    - Macrocytic—RBC maturation defect
- MCHC
    - Low—iron deficiency
    - High—spherocytosis, unstable Hgb
- Red cell distribution width (RDW)—size variability
- RBC count
- Peripheral blood smear (see Table 15-3)
    - RBC size, morphology, inclusion bodies
    - Platelet and white blood cell (WBC) size, morphology
- Possible bone marrow aspirate/biopsy—cellularity, morphology, stroma
- Chemistry—liver function tests (LFTs), lactic dehydrogenase (LDH), creatinine (Cr), uric acid
- Imaging as appropriate
- Other special tests—serum ferritin, B_{12}, folate, reticulocyte count, Coombs' test, osmotic fragility, etc.

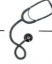

- **Poikilocytosis** is variation in *shape* of RBCs.
- **Anisocytosis** is variation in *size* of RBCs.

TREATMENT

- Supplement or remove causative factor.
- Support hemodynamics as appropriate.

Physiologic Anemia of Infancy

DEFINITION

- Normal newborns have higher hemoglobin
- Remains unchanged until third week
- Decreases to 11 g/dL at 8 to 12 weeks

ETIOLOGY

- Abrupt cessation of erythropoiesis with the onset of respiration
- Decreased survival of fetal RBCs
- Expansion of blood volume in first 3 months

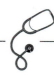

Normal newborn Hgb is 14 to 20 g/dL.

PATHOPHYSIOLOGY

Physiologic adaptation to extrauterine life.

TREATMENT

- No therapy needed
- Essential nutrients for hematopoiesis (folic acid and iron)

Transient Erythroblastopenia of Childhood

DEFINITION

Transient failure of the bone marrow to produce RBCs.

TABLE 15-3. Some erythrocyte morphology and inclusion bodies.

Cell	Spherocyte	Target Cell	Echinocyte (Burr)	Acanthocyte	Dacrocyte
Description	Round, no central clearing	Concentric circles	Evenly spaced projections (spikes)	Irregularly spaced projections	Teardrop shape
Mechanism	Defective RBC membrane	Increase in membrane to Hgb ratio	Spiculed, crenated	Excess lipid in membrane	Extramedullary hematopoiesis
Etiologies	Hereditary spherocytosis Autoimmune hemolytic anemia	Liver disease Hemoglobino-pathies (e.g., Hgb C, S) Postsplenectomy Thalassemia	Liver disease Postsplenectomy Azotemia/uremia Gastric carcinoma	Liver disease Renal failure Splenic disease DIC Pyruvate kinase deficiency	Myelofibrosis

Cell	Schistocyte	Sickle Cells	Basophilic Stippling	Howell–Jolly Body	Heinz Bodies
Description	"Bite cell"	Pointed	Round, dark-blue granules in the cell	Densely blue cytoplasmic inclusions	Round protuberances deforming the cell
Mechanism	Mechanical damage		Aggregated ribosomes	Nuclear fragments	Oxidized/denatured Hgb
Etiologies	G6PD deficiency DIC HUS Vasculitis	Sickle cell disease	Sideroblastic anemia Myelodysplastic syndrome Heavy metal poisoning	Hemolytic anemia Megaloblastic anemia Hyposplenism Postsplenectomy	Oxidative medications, chemicals Abnormal Hgb (H, Köln) Enzyme deficiencies (G6PD)

RBC, red blood cell; G6PD, glucose-6-phosphate dehydrogenase; DIC, disseminated intravascular coagulation; HUS, hemolytic–uremic syndrome.

Typical Scenario

A previously healthy 1-year-old male infant had a cold 8 weeks ago. He now is pale and irritable and refuses to eat. A CBC shows Hgb 5.0, Hct 10%, MCV 80, retic count 0%, WBC 9, platelets 400K. *Think:* Transient erythroblastosis of childhood.

ETIOLOGY

- Unknown
- Linked possibly to parvovirus B19

SIGNS AND SYMPTOMS

Gradual pallor and fatigue.

DIAGNOSIS

CBC, smear.

TREATMENT

- RBC production should return spontaneously in 30 to 60 days.
- In the meantime, supportive transfusions.
- If it does not, different causes of the anemia must be investigated.

Iron Deficiency Anemia

DEFINITION

Microcytic anemia.

ETIOLOGY

- Inadequate intake (whole cow's milk has no iron)
- Loss of iron
  - Bleeding
  - Rapid growth spurts (early infancy and adolescence)
  - Prematurity (decreased iron stores)
  - Chronic diseases (juvenile rheumatoid arthritis [JRA], cystic fibrosis [CF])

EPIDEMIOLOGY

- Most common anemia in children
- 6 months to 3 years old especially

SIGNS AND SYMPTOMS

- Usual symptoms of anemia
- Cheilosis/angular stomatitis, glossitis
- Koilonychia (spoon nails)
- Esophageal web
- Blue sclera
- Splenomegaly

DIAGNOSIS

- Decreased serum ferritin (< 10 ng/mL)
- Decreased serum iron
- Increased iron-binding capacity
- Microcytic and hypochromic
- Increased RDW
- Increased platelet count (> 600,000/mm^3)
- Hypercellular marrow with erythroid hyperplasia
- Decreased stainable iron

TREATMENT

- Ferrous sulfate 3 to 6 mg/kg/day for at least 8 weeks after a normal Hgb level is obtained
- Retic response to oral iron within 4 days
- Iron supplementation:
  - Term infants no later than 4 months (1 mg/kg/day)
  - Preterm infants no later than 2 months (2 mg/kg/day, max 15 mg/day)

Lead Poisoning

DEFINITION

Variant of iron deficiency anemia.

ETIOLOGY

- Environmental (aerosolized and oral)
- Lead-containing paint
- Pica

Typical Scenario

A 9-month-old child who has been fed whole milk from early infancy presents with the following lab values: Hgb 7.5 g, MCV 62, RBC 3.2. *Think:* Iron deficiency anemia.

Mentzer Index
MCV/RBC
≥ 13 Iron deficiency
≤ 13 Thalassemia trait

Iron Deficiency Anemia
- Microcytic
- Hypochromic
- Low reticulocyte count
- Elevated RDW

HIGH-YIELD FACTS

Hematologic Disease

Chronic lead poisoning interferes with iron utilization and hemoglobin synthesis.

Screening for lead poisoning occurs at 10 to 14 months and at 2 years of age.

Typical Scenario

2½-year-old boy with hyperactivity lives in old apartment building with peeling paint on the walls. His gait has become ataxic and his speech has regressed. His Hgb is 8.5 g. *Think:* Lead poisoning.

Goat's milk is folate deficient.

Green vegetables, fruits, liver, and kidneys contain folate.

PATHOPHYSIOLOGY

- Lead is a nonessential metal.
- Irreversible binding with sulfhydryl group of proteins.
- Inhibits enzymes involved in heme production.
- Impairs iron utilization.

SIGNS AND SYMPTOMS

- Acute encephalopathy
- Lead lines—thick transverse radiodense lines in the metaphyses of growing bones on radiographs

DIAGNOSIS

- Microcytic hypochromic anemia
- Basophilic stippling
- Increased serum lead and free erythrocyte protoporphyrin (FEP) level
- Increased urine coproporphyrin

TREATMENT

- Environment control
- 70 μg/dL—medical emergency
  - Dimercaprol (BAL) followed by ethylenediaminetetraacetic acid (EDTA)—5 days' treatment
- 45 to 69 μg/dL
  - EDTA—5 days' treatment
  or
  - Succimer (DMSA) orally 350 mg/m^2 q8h for 5 days then q12h for 19 days
- 20 to 45 μg/dL
  - EDTA-provocative chelation test
- 10 to 19 μg/dL
  - Education

Folate Deficiency

DEFINITION

Megaloblastic anemia.

ETIOLOGY

- Deficient intake or absorption
- Pregnancy (increased requirement)
- Very-low-birth-weight (VLBW) infants
- Drugs (phenytoin, methotrexate)
- Vitamin C deficiency

EPIDEMIOLOGY

Peak age 4 to 7 months.

SIGNS AND SYMPTOMS

- Features of anemia
- Failure to gain weight
- Chronic diarrhea

DIAGNOSIS

- Macrocytic anemia
- Low reticulocyte count
- Increased LDH

- Neutropenia (hypersegmented neutrophils)
- Thrombocytopenia
- Bone marrow hypercellular and megaloblastic changes
- Serum and RBC folate levels

TREATMENT

- Parenteral folic acid 2 to 5 mg/24 hr only after confirmation.
- Folic acid is contraindicated in vitamin B_{12} deficiency, because it will mask anemia yet B_{12} deficiency neurologic symptoms will progress.

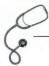

Normal values:
- Serum folate 5 to 20 ng/mL
- RBC folate 150 to 600 ng/mL

Vitamin B_{12} Deficiency

DEFINITION

Megaloblastic anemia.

ETIOLOGY

- Inadequate intake (strict vegetarians)
- Pernicious anemia
- Surgery of stomach or terminal ileum

PATHOPHYSIOLOGY

Deficiency of intrinsic factor due to autoimmunity or gastric mucosal atrophy prevents adequate B_{12} absorption.

RBC folate is the best indicator of chronic deficiency.

SIGNS AND SYMPTOMS

- Juvenile pernicious anemia
- Red, beefy tongue
- Premature graying, blue eyes, vitiligo
- Myxedema, gastric atrophy
- Weakness, irritability, anorexia
- Neurologic (ataxia, paresthesias, hyporeflexia, Babinski response, clonus)

DIAGNOSIS

- Macrocytic anemia
- Macro-ovalocytosis
- Large, hypersegmented neutrophils
- Increased LDH
- Methylmalonic acid in urine
- Anti-intrinsic factor antibody
- Schilling test (vitamin B_{12} absorption)

Subacute combined systems disease in B_{12} deficiency — demyelination of dorsal and lateral columns of spinal cord:
- Decreased vibration sense
- Decreased proprioception
- Gait apraxia
- Spastic paraparesis
- Paresthesias
- Incontinence
- Impotence

TREATMENT

- Vitamin B_{12} IM monthly.
- Oral therapy is contraindicated.

Copper Deficiency

PATHOPHYSIOLOGY

Copper is essential for production of red blood cells, transferrin, and hemoglobin.

SIGNS AND SYMPTOMS

- Refractory anemia, neutropenia
- Osteoporosis
- Ataxia

Dietary copper is found in liver, oysters, meat, fish, whole grains, nuts, and legumes.

Anemia of Chronic Disease

ETIOLOGY

- JRA, systemic lupus erythematosus (SLE), ulcerative colitis
- Malignancies
- Renal disease

DIAGNOSIS

- Can be normochromic and normocytic or hypochromic and microcytic
- Hgb ranges 7 to 10 g/dL
- Low serum iron with normal or low total iron-binding capacity (TIBC)
- Elevated serum ferritin

TREATMENT

- Treat underlying cause
- Iron if concomitant iron deficiency is present

HEMOLYTIC ANEMIAS

See Figure 15-1.

SIGNS AND SYMPTOMS

- Can vary from asymptomatic to generalized symptoms to severe pain crises.
- Icterus, fever, splenomegaly.
- Increased products of RBC destruction.
- Compensatory increase in hematopoiesis–reticulocytosis.
- See Table 15-4.

DIAGNOSIS

- Increased direct bilirubin
- Decreased haptoglobin (intravascular especially)

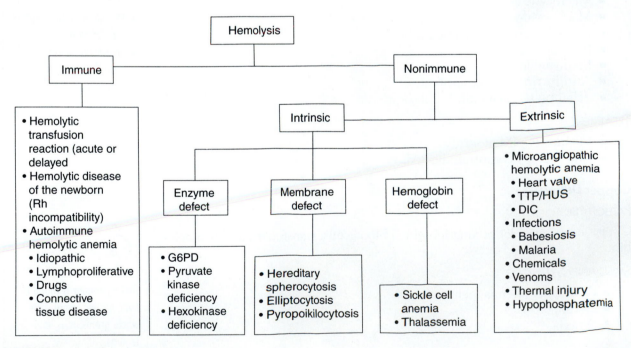

FIGURE 15-1. Hemolytic anemias.

TABLE 15-4. Hemolysis.

Feature	Extravascular	Intravascular
RBC morphology	Abnormal	Normal
Hemoglobinemia/uria	–	+
Hemosiderinuria	–	+
Serum haptoglobin	Normal	↓
Splenomegaly	+	–
Examples		Transfusion reactions Microangiopathic hemolytic Infections: babesiosis, malaria G6PD Paroxysmal nocturnal hemoglobinuria

RBC, red blood cell; G6PD, glucose-6-phosphate dehydrogenase.

- Increased hemoglobinuria/hemosiderinuria (intravascular)
- Increased LDH

Hemolytic Disease of the Newborn

DEFINITION

Erythroblastosis fetalis.

ETIOLOGY

Maternal sensitization to Rh, ABO, or other blood system antigens (Kell, Duffy).

PATHOPHYSIOLOGY

- Paternal heterozygosity allows an Rh-positive (or other alloantibody) infant to be carried by an Rh-negative mother.
- Maternal blood comes into contact with fetal blood cells.
- Maternal antibodies are produced against the Rh antigen.
- During a subsequent pregnancy with an Rh-positive infant, maternal antibodies cross the placenta and bind to fetal RBCs, leading to hemolysis.
- Destruction of RBCs causes increased unconjugated bilirubin, becoming clinically apparent only after delivery as the placenta effectively metabolizes it.
- Severe anemia leads to increased extramedullary erythropoiesis, with potential replacement of hepatic parenchyma.

EPIDEMIOLOGY

- Severe Rh disease is rare in the United States nowadays.
- Rh sensitization occurs in 11 of 10,000 pregnancies.
- < 1% of births are associated with significant hemolysis.
- Approximately 50% of affected newborns do not require treatment, 25% are term but die or develop kernicterus, 25% become hydropic in utero.

SIGNS AND SYMPTOMS

- Hemolytic anemia
- Fetal hydrops:
  - Large placenta
  - Increased unconjugated hyperbilirubinemia—rapidly progressive jaundice after birth, kernicterus
  - Abdominal distention—hepatosplenomegaly, ascites, hepatic dysfunction
  - Abduction of limbs, loss of flexion
  - Scalp edema
  - Purpura
  - Cyanosis

DIAGNOSIS

Positive direct Coombs' test.

TREATMENT

- Know blood types of both parents early in the pregnancy.
- Prophylaxis (RhoGam) during and immediately after delivery for mothers at risk for alloimmunization.
- Exchange transfusion to infant of Rh-negative blood.

SICKLE CELL DISEASE

DEFINITION

Chronic hemolytic anemia due to premature destruction of red cells.

ETIOLOGY

Defect in β-globin–hemoglobin S (HgbS)—substitution of glutamic acid at sixth position of β chain by valine.

PATHOPHYSIOLOGY

- Unusual solubility problem in the deoxygenated state.
- HgbS is a low-affinity hemoglobin.

EPIDEMIOLOGY

- Autosomal recessive.
- 1:500 African-Americans.
- Eight percent of African-Americans are carriers.

SIGNS AND SYMPTOMS

- Newborn screening
- Appears after 6 months of age (when HbF is decreased)
- Anemia (due to hemolysis)
- Vaso-occlusive crisis:
  - Hand–foot syndrome
  - Extremities and spine
  - Tissue ischemia and infarction (leg ulcers)
- Infection (encapsulated organisms):
  - *Streptococcus pneumoniae* (30%)
  - *Haemophilus influenzae*
  - *Salmonella* osteomyelitis
- Priapism (prolonged, painful erection)
- Splenomegaly
- Cardiac enlargement
- Short stature, delayed puberty

- Direct Coombs' tests for antibodies on patient's RBCs.
- Indirect Coombs' tests for antibodies in patient's serum.

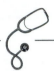

Mutation causing sickle cell disease: Glu-6-val.

As part of a routine genetic screening, a term black newborn has Hgb F, A, and S. Possible diagnoses on quantitative testing could be HgbAS trait or HgbS-thalassemia.

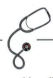

4 sickle cell crises
- Vaso-occlusive crisis
- Aplastic crisis (parvovirus)
- Sequestration crisis
- Hemolytic crisis

The most common cause of fatal sepsis in patients with sickle cell disease is *Streptococcus pneumoniae.*

- Gallstones

DIAGNOSIS

- Hgb electrophoresis (definitive test)
- HgbS 90%
- HgbF 2–10%
- No HgbA
- Hgb ranges 5 to 9 g/dL
- Peripheral smear—target cells and sickled cells
- Increased WBCs and platelets

TREATMENT

- Pneumococcal vaccine (at 2 and 5 years)
- Prophylactic penicillin by 4 months of age:
  - 125 mg/12 hr (< 5 years)
  - 250 mg/12 hr (> 5 years)
- Painful crisis—hydration and analgesics
- Priapism—exchange transfusion

There now exists universal newborn screening for sickle cell disease.

Typical Scenario

A 15-year-old African-American girl is limping. *Think:* Sickle cell disease.

Thalassemia

DEFINITION

Hereditary hemolytic anemia.

ETIOLOGY

Total or partial deletions of globin chain

α-Thalassemia (gene deletion)
- Hgb Bart's (four-gene- deletion)
- HgbH (three-gene deletion)
- α-thalassemia minor (two-gene deletion)
- Silent carrier (one-gene deletion)

β-Thalassemia
- Homozygous (β-thalassemia major)
- Heterozygous (β-thalassemia minor)

SIGNS AND SYMPTOMS

- Severe hemolytic anemia
- Hepatosplenomegaly
- Extramedullary hemopoiesis (classic facies–maxillary overgrowth and skull bossing)

DIAGNOSIS

- Hypochromic, microcytic anemia
- Hgb < 5 g/dL
- Reticulocytopenia
- Markedly increased LDH (ineffective erythropoiesis)
- Hgb electrophoresis:
  - HgbA markedly decreased or absent
  - HgbF marked elevation (30–90%)
  - Increased HgbA$_2$ (> 3.5%)

TREATMENT

- Monthly transfusion of packed RBCs to maintain Hgb > 10 g/dL
- Splenectomy if requiring > 240 mL/kg of packed RBCs/year

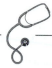

β-thalassemia major is fatal without regular transfusion.

Typical Scenario

A 9-year-old boy has required transfusion since early infancy. *Think:* β-Thalassemia major.

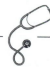

Hemosiderosis
- Cardiomyopathy
- Cirrhosis
- Diabetes

Glucose-6-Phosphate Dehydrogenase (G6PD) Deficiency

DEFINITION

Enzyme defect of hexose monophosophate (HMP) pathway resulting in hemolysis when exposed to stresses such as infection or certain drugs.

ETIOLOGY

Hereditary decrease of G6PD that normally maintains adequate level of glutathione in a reduced state in RBCs.

PATHOPHYSIOLOGY

- Oxidized glutathione complexes with Hgb, forming Heinz bodies.
- RBC less deformable.
- Splenic macrophages "bite out" RBCs.

EPIDEMIOLOGY

- Most common hemolytic enzymopathy
- X-linked
- Higher incidence in black, Middle Eastern, and Mediterranean populations

SIGNS AND SYMPTOMS

- Episodic intravascular hemolysis secondary to oxidant stress (drugs, fava beans, etc.)
- Spontaneous chronic nonspherocytic hemolytic anemia
- Jaundice, dark urine
- Splenomegaly

DIAGNOSIS

- Reduced G6PD activity in RBCs
- Anemia, Heinz bodies, and bite cells on peripheral smear
- Reticulocytosis
- Elevated serum bilirubin and LDH
- Decreased serum haptoglobin
- Hemoglobinuria

TREATMENT

- Admit
- Removal of oxidant stressor
- Oxygen
- Transfusion of packed RBC if:
  - Hemodynamic instability
  - Hgb < 6 g/dL
  - Ongoing hemolysis

Pyruvate Kinase (PK) deficiency

DEFINITION

Congenital hemolytic anemia (decreased RBC PK).

PATHOPHYSIOLOGY

Pyruvate kinase catalyzes the final step in the glycolytic pathway.

EPIDEMIOLOGY

- Second most common hemolytic enzymopathy
- Autosomal recessive

> **Typical Scenario**
>
> A previously well 2-year-old black male child is treated with sulfonamide. Two days later, he develops fever, back pain, dark urine, and anemia. Blood smear shows fragmented erythrocytes. *Think:* G6PD deficiency.

> **Typical Scenario**
>
> A healthy-appearing 14-year-old girl of Greek ancestry has a microcytic, hypochromic anemia. Her development has been normal. *Think:* Iron deficiency anemia (don't let the ethnic information throw you off).

> Drugs causing hemolysis in G6PD deficiency:
> - Aspirin
> - Sulfonamides
> - Ciprofloxacin
> - Antimalarials

> Ingestion of fava beans can cause hemolysis in patients with G6PD deficiency ("favism").

SIGNS AND SYMPTOMS

- Chronic hemolytic anemia
- Hyperbilirubinemia/failure to thrive (FTT) in newborn
- Decreased reticulocytes (selective destruction)

DIAGNOSIS

Decreased RBC PK activity.

TREATMENT

- Avoid oxidant stresses.
- Exchange transfusion (hyperbilirubinemia).
- Transfusion of packed RBCs if severe anemia or aplastic crisis.
- Splenectomy (after 5–6 years of age) if persistently severe anemia or frequent transfusion requirement.
- Folate supplementation.

Hexokinase Deficiency

DEFINITION

Hereditary nonspherocytic hemolytic anemia.

PATHOPHYSIOLOGY

Hexokinase binds to glucose and catalyzes its phosphorylation to glucose-6-phosphate.

EPIDEMIOLOGY

Rare.

SIGNS AND SYMPTOMS

Hemolytic anemia.

HEMOLYTIC MEMBRANE DEFECTS

Hereditary Spherocytosis

DEFINITION

Red cell membrane defect leading to abnormally shaped erythrocytes and hemolysis.

ETIOLOGY

Genetic defect in erythrocyte membrane proteins, such as ankyrin.

PATHOPHYSIOLOGY

- Abnormal proteins cause destabilized RBC membrane—spherocytes.
- Abnormal RBCs become sequestered in the spleen and hemolyze.

EPIDEMIOLOGY

Autosomal dominant.

SIGNS AND SYMPTOMS

- Commonly asymptomatic
- Evidence of hemolysis
- Aplastic/hemolytic crisis
- Splenomegaly
- Gallstones
- Leg ulcers
- Positive family history

Typical Scenario

A male child has sudden onset of dark urine, pallor, and jaundice after an exposure to an oxidant stress. *Think:* G6PD deficiency.

Parents of a child with G6PD deficiency should be provided a list of drugs and foods to avoid.

Splenectomy for PK deficiency will raise reticulocyte count.

HIGH-YIELD FACTS

Hematologic Disease

Typical Scenario

A 4-year-old boy has pallor and a family history of gallstone surgery. His Hgb is 8 g, retics 11, bili 2. *Think:* Hereditary spherocytosis.

DIAGNOSIS

- Increased osmotic fragility
- Spherocytes on peripheral film
- Reticulocytosis
- Hyperbilirubinemia

TREATMENT

- Splenectomy (avoid or at least delay until > 5 years old).
- Pneumococcal, meningococcal, and *Haemophilus influenzae* Hib vaccines before splenectomy.
- Treatment does not fix underlying RBC defect.

Paroxysmal Nocturnal Hemoglobinuria

DEFINITION

- Abnormality of stem cell
- Acquired defect of red cell membrane

SIGNS AND SYMPTOMS

- Hemolysis worse during sleep leading to morning hemoglobinuria.
- Marrow failure.
- Intermittent or chronic hemolytic anemia.
- Leukopenia, thrombocytopenia.
- Complications can include thromboembolic phenomenon and acute myelogenous leukemia.

DIAGNOSIS

- Positive result in acid serum
- Sucrose lysis test

TREATMENT

- Prednisone (2 mg/kg/24 hr).
- Bone marrow transplantation.
- Splenectomy is not indicated.

APLASTIC ANEMIA

Definition

Rare group of closely related disorders leading to decreased numbers of blood cells in each of the lines—RBCs, WBCs, and platelets.

ETIOLOGY

- Exact cause is unknown
- Chemical exposure
- Viral infection
- Genetic causes (e.g., Fanconi's anemia)

SIGNS AND SYMPTOMS

- Fatigue (fewer RBCs)
- Infections (fewer WBCs)
- Bleeding (fewer platelets)
- Increased risk of leukemia

DIAGNOSIS

- CBC—suspicious if at least two of the three cell lines are decreased.
- Bone marrow biopsy is definitive.

TREATMENT

- Platelet and RBC transfusions

Hereditary spherocytosis has the following characteristics: increased osmotic fragility, increased retic count, positive family history, and splenomegaly. Coombs' test is *not* positive.

Splenectomy predisposes patients to overwhelming postsplenectomy infections (OPSIs) caused by encapsulated organisms:

- *Streptococcus pneumoniae*
- *Neisseria meningitidis*
- *Haemophilus influenzae*

Onset of paroxysmal nocturnal hemoglobinuria is in late childhood.

- Immunosuppressive drugs—antilymphocyte globulin (ALG), antithymocyte globulin (ATG), cyclosporine
- Growth factors—erythropoietin (EPO), granulocyte colony stimulating factor (G-CSF), granulocyte macrophage colony stimulating factor (GM-CSF)
- Stem cell transplantation is definitive cure, but requires chemotherapy and/or radiation in preparation

FANCONI SYNDROME

DEFINITION

Rare disorder characterized by wasting of variable amounts of phosphate, glucose, amino acid, and bicarbonate by the proximal renal tubule.

ETIOLOGY

- Inherited
  - Cystinosis (defect of cystine metabolism that results in deposition of cystine in major organs of body, especially kidney, liver, eye, and brain)
  - Galactosemia
  - Fanconi-Bickel syndrome (disorder of carbohydrate metabolism due to defect of glucose transporter-2)
  - Fructosemia
  - Lowe syndrome (x-linked disorder with congenital cataracts, mental retardation, and Fanconi syndrome)
  - Tyrosinemia
  - Wilson's disease
  - X-linked nephrolithiasis (Dent disease)
- Acquired secondary to exposure to:
  - Chemotherapeutic/immunosuppressive agents (ifosfamide, tacrolimus, cyclosporine)
  - Heavy metals
  - Gentamicin
  - Outdated tetracycline

SIGNS AND SYMPTOMS

- Growth retardation
- Rickets
- Polyuria
- Dehydration
- Anorexia
- Vomiting

DIAGNOSIS

- Elevated levels of glucose and electrolytes (phosphate, sodium, potassium, bicarbonate) in the urine
- Evidence of renal insufficiency

TREATMENT

- Bicarbonate therapy is mainstay
- Replacement of phosphate

THROMBOTIC THROMBOCYTOPENIC PURPURA (TTP)

DEFINITION

Hemolytic anemia that results from deposition of abnormal VWF multimors into microvasculature.

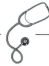

Cystinosis is the most common cause of Fanconi syndrome.

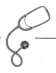

Fanconi syndrome is one of the causes of proximal RTA.

It is important to distinguish Fanconi *syndrome* from Fanconi's *anemia*. Fanconi's anemia is an inherited disorder of bone marrow failure, whereas Fanconi's syndrome is a disorder of renal tubules.

Typical Scenario

Ten days after an episode of viral diarrhea, a 2-year-old boy has pallor and icterus and petechiae of the skin and mucous membranes. His mother reports that he has not urinated for 24 hours. Characteristic lab findings include fragmented erythrocytes on smear, increased blood urea nitrogen (BUN), increased retic count, indirect hyperbilirubinemia, and normal platelet count. *Think:* HUS.

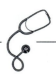

ITP is the most common thrombocytopenia of childhood.

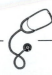

Purpuric lesions do not blanch.

SIGNS AND SYMPTOMS

- Fever
- Microangiopathic hemolytic anemia
- Thrombocytopenia
- Abnormal renal function
- Neurologic signs

DIAGNOSIS

- Normal prothrombin time (PT) and activated partial thromboplastin time (aPTT)
- Microangiopathic hemolytic anemia
- Abnormal red cell morphology with schistocytes, spherocytes, helmet cells
- Increased reticulocyte count
- Thrombocytopenia

TREATMENT

- Plasmapheresis
- Corticosteroids
- Splenectomy

HEMOLYTIC–UREMIC SYNDROME (HUS)

ETIOLOGY

Acute gastroenteritis *Escherichia coli* 0157H7.

SIGNS AND SYMPTOMS

- Hemolytic anemia
- Thrombocytopenia
- Acute renal failure (ARF)

DIAGNOSIS

- Abnormal red cell morphology
- Thrombocytopenia with normal megakaryocytes in marrow
- Urine—protein, RBCs, and casts

TREATMENT

- Fluid management
- Dialysis
- Plasmapheresis (neurologic complications)

IDIOPATHIC THROMBOCYTOPENIC PURPURA (ITP)

DEFINITION

- Acquired hemorrhagic disorder that results from excessive destruction of platelets
- Acute (remission within 6 months)
- Chronic (> 6 months)

ETIOLOGY

Viral illnesses (varicella, rubella, mumps, infectious mononucleosis)—50–65%.

PATHOPHYSIOLOGY

- Immune mechanism—autoantibodies
- Sensitization

DIAGNOSIS

- Diagnosis of exclusion

- WBC and Hgb levels normal
- Normal peripheral smear except thrombocytopenia
- Bone marrow (not always indicated)
- Normal erythrocytic and granulocytic series
- Normal or increased megakaryocytes

TREATMENT

- Intravenous immune globulin (IVIG)
- Intravenous methylprednisolone
- Splenectomy
  - Older children (> 4 years)
  - Severe ITP
  - Chronic ITP (> 1 year)
- Platelet transfusion generally not helpful

Don't give prednisone in ITP without a marrow examination.

DISSEMINATED INTRAVASCULAR COAGULATION (DIC)

DEFINITION

Increased fibrinogenesis and fibrinolysis.

ETIOLOGY

- Septic shock (meningococcemia)
- Incompatible transfusion
- Rickettsial infection
- Snake bite
- Acute promyelocytic leukemia

PATHOPHYSIOLOGY

- Hypoxia
- Acidosis
- Tissue necrosis
- Shock
- Endothelial damage

SIGNS AND SYMPTOMS

- Bleeding
- Petechiae and ecchymoses
- Hemolysis

DIAGNOSIS

- Increased PT and aPTT
- Decreased fibrinogen and platelets
- Increased fibrin degradation products and D-dimer

TREATMENT

- Treat underlying cause.
- Replacement therapy:
  - Platelets (thrombocytopenia)
  - Cryoprecipitate (hypofibrinogenemia)
  - Fresh frozen plasma (FFP) (replacement of coagulation factors)
- Heparin prevents consumption of coagulation factors.

Typical Scenario

A 4-year-old previously healthy girl with purple skin lesions had a visit to the ED with an upper respiratory infection (URI) a month ago. CBC is normal except for low platelets. *Think:* ITP.

DIC is frequently associated with purpura fulminans and acute promyelocytic leukemia.

COAGULATION DISORDERS

- Bleeding due to platelet problems usually occurs immediately and is mucocutaneous. Bleeding due to factor deficiencies is often "deeper" bleeding (intra-articular, intramuscular).
- See Table 15-5.

HIGH-YIELD FACTS

Hematologic Disease

TABLE 15-5. Coagulation tests.

Test	Purpose	
PT (INR)	Extrinsic system	Elevated in DIC, warfarin use, liver failure, myelofibrosis, vitamin K deficiency, fat malabsorption, circulating anticoagulants, factor deficiencies
aPTT	Intrinsic	Elevated in factor deficiencies, circulating anticoagulants, heparin use
Bleeding time	Surgical	Related to platelet count If lengthened and platelet count is normal, consider qualitative platelet defect
Platelet count	Related to bleeding time	< 100,000/mm³—mild prolongation of bleeding time < 50,000—easy bruising < 20,000—increased incidence of spontaneous bleeding
Platelet aggregation	Qualitative	May be abnormal even with normal platelet count—qualitative platelet disorders (Glanzman's thrombasthenia), von Willebrand factor deficiency
Fibrin degradation products	Fibrin activation	Elevated in DIC, trauma, inflammatory disease
D-dimer	Intravascular fibrinolysis	Present in most individuals, especially with cancer, trauma Sensitive for active clotting, but not specific
Assays for specific factors	Quantitative	Hemophilia A (VIII), hemophilia B (IX), von Willebrand factor deficiency (VIII, vWF)

PT, prothrombin time; INR, international normalized ratio; aPTT, activated partial thromboplastin time.

Typical Scenario

A child presents with epistaxis, prolonged bleeding time, and a normal platelet count. *Think:* von Willebrand's disease.

vWF does not cross placenta.

von Willebrand Disease

DEFINITION
Most common hereditary bleeding disorder.

ETIOLOGY
- Autosomal dominant—chromosome 12
- Deficiency of factor VIII-R

PATHOPHYSIOLOGY
- Defective platelet function due to decrease in level or function of von Willebrand cofactor
- Three types:
  - Type I—low levels of von Willebrand factor (vWF) (and factor VIII)
  - Type II—abnormal vWF
  - Type III—may have total absence of vWF (and < 10% factor VIII levels)

SIGNS AND SYMPTOMS
- Easy bruising
- Heavy or prolonged menstruation
- Frequent or prolonged epistaxis
- Prolonged bleeding after injury, surgery (circumcision), or invasive dental procedures

DIAGNOSIS

- Increased aPTT and bleeding time
- Abnormal factor VIII clotting activity
- Quantitative assay for vWF antigen
- Reduced ristocetin co-factor activity
- Abnormal platelet aggregation tests
- Normal platelet count

TREATMENT

- Avoid unnecessary trauma
- Desmopressin
- Replacement therapy:
  - Factor VIII concentrate
  - Weight (kg) × desired % replacement × 0.5
- Cryoprecipitate recommended only in life-threatening emergencies due to the risk of human immunodeficiency virus (HIV) and hepatitis infection

Bleeding time	Desired level (%) VIII
Hematoma	20–40%
Dental extraction	50%
Head injury	100%
Major surgery	100%

Hemophilia

DEFINITION

- Inherited coagulation defects
- Hemophilia A: factor VIII deficiency
- Hemophilia B: factor IX deficiency

PATHOPHYSIOLOGY

Slowed rate of clot formation.

SIGNS AND SYMPTOMS

- Easy bruising
- Intramuscular hematomas
- Hemarthroses (ankles, then knees and elbows) leading to joint destruction if untreated
- Spontaneous hemorrhaging if levels < 5%

DIAGNOSIS

- Family history
- aPTT 2 to 3 times upper limit of normal

TREATMENT

- Early diagnosis.
- Prevent trauma.
- Recombinant factors.
- Cryoprecipitate.
- Beware of transfusion complications, including disease transmission.

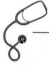

Avoid aspirin and nonsteroidal anti-inflammatory drug (NSAID) use in patients with von Willebrand disease.

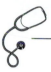

Patients with hemophilia may lose large amounts of blood into an iliopsoas hematoma.

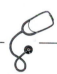

Only 30% of male infants with hemophilia bleed at circumcision.

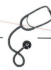

- 1 unit of VIII/kg — increase 2%
- 1 unit of IX/kg — increase 1%

DEFINITION

Predisposition to thrombosis.

PATHOPHYSIOLOGY

Primary (inherited) or secondary (acquired) disturbances in the three areas of Virchow's triad:

- Endothelial damage (e.g., inflammation, trauma, burns, infection, surgery, central lines, artifical heart valves)
- Change in blood flow (e.g., immobilization, local pressure, congestive heart failure [CHF], hypovolemia, hyperviscosity, pregnancy)
- Hypercoagulability (e.g., factor release secondary to surgery, trauma, malignancy); antiphospholipid antibodies, lupus, oral contraceptive use; genetic predispositions such as deficiencies of protein S, protein C, antithrombin III, or factor V Leiden; nephrotic syndrome, polycythemia vera, sickle cell anemia, homocystinemia, fibrinogenemia

SIGNS AND SYMPTOMS

- Deep vein thrombosis (DVT)
- Pulmonary embolism (PE)
- Myocardial infarction (MI)
- Stroke

DIAGNOSIS

- Family history
- Patient history of recurrent, early, unusual, or idiopathic thromboses
- Appropriate screening
- Risk factor assessment

TREATMENT

- Reduce risk factors—mobilize patients, encourage to quit smoking and alcohol, hydrate
- Aspirin, heparin, warfarin, etc., as appropriate

MALARIA

DEFINITION

Bloodborne parasite infection.

ETIOLOGY

- Transmitted by female *Anopheles* mosquito
- Four species of *Plasmodium:*
  - *P. falciparum*
  - *P. malariae*
  - *P. ovale*
  - *P. vivax*

EPIDEMIOLOGY

Most frequent cause of hemolysis worldwide.

SIGNS AND SYMPTOMS

- Fever
- Chills
- Jaundice
- Splenomegaly
- Sweats

HgbS confers resistance against *Plasmodium falciparum*.

Typical Scenario

An 8-year-old American born boy of Somali parents presents with fever for 1 week after returning from his vacation. On examination he has splenomegaly. *Think:* Malaria.

DIAGNOSIS

- Traditional method: identification of organisms on thick and thin peripheral blood smears obtained when patient is acutely febrile.
- Newer methods include polymerase chain reaction (PCR) and immunoassays.

TREATMENT

- See CDC Web site for specific guidelines.
- Chloroquine is used for *P. ovale*, *P. vivax*, *P. malariae*, and chloroquine-sensitive *P. falciparum*.
- Significant areas of chloroquine-resistant *P. falciparum* exist. In these places, mefloquine or atovaquone–proguanil should be used.

TRANSFUSION REACTIONS

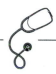

Children rarely have febrile reactions to initial transfusion unless they are immunoglobulin A (IgA) deficient.

EPIDEMIOLOGY

- Approximately 4% of transfusions are associated with some form of adverse reaction.
- Most are febrile nonhemolytic or urticarial.
- See Table 15-6.

INDICATIONS FOR TRANSFUSION OF BLOOD PRODUCTS

- Packed RBCs—Hgb < 8 or 8 to 10 if symptomatic
- Platelets—< 10,000/μL; 10,000 to 50,000 if bleeding; < 75,000 in preparation for surgery
- FFP—treatment of bleeding from vitamin K deficiency, increased international normalized ratio (INR), liver disease, or during plasma exchange for TTP
- Cryoprecipitate—hypofibrinogenemia, hemophilia A, von Willebrand factor deficiency, factor XIII deficiency

One unit of whole blood is 450 mL and should increase the hemoglobin by 1 g/dL and the hematocrit by 3%.

COMPLICATIONS

- Hemolytic, febrile, and allergic reactions
- Transfusion-related acute lung injury (TRALI)
- Disease transmission (e.g., HIV, hepatitis B virus [HBV], hepatitis C virus [HCV], human T-lymphotropic virus [HTLV], cytomegalovirus [CMV], parvovirus)
- Iron overload, electrolyte disturbances
- Fluid overload, hypothermia

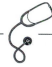

Life-threatening transfusion reactions are nearly always due to clerical errors (wrong ABO blood type).

METHEMOGLOBINEMIA

ETIOLOGY

- Inherited:
  - Deficiency of cytochrome b5 reductase
  - Hgb M disease—inability to convert methemoglobin back to hemoglobin
- Acquired—increased production of methemoglobin:
  - Nitrites (contaminated water), xylocaine/benzocaine (teething gel), sulfonamides, benzene, aniline dyes, potassium chlorate

PATHOPHYSIOLOGY

- Hgb iron in ferrous form.
- Methemoglobin iron is in ferric form (< 2%) and is unable to transport oxygen.

257

TABLE 15-6. Transfusion reactions.

Type	Etiology	Signs and Symptoms	Treatment	Prevention
Acute hemolytic (1 in 15,000–36,000) (fatal 1 in 630,000)	RBC incompatibility Damaged RBCs Hypotonic solution	Fever, chills, nausea Chest/arm/back pain Hemoglobinuria, oliguria Shock, hypotension DIC Dyspnea	Stop transfusion Manage blood pressure and renal perfusion Control DIC	Pretransfusion testing Accurate labeling, unit inspection Proper patient identification
Delayed hemolytic	Antibodies to minor blood group antigens during prior transfusion (Kidd, Duffy, Rh, Kell)	3–10 days post-transfusion Falling hematocrit, fever, hyperbilirubinemia/uria	Usually self-limited Supportive	Chronically transfused patients should received leukocyte reduced products
Allergic (1 in 30–100)	Antibodies to plasma proteins	Hives, itching, local erythema	Antihistamines	Pretransfusion antihistamines Washed cellular blood products
Anaphylactic (1 in 18,000–170,000)	Antibodies to IgA	Cough, respiratory distress, bronchospasm Nausea, vomiting, abdominal cramps, diarrhea Shock, vascular instability, loss of consciousness	Stop transfusion Epinephrine Supportive care	IgA-deficient plasma products Washed cellular blood products
Febrile nonhemolytic (1 in 50–100)	Antibodies to granulocytes Cytokines in plasma	Fever, chills Dyspnea, anxiety	Stop transfusion Demerol Antipyretics	Pretransfusion antipyretics Leukocyte-reduced blood products
Transfusion-related acute lung injury (TRALI) (1 in 5,000–10,000)	Antigranulocyte antibodies in donor product	Bilateral pulmonary edema Cyanosis, hypoxemia Respiratory distress, cough Hypotension, normal central venous pressure ARDS-like picture Fever, chills	Supportive	Do not use plasma products from implicated donor
Circulation overload	Hypervolemia Rapid infusion CHF	Dyspnea, cyanosis, hypoxemia Tachycardia, hypertension Pulmonary edema, cough	Diuretics Oxygen Phlebotomy	Pretransfusion diuretics Slow infusion Limit volume

RBC, red blood cell; IgA, immunoglobulin A; CHF, congestive heart failure; DIC, disseminated intravascular coagulation; ARDS, adult respiratory distress syndrome.

Suspect methemoglobinemia if:
- Oxygen-unresponsive cyanosis
- Chocolate brown blood

SIGNS AND SYMPTOMS

Depends on the concentration:
- 10–30%: cyanosis
- 30–50%: dyspnea, tachycardia, dizziness
- 50–70%: lethargy, stupor
- > 70%: death

DIAGNOSIS

Methemoglobin level.

TREATMENT

- Again, depends on concentration
- < 30%: treatment not needed
- 30–70%: IV methylene blue
- If no response: hyperbaric O_2
- Oral ascorbic acid (200–500 mg)

PORPHYRIA

DEFINITION AND ETIOLOGY

Protoporphyrin is essential molecule of heme proteins. Porphyria refers to a group of disorders characterized by an inherited deficiency of the heme biosynthetic pathway.

SIGNS AND SYMPTOMS

- Photosensitivity (with edema and blister formation)
- Neurologic (myalgias, numbness, tingling, back and extremity pain, loss of deep tendon reflexes)
- Red urine
- Severe crampy abdominal pain
- Tachycardia

DIAGNOSIS

- Hyponatremia
- Renal insufficiency
- Serum/urine porphyrin levels

TREATMENT

- For acute attacks: analgesia, hydration, maintain electrolytes, IV hematin
- Long-term management:
  - Avoid alcohol and all drugs that can precipitate an attack
  - High-carbohydrate diet
  - Sunscreen

POLYCYTHEMIA

DEFINITION

Abnormal elevation of Hct (> 55%).

ETIOLOGY

- Absolute/primary (defect of hematopoietic stem cell):
  - Polycythemia vera (increase in all cell lines)—mean age 60 years
  - Elevated erythropoeitin level (hypoxia, e.g., cyanotic congestive heart disease, renal tumors)
- Relative/secondary (e.g., dehydration, burns)

EPIDEMIOLOGY

Very rare in children.

SIGNS AND SYMPTOMS

- Headache, weakness, dizziness
- Hepatosplenomegaly

DIAGNOSIS

- Increased RBC mass
- Arterial oxygen saturation > 92%

- Splenomegaly or two of the following:
  - Thrombocytosis
  - Leukocytosis
  - Increased leukocyte alkaline phosphatase activity without fever or infection
  - Increased serum vitamin B_{12} or unsaturated B_{12} binding capacity

TREATMENT
- Phlebotomy (Hct ≤ 45%)
- Chemotherapy

COMPLICATION
Acute myelogenous leukemia (AML).

DISORDERS OF WHITE BLOOD CELLS

Neutropenia

DEFINITION
Absolute neutrophil count (ANC) < 1,500/mm³:
- Mild 1,000–1,500
- Moderate 500–1,000
- Severe < 500

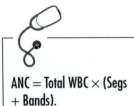

ANC = Total WBC × (Segs + Bands).

ETIOLOGY
- Congenital
- Kostmann syndrome
- Schwachmann syndrome
- Fanconi syndrome
- Acquired
- Infection
- Immune
- Hypersplenism
- Drugs
- Aplastic anemia
- Vitamin B_{12}, folate, or copper deficiency

SIGNS AND SYMPTOMS
- Increased susceptibility for infection
- Stomatitis, gingivitis, recurrent otitis media, cellulitis, pneumonia, and septicemia

LEUKEMIA

EPIDEMIOLOGY
- Leukemia is the most common malignancy, followed by brain tumors.

RISK FACTORS
- Trisomy 21
- Fanconi's anemia
- Bloom's syndrome
- Immune deficiency
- Wiskott–Aldrich syndrome
- Agammaglobulinemia
- Ataxia–telangiectasia

Typical Scenario

A 3-year-old girl has had fever, anorexia, and fatigue for the past month. She has lost 5 kg. She has pallor, cervical adenopathy, splenomegaly, skin ecchymoses, and petechiae. *Think:* Acute leukemia.

- Fever
- Pallor
- Bleeding
- Bone pain
- Abdominal pain
- Lymphadenopathy
- Hepatosplenomegaly

Acute Lymphoblastic Leukemia (ALL)

DEFINITION

Malignant disorder of lymphoblasts.

EPIDEMIOLOGY

- Most common malignancy in children
- 80% of leukemia in children

SIGNS AND SYMPTOMS

- Fatigue, anorexia, lethargy, pallor
- Bone pain
- Fever
- Bleeding, bruising, petechiae
- Lymphadenopathy
- Hepatosplenomegaly
- Bone tenderness
- Testicular swelling
- Septicemia

DIAGNOSIS

- CBC: anemia, abnormal white count, low platelet count
- Electrolytes, calcium, phosphorus, uric acid, lactic dehydrogenase (LDH)
- Chest x-ray (mediastinal mass)
- Bone marrow—hypercellular, increased lymphoblasts
- Cerebrospinal fluid (CSF)—blasts

Marrow exam is essential to confirm the diagnosis of ALL.

TREATMENT

- Four phases:
  - Remission induction: cytoxan, vincristine, prednisone, L-asparaginase, and/or doxorubicin.
  - Consolidation: may add 6MP, 6TG, or cytosine arabinoside
  - Maintenance therapy: 2 years—methotrexate and 6MP, may add vincristine and prednisone
  - CNS prophylaxis: Methotrexate to CSF, may have radiation to the head
- Infection prevention—antibiotics, isolation if necessary

Acute Myelogenous Leukemia (AML)

DEFINITION

Malignant proliferation of immature granular leukocytes.

EPIDEMIOLOGY

- 15–20% of leukemia cases
- Occurs primarily in children < 1 year old
- 1 in 10,000 people

ETIOLOGY

Predisposing factors
- Trisomy 21
- Diamond–Blackfan syndrome
- Fanconi's anemia
- Bloom syndrome
- Kostmann's syndrome
- Toxins such as benzene
- Immunosuppression
- Polycythemia vera

SIGNS AND SYMPTOMS

- Manifestations of anemia, thrombocytopenia or neutropenia, including fatigue, bleeding, and infection
- Chloroma—localized mass of leukemic cells
- Bone/joint pain
- Hepatosplenomegaly
- Lymphadenopathy

DIAGNOSIS

- > 25% myeloblasts in the bone marrow, hypercellular
- Abnormal white count, platelet count, and anemia
- Bone destruction and periosteal elevation on x-ray

TREATMENT

- Two phases:
  - Remission induction: 1 week—anthracycline (daunorubicin) and cytosine arabinoside (cytarabine)
  - Postremission therapy: several more courses of high-dose cytarabine chemotherapy, allogenic stem cell transplant, or autologous stem cell transplant
- Infection prevention—isolation, antibiotics
- RBC transfusions for anemia
- Platelet transfusions for bleeding
- Complete remission in 70–80%

Chronic Myelogenous Leukemia (CML)

DEFINITION

Clonal disorder of the hematopoietic stem cell with specific translocation.

ETIOLOGY

Philadelphia chromosome t(9;22)(q34;q11).

EPIDEMIOLOGY

Tends to occur in middle-aged people.

SIGNS AND SYMPTOMS

- Insidious onset
- Splenomegaly (massive)
- Fever, bone pain, sweating

TREATMENT

- Hydroxyurea
- α-Interferon
- Bone marrow transplant
- Radiation

CML often gets diagnosed when CBC is performed for other reasons.

Juvenile Chronic Myelogenous Leukemia (JCML)

DEFINITION

- Clonal condition involving pluripotent stem cell
- < 2 years

EPIDEMIOLOGY

Ninety-five percent diagnosed before age 4.

SIGNS AND SYMPTOMS

- Skin lesions (eczema, xanthoma, café au lait spots)
- Lymphadenopathy
- Hepatosplenomegaly

DIAGNOSIS

- Monocytosis
- Increased marrow monocyte precursors
- Philadelphia chromosome absent
- Blast count
- < 5% (peripheral blood)
- < 30% (marrow)

TREATMENT

- Complete remissions have occurred with stem cell transplant.
- Majority relapse, with overall survival of 25%.

Congenital Leukemia

DEFINITION

Serious neonatal malignancy.

EPIDEMIOLOGY

- Rare
- AML more common, unlike the predominance of ALL in later childhood

Lymphoma

DEFINITION

- Lymphoid malignancy arising in a single lymph node or lymphoid region (liver, spleen, bone marrow)
- Hodgkin's
  - Nodular sclerosing (46%—most common)
  - Mixed cellularity (31%)
  - Lymphocyte predominance (16%)
  - Lymphocyte depletion (7%)
- Non-Hodgkin's (10% of all pediatric tumors)
  - Lymphoblastic
  - Burkitt's (39%)
  - Large cell or histiocytic

SIGNS AND SYMPTOMS

- Fever, night sweats
- Weight loss, loss of appetite
- Cough, dysphagia, dyspnea
- Lymphadenopathy—lower cervical, supraclavicular
- Hepatosplenomegaly

Neurofibromatosis is associated with an increased incidence of JCML and leukemia.

Reed—Sternberg cells are characteristic of Hodgkin's lymphoma.

Suspicious lymph nodes are:
- Painless, firm, and rubbery
- In the posterior triangle

DIAGNOSIS

Diagnosis and staging
- CBC, erythrocyte sedimentation rate (ESR)
- Serum electrolytes, uric acid, LDH
- Chest x-ray
- Computed tomography (CT) of chest, abdomen, and pelvis
- Lymph node or bone marrow biopsy

STAGING

- Stage I—One lymph node involved
- Stage II—Two lymph nodes on same side of diaphragm
- Stage III—lymph node involvement on both sides of diaphragm
- Stage IV—bone marrow or liver involvement

TREATMENT

- Radiation for stage I or II disease
- Chemotherapy for stage III or IV

Endocrine Disease

DIABETES

See Table 16-1.

DEFINITION

Syndrome characterized by disturbance of metabolism of carbohydrate, protein, and fat, resulting from deficiency in insulin secretion or its action.

EPIDEMIOLOGY

Diabetes is the most common endocrine disorder of the pediatric age group.

PATHOPHYSIOLOGY

- Decreased glucose utilization
- Increased glucose production

SIGNS AND SYMPTOMS

- Triad of polyuria, polydipsia, and polyphagia.
- Weight loss and enuresis are common symptoms.
- Vomiting, dehydration, abdominal pain.

Think of testing urine glucose with the onset of enuresis in a previously toilet-trained child.

TABLE 16-1. Diabetes	
Type I (Insulin Dependent)	**Type II (Non–Insulin Dependent)**
Severe insulin deficiency	Insulin increased, normal, or decreased Insulin resistance
Juvenile onset	Adult onset or maturity onset Increased risk with obesity
Ketosis common	Ketosis infrequent Hyperosmolar coma
HLA-DR3 and -DR4 (chromosome 6)	
Glucosuria, ketonuria, random glucose > 200 mg/dL	Fasting glucose > 140 mg/dL Impaired glucose tolerance

HLA, human leukocyte antigen.

Insulin-dependent diabetes mellitus in children is associated with blood islet–cell antibodies and increased prevalence of human leukocyte antigen (HLA)-DR3 and -DR4 or both.

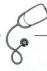

Dehydration in DKA is primarily intracellular and is often underestimated.

Serum Na decreases 1.6 mEq/L for each 100 mg/dL rise in glucose.

Total body potassium may be considerably depleted even when serum K+ is normal or increased.

DIAGNOSIS

- Fasting blood glucose > 126 mg/dL
- Random blood glucose > 200 mg/dL

TREATMENT

- Diet
- Insulin (0.5–1 U/kg)
- Exercise
- Patient education and counseling

DIABETIC KETOACIDOSIS (DKA)

DEFINITION

- Hyperglycemia > 300 mg/dL
- Acidosis pH < 7.30
- Bicarbonate < 15 mEq/L

ETIOLOGY

- Relative or absolute insulin deficiency
- Precipitating factors—stress, infection, trauma

SIGNS AND SYMPTOMS

Polyuria, polydipsia, fatigue, headache, nausea, vomiting, tachycardia, air hunger.

LABORATORY FINDINGS

- Increased hemoglobin (Hgb) and hematocrit (Hct) (hemoconcentration)
- Increased white blood cell (WBC) count
- Decreased serum sodium (Na) (pseudohyponatremia)
- Normal or increased potassium (K)
- Decreased HCO_3

TREATMENT

- Slow fluid and electrolyte replacement
- Insulin regular (0.1 U/kg/hr)
- Glucose (add glucose when blood glucose is 250–300 mg/dL)

COMPLICATIONS

- Hypoglycemia
- Hypokalemia
- Cerebral edema: cause of death in patients with DKA (get a head CT plus electrolytes and glucose for mental status changes)

HYPERINSULINISM

EPIDEMIOLOGY

Sixty percent develop hypoglycemia during the first month of life, 30% in the first year.

Transient Hyperinsulinemia

ETIOLOGY

- Excessive insulin secretion in infants
- Small-for-gestational-age (SGA) or premature infants

- Fetal hypoxia
- Born to mother with poorly controlled diabetes
- Surreptitious insulin administration

TREATMENT

- Feed every 3 to 4 hours
- IV glucose if necessary
- In severe, prolonged cases, diazoxide

Permanent Hyperinsulinemia

- Can be caused by genetic mutations
- Also may be caused by a β-cell dysregulation, such as due to an isolated islet cell adenoma

HYPOGLYCEMIA

- Poisons/drugs
- Liver disease
- Metabolic disorders
- Systemic disease—sepsis, burns, cardiogenic shock

HEMOCHROMATOSIS

DEFINITION

- Increased storage of iron in the form of hemosiderin in parenchymal cells
- Liver, heart, gonad, skin, and joints

ETIOLOGY

- Hereditary
- Neonatal
- Transfusion induced

SIGNS AND SYMPTOMS

- Cirrhosis
- Bronzing of skin
- Diabetes mellitus

LABORATORY FINDINGS

- Increased serum ferritin
- Increased transferrin saturation

TREATMENT

Chelation with desferoxamine.

HYPERTHYROIDISM

DEFINITION

Increased secretion of thyroid hormone.

Typical Scenario

A 2-hour-old newborn has a plasma glucose of 20 mg/dL. Physical exam shows a large plethoric newborn with macrocephaly. Birth weight is > 90th percentile and head circumference is at the 50th percentile. *Think:* Hyperinsulinism.

Typical Scenario

A 14-year-old boy with an 8-year history of diabetes mellitus has had frequent admissions for DKA in the past 18 months. His school performance has been deteriorating. Recently, he has had frequent episodes of hypoglycemia. He is Tanner stage 2 in pubertal development, is growing at a normal rate, and has mild hepatomegaly. *Think:* Surreptitious administration of insulin.

Typical Scenario

A 3½-year-old boy is found unconscious. He has a flushed face, pulse of 160/min, respiratory rate of 16/min, blood pressure 40/20 mm Hg, rectal temperature of 36.2, and an unusual odor on his breath. He has a generalized tonic–clonic seizure. *Think:* DKA, and check a serum glucose.

Juvenile Graves' Disease

Triad of:
- Hyperthyroidism with diffuse goiter
- Ophthalmopathy
- Dermopathy

ETIOLOGY
- Immunogenetic disorder with thyroid-stimulating immunoglobulin
- Antithyroglobulin antibodies
- Antimicrosomal antibodies
- Thyroid-stimulating hormone (TSH) receptor antibody

SIGNS AND SYMPTOMS
- Gradual onset (6–12 months)
- Emotional disturbance
- Increased appetite with decrease or no change in weight
- Goiter
- Fatigue, myopathy, increased sweating
- Heat intolerance
- Fine tremors
- Exophthalmos
- Menstrual irregularities
- **Thyroid storm:**
  - Hyperthermia
  - Severe tachycardia leading to cardiogenic shock
  - Central nervous system (CNS) manifestations

Early diagnosis of congenital hypothyroidism is crucial to prevent or minimize cognitive impairment.

LABORATORY FINDINGS
- Elevated thyroxine (T_4), free T_4, and triiodothyronine (T_3)
- Decreased TSH
- Elevated TSH receptor–stimulating antibodies

TREATMENT
- Pediatric endocrine consultation
- Medical (preferred):
  - Propylthiouracil 5 to 10 mg/kg/day q8h PO
  - Propranolol 0.5 to 1 mg/kg/day PO (0.01–0.15 mg/kg/dose IV)
- Surgical—thyroidectomy

HYPOTHYROIDISM

DEFINITION

Decreased production of thyroid hormone or defect in thyroid receptor activity.

Classic findings of congenital hypothyroidism are rare in the early neonatal period due to placental transfer of maternal thyroid hormone.

Congenital Hypothyroidism

ETIOLOGY
- Hereditary
- Prenatal exposure to radioiodine or antithyroid medications

SIGNS AND SYMPTOMS
- Most cases are asymptomatic at birth.
- Wide fontanelle.
- Prolonged jaundice.

Look for hypothyroidism in Down's syndrome, Turner's syndrome, and Klinefelter's syndrome.

- Macroglossia.
- Hoarse cry.
- Abdominal distention, constipation.
- Umbilical hernia.
- Hypotonia.
- Goiter.
- Slowed development, late teeth, late milestones, small size.
- Eventual mental retardation if left untreated.

DIAGNOSIS

Newborn screening (TSH, T_4).

Acquired Hypothyroidism

- Lymphocytic thyroiditis (Hashimoto's) is the most common cause.
- Growth deceleration.

TREATMENT

L-thyroxine 10 µg/kg/day.

THYROID NEOPLASM

EPIDEMIOLOGY

- Rare in children
- Family history
- Prior irradiation

TYPES

- Thyroid adenoma
- Thyroid carcinoma
- Papillary carcinoma
- Medullary carcinoma

SIGNS AND SYMPTOMS

- Nodular enlargement
- Hypo- or hyperthyroidism

DIAGNOSIS

- Thyroid profile
- Definite diagnosis by needle biopsy or surgical excision

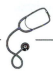

Incidence of malignancy of a thyroid neoplasm is higher in children than in adults.

The risk of malignancy is higher in solitary thyroid nodules.

HYPERPARATHYROIDISM

DEFINITION

Increased parathyroid hormone (PTH).

EPIDEMIOLOGY

Uncommon in children.

ETIOLOGY

- Primary (defect of parathyroid gland)
- Secondary:
  - Chronic renal failure
  - Liver disease
  - Vitamin D deficiency

Rapid and painless enlargement of a thyroid growth may suggest neoplasia.

HIGH-YIELD FACTS

Endocrine Disease

SIGNS AND SYMPTOMS

- Clinical manifestation of hypercalcemia
- Muscle weakness, anorexia, nausea, vomiting, constipation, polydipsia, polyuria, loss of weight, fever

DIAGNOSIS

- Increased serum Ca
- Decreased P
- Increased PTH
- Subperiosteal absorption

TREATMENT

- Treatment of underlying cause
- Hydration
- Furosemide (increased Na and Ca excretion)
- Prednisone (decreased intestinal absorption of Ca)

HYPOPARATHYROIDISM

DEFINITION

Decreased PTH.

ETIOLOGY

- Autoimmune
- DiGeorge syndrome
- Acute illness
- Hypomagnesemia

SIGNS AND SYMPTOMS

Most common presentation is seizure, tetany, numbness, and carpopedal spasm.

DIAGNOSIS

- Decreased serum Ca
- Increased serum P
- Markedly decreased PTH

DIFFERENTIAL DIAGNOSIS

Pseudohypoparathyroidism (markedly increased PTH—PTH unresponsiveness).

TREATMENT

- Correction of hypocalcemia
- Intravenous (IV) 10% calcium gluconate
- 1 to 2 mL/kg (neonates)
- 5 to 10 mL (older children)
- Vitamin D

CONGENITAL ADRENAL HYPERPLASIA

DEFINITION

Genetic defect of adrenal corticosteroid synthesis.

EPIDEMIOLOGY

- Most common cause of ambiguous genitalia
- 1:15,000 live births

Typical Scenario

A 10-year-old girl has severe abdominal pain and gross hematuria. She passes a calculus in her urine. She had received no medication and has no family history of renal stones. *Think:* Primary hyperparathyroidism.

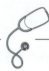

Patients with hyperparathyroidism can develop nephrocalcinosis.

Hypoparathyroidism can be seen with polyglandular failure: thyroiditis, diabetes, adrenal insufficiency, mucocutaneous candidiasis.

Pay attention to heart rate with treatment for hypoparathyroidism: Bradycardia is an indication to stop calcium infusion.

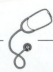

A newborn with ambiguous genitalia is a medical and social emergency.

ETIOLOGY

- 21-hydroxylase deficiency (90%)
- 11 β-hydroxylase deficiency
- 3 β-hydroxysteroid dehydrogenase

SIGNS AND SYMPTOMS

- Ambiguous genitalia in female
- Normal genitalia at birth in males, develop premature isosexual development
- Salt wasting (two thirds of cases)
- Vomiting, dehydration, and shock at 2 to 4 weeks of age

DIAGNOSIS

- Normal karyotype
- Hyponatremia, hypochloremia, hyperkalemia, hypoglycemia
- Markedly increased 17-hydroxyprogesterone

TREATMENT

- Fluid and electrolyte replacement
- Normal saline (NS) 20 mL/kg bolus, then maintenance plus ongoing fluid losses
- Management of hypoglycemia
- Hydrocortisone 25 mg IV bolus, then 50 mg/m²/24 hr
- Fludrocortisone 0.1 mg/day

Combination of hyperkalemia and hyponatremia clue to diagnosis of congenital adrenal hyperplasia.

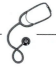

Most urgent tests for congenital adrenal hyperplasia:
1. Serum glucose
2. Serum electrolytes
Other tests: cortisol, testosterone, 17-OH progesterone.

CUSHING'S SYNDROME

DEFINITION

Characteristic pattern of obesity with hypertension (HTN) due to abnormally high level of cortisol.

ETIOLOGY

- Bilateral adrenal hyperplasia (Cushing's disease)—pituitary tumor
- Adrenal tumors (adenoma, carcinoma)

SIGNS AND SYMPTOMS

- Truncal obesity, rounded moon facies, buffalo hump, purple striae, acne
- HTN, muscle weakness

DIAGNOSIS

- Elevated serum cortisol
- Elevated 24-hour urine test for free cortisol
- Dexamethasone suppression test
  - Normal if a single dose of 0.3 mg/m² at 11 P.M. results in plasma cortisol of < 5 g/dL at 8 A.M. the next morning
- Polycythemia, lymphopenia, and eosinopenia
- Abdominal computed tomography (CT) (adrenal tumors)
- Pituitary magnetic resonance imaging (MRI) (pituitary adenoma)

DIFFERENTIAL DIAGNOSIS

- Exogenous obesity
- Normal growth rate
- Urinary corticosteroids suppressed by dexamethasone

In congenital adrenal hyperplasia, blood should be drawn for steroid profile before the administration of hydrocortisone.

Cushing's disease is a state of hypercortisolism secondary to adrenocorticotropic hormone (ACTH)-producing pituitary adenoma.

Growth retardation may be the early manifestation of Cushing's syndrome. Virilization may indicate adrenal carcinoma.

TREATMENT

- Pediatric endocrine, surgical, and neurosurgical consultation
- Adrenalectomy and radiotherapy (adrenal tumors)
- Transsphenoidal resection of pituitary adenoma

ACUTE ADRENAL INSUFFICIENCY

DEFINITION

- Adrenal cortex fails to produce enough glucocorticoid and mineralocorticoids in response to stress.
- May be primary adrenal disorder or secondary to hypopituitarism.
- **Addison's disease:**
  - Primary adrenal insufficiency
  - Destruction of adrenal cortex
    - Autoimmune
    - Tuberculosis

ETIOLOGY

Primary

- Autoimmune destruction (80%)
- Congenital adrenal hyperplasia (CAH)
- Tuberculosis (TB)
- Meningococcal septicemia

Secondary

- Adrenal suppression
- Pituitary or hypothalamic tumors
- Septo-optic dysplasia
- Congenital hypopituitarism

SIGNS AND SYMPTOMS

- Weakness, nausea, vomiting, weight loss, salt craving
- Postural hypotension
- Hyperpigmentation
- Adrenal crisis (fever, vomiting, dehydration, and shock precipitated by infection, trauma or surgery in susceptible patient)

DIAGNOSIS

- Hyponatremia, hyperkalemia, hypoglycemia
- Chest x-ray (small heart)
- Decreased cortisol level (< 5 g/dL) that fails to rise after ACTH administration

TREATMENT

- Volume replacement
- Hydrocortisone 50 to 100 mg IV, then 50 mg/m²/24 hr or methylprednisolone 7.5 mg/m²/24 hr

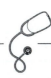

DEFINITION

- Catecholamine-secreting (functional) adrenomedullary tumor of chromaffin tissue
  - Adrenal medulla (70%)
  - Extra-adrenal (30%)
- Usually benign, well encapsulated

ETIOLOGY

- Unknown
- May occur in isolation
- Also seen in the MEN II (bilateral), von Hippel–Lindau, neurofibromatosis type I, and familial carotid body tumor syndromes

SIGNS AND SYMPTOMS

- Nonspecific symptoms
- Headache, palpitations, increased sweating
- Tremor, fatigue, chest or abdominal pain, and flushing
- HTN

DIAGNOSIS

- Increased urinary catecholamines or metabolites
- Metanephrine
- Normetanephrine
- Vanillylmandelic acid (VMA)
- Abdominal ultrasound (US)
- Abdominal CT and MRI

DIFFERENTIAL DIAGNOSIS

- Ganglioneuroma
- Neuroblastoma
- Ganglioneuroblastoma

TREATMENT

Surgical excision.

ETIOLOGY

Primary (Pituitary Adenoma)
- Growth hormone (GH)-secreting adenoma
- Prolactin-secreting adenoma

Secondary
- Primary hypogonadism
- Primary hypoadrenalism
- Primary hypothyroidism

Tumors arising in the adrenal medulla produce both epinephrine and norepinephrine. Extra-adrenal tumors produce only norepinephrine.

Siblings of a patient with a pheochromocytoma should be periodically evaluated because of increased familial incidence.

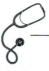

The most useful screening test for pheochromocytoma is blood pressure. Hypertensive paroxysms are an important diagnostic clue.

Increased urinary norepinephrine indicates an extra-adrenal site of a pheochromocytoma, whereas increased epinephrine indicates an adrenal lesion.

After successful surgery of a pheochromocytoma, catecholamine excretion returns to normal in about 1 week.

HIGH-YIELD FACTS

Endocrine Disease

HYPOPITUITARISM

DEFINITION
Deficiency of more than one pituitary hormone.

PHYSIOLOGY
- ACTH → adrenal glucocorticoids
- TSH → thyroid hormone
- Luteinizing hormone (LH) and follicle-stimulating hormone (FSH) → gonadal function
- Prolactin → lactation
- GH → growth

ETIOLOGY
- Midline anomalies (septo-optic dysplasia, cleft palate)
- Craniopharyngioma
- Head trauma
- CNS surgery
- CNS irradiation

SIGNS AND SYMPTOMS
- Depends on missing hormone
- GH deficiency (poor linear growth, hypoglycemia)
- In neonates (hypoglycemia and micropenis)
- LH and FSH (pubertal delay)

TREATMENT
Replacement directed toward the hormonal deficiency.

Typical Scenario

An infant has hypoglycemia and a micropenis. *Think:* Hypopituitarism.

Cortisol and GH are insulin counter-regulatory hormones.

Prolactin secretion tonically inhibited by dopamine in pituitary—prolactinomas respond to dopamine agonists such as bromocriptine.

PITUITARY TUMOR

MOST COMMON
Prolactinoma.

SIGNS AND SYMPTOMS
- Headache
- Amenorrhea
- Galactorrhea

DIAGNOSIS
Increased prolactin (up to 1,000 ng/mL).

TREATMENT
Surgical resection except if isolated prolactinoma, then try medical treatment first.

SHORT STATURE

DEFINITION
Height below the 5th percentile (2 standard deviations below the mean).

NORMAL
- Chronological age (CA) = Bone age (BA) = Height age (HA)
- Normal growth 5 cm/year

FAMILIAL

- Most common cause of short stature
- Normal variant of growth
- Normal rate of growth
- Normal bone age
- Puberty at average age
- Usually at least one parent has short stature

CONSTITUTIONAL

- Normal variant of growth
- Normal at birth, then decelerate between 6 months and 1 year old
- Resume growth rate by 2 to 3 years
- Delayed puberty
- Delayed bone age (bone age = height age)

NUTRITIONAL

- Irritable bowel disease
- Celiac disease
- Anemia

PSYCHOSOCIAL DEPRIVATION

Children with psychosocial deprivation clinically resemble children with GH deficiency with retardation of bone age and similar findings on GH stimulation testing; however, testing and growth revert to normal when the child is removed from the deprived environment.

GROWTH HORMONE DEFICIENCY

- Pathologic cause of short stature
- Decreased growth velocity
- Delayed bone age
- Pubertal delay
- Causes—idiopathic, hypothalamic/pituitary tumor
- Diagnosis—inadequate response to GH stimulation
- Treatment—biosynthetic human GH

HYPOTHYROIDISM

- Pathologic cause of short stature
- Decreased growth velocity
- Delayed bone age
- Diagnosis—elevated TSH, decreased T_4
- Treatment—Synthroid (T_4)

PITUITARY

- Panhypopituitarism—hypoglycemia and micropenis
- Normal at birth
- Height age is delayed, as is bone age

CUSHING'S SYNDROME

- Pathologic cause of short stature.
- Increased cortisol inhibits growth.
- Causes—endogenous or exogenous steroids.
- Diagnosis—ACTH and cortisol levels.

CHROMOSOMAL DISORDERS

- Turner's syndrome
- Down's syndrome
- Silver–Russell syndrome

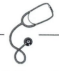

The most common causes of short stature are normal variants including familial short stature and constitutional delay.

Children with constitutional delay are the so-called "late-bloomers."

There is an increased risk of leukemia with GH therapy.

TALL STATURE

DEFINITION

Height more than 2 standard deviations above the mean.

FAMILIAL

Most common.

HORMONAL

- Increased adrenal androgen steroids (congenital adrenal hyperplasia [CAH])
- Increased sex steroids
- Increased GH

SYNDROMES

- Marfan syndrome
- Homocystinuria
- Klinefelter's syndrome
- Sotos' syndrome (not truly endocrine, associated mental retardation)

GIGANTISM/ACROMEGALY

DEFINITION

- Increased GH
- If occurs before epiphyses close, leads to gigantism
- If after epiphyses close, leads to acromegaly

ETIOLOGY

Pituitary adenoma.

SIGNS AND SYMPTOMS

- Gigantism
- Rapid linear growth
- Coarse facial features
- Enlarging hands and feet
- Acromegaly
- Enlargement of distal parts
- Increased GH (may reach 400 ng/mL)

> **Beckwith–Weidemann Syndrome**
> Large babies due to overproduction of insulin-like growth factor II.

DIABETES INSIPIDUS

DEFINITION

Inability of kidneys to concentrate urine.

EPIDEMIOLOGY

Central	**Nephrogenic**
Acquired	X-linked recessive
Any age	Males—early infancy

ETIOLOGY

Central (Decreased Antidiuretic Hormone (ADH)	**Nephrogenic (Renal Unresponsiveness to ADH)**
Idiopathic	Idiopathic
Head injury	Renal diseases
Meningitis	Hypercalcemia

Suprasellar tumors
   (craniopharyngioma)
Septo-optic dysplasia
Histiocytosis

Hypokalemia
Toxins (lithium, demeclocycline)

SIGNS AND SYMPTOMS

Central
Polyuria (both volume and
   frequency)
Excessive thirst
Enuresis

Nephrogenic
Polyuria, failure to thrive (FTT),
   hyperpyrexia, vomiting
Hypernatremic dehydration

DIAGNOSIS

- Increased serum osmolality (N < 290 mOsm/L)
- Increased serum Na (N < 145 mmol/L)
- Dilute urine (N > 150 mOsm/L)

TREATMENT

Central
Fluids
Desmopressin (DDAVP) (5–10
   µg intranasally or 0.2—0.4 g/kg
   subcutaneously)

Nephrogenic
Fluids
Thiazide diuretic (paradoxical effect)

In diabetes insipidus, there is high urine output despite significant dehydration.

SYNDROME OF INAPPROPRIATE SECRETION OF ANTIDIURETIC HORMONE (SIADH)

DEFINITION

Increased ADH.

ETIOLOGY

- Bacterial meningitis
- Positive pressure ventilation
- Rocky Mountain spotted fever
- Pneumonia

SIGNS AND SYMPTOMS

- Asymptomatic until Na < 120
- Headache, nausea, vomiting, irritability, seizure

DIAGNOSIS

- Hyponatremia
- Decreased serum osmolality
- Increased urine osmolality
- Increased urine Na (> 18 mEq/L)
- Normal renal, adrenal, and thyroid function

TREATMENT

- Symptomatic: hypertonic (3%) saline 3 mL/kg
- Asymptomatic:
  - Fluid restriction
  - Demeclocycline if resistant (rarely used)

In SIADH, there is an absence of edema and dehydration.

Urine osmolality < 100 mOsm/kg excludes diagnosis of SIADH.

- Pubertal events are classified by Tanner staging.
- See Table 16-2 and Figure 16-1.

NORMAL FEMALE PROGRESSION

Thelarche → height growth spurt → pubic hair → menarche (13 years).

NORMAL MALE PROGRESSION

Testicular enlargement → penile enlargement → height growth spurt (14 years) → pubic hair.

Precocious Puberty

DEFINITION

- Onset of secondary sexual characteristics
- < 8 years (girls)
- < 9 years (boys)
- Premature breast development (thelarche)
- Premature pubic hair development (adrenarche)

ETIOLOGY

- Premature activation of the hypothalamic–pituitary–gonadal axis
  - Gonadotropin dependent—increased FSH and LH
  - Gonadotropin independent—excess sex steroids (decreased FSH and LH)
  - Male:
    - Bilateral testicular enlargement
      - Gonadotropin from brain tumor (glioma, pinealoma, hamartoma), head injury, hydrocephalus
    - Unilateral testicular enlargement
      - Gonadal tumor—testicular Leydig cell tumor
    - Prepubertal testes
      - Adrenal CAH
  - Female:
    - Premature onset of normal puberty
    - Organic causes rare

> The increase in height velocity in boys occurs at a later chronologic age than in girls.

> Most normal 11-year-old girls have pubic hair.

> Precocious puberty in girls is usually idiopathic, while in boys it usually has an organic cause.

TABLE 16-2. Tanner stages.

Stage	Breast Development (Female)	Genital Development (Male)	Pubic Hair (Female and Male)
I	Preadolescent	Preadolescent	Preadolescent
II	Breast bud (11 years)	Enlargement of scrotum and testes, darkening of scrotum and texture change (12 years)	Sparse, long, slightly pigmented downy hair (female 12, male 13.5)
III	Continued enlargement, no contour separation (12 years)	Enlargement of penis (13 years)	Darker, coarser, and more curled (female 12.5, male 14)
IV	Secondary mound, projection of areola and papilla (13 years)	Increase in penis breadth and development of glans (14 years)	Hair resembles adult, distributed less than adult and not to medial thighs (female 13, male 14.5)
V	Mature stage (15 years)	Mature stage (15 years)	Mature stage (female 14.5, male 15)

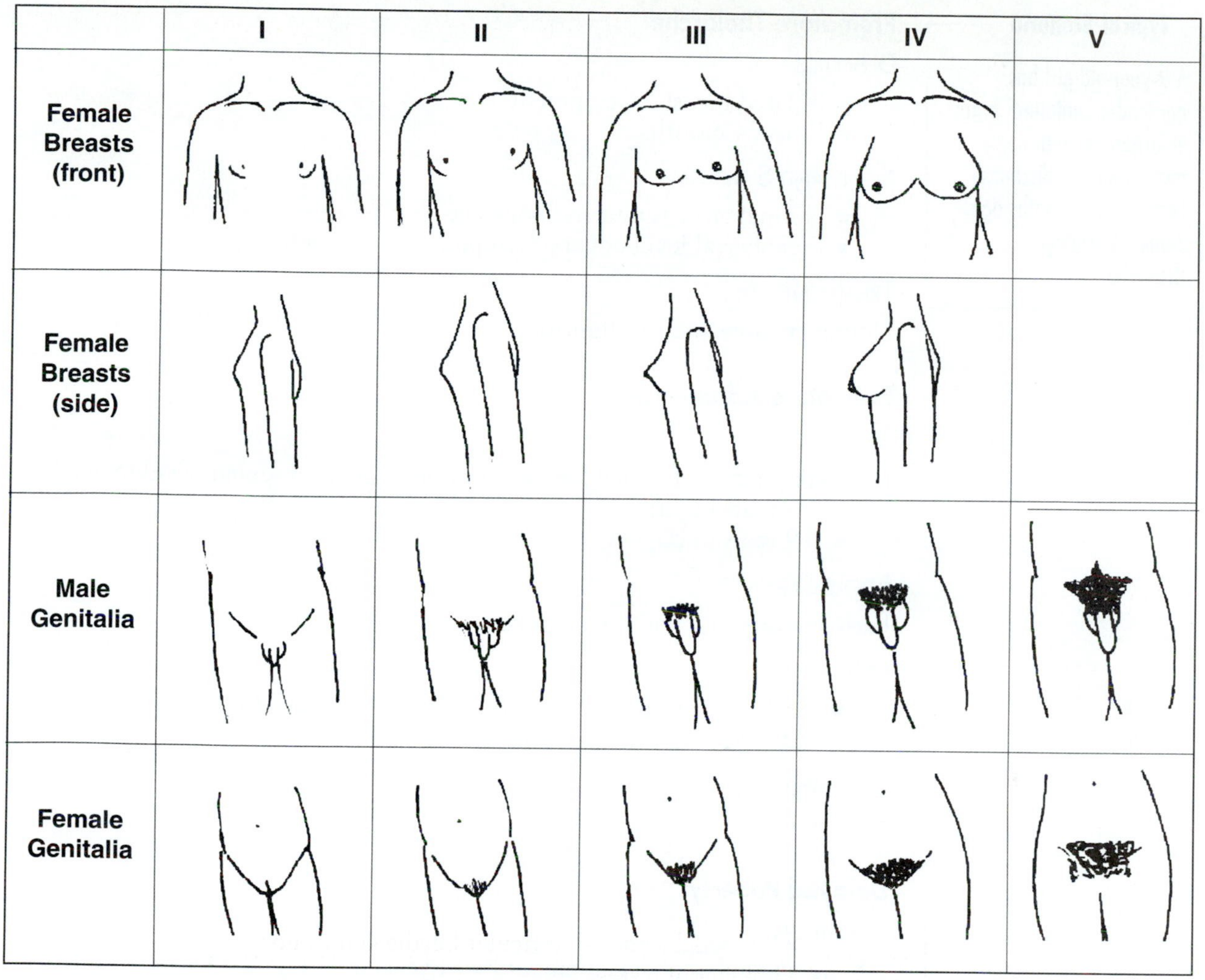

	I	II	III	IV	V
Female Breasts (front)					
Female Breasts (side)					
Male Genitalia					
Female Genitalia					

FIGURE 16-1. Tanner stages. (Artwork by Elizabeth N. Jacobson.)

- McCune–Albright syndrome—ovarian cysts secreting estrogen
  - Adrenal—CAH
  - Ovarian granulosa cell tumor
- Exogenous sex steroids

SIGNS AND SYMPTOMS

- Growth acceleration
- Significantly advanced bone age

DIAGNOSIS

- Pubertal levels of gonadotropins (low) and estrogen or testosterone
- No increase in gonadotropins after gonadotropin-releasing hormone (GnRH)

TREATMENT

- Treatment of underlying cause
- GnRH analogues

Typical Scenario

A 7-year-old girl develops enlarged breasts. Six months later she begins to develop pubic and axillary hair. Her menses began at age 8. *Think:* Idiopathic precocious puberty.

Premature Thelarche

DEFINITION
- Isolated breast development
- 12 to 24 months

SIGNS AND SYMPTOMS
- Normal growth rate and bone age
- Prepubertal level of gonadotropins and estrogen

TREATMENT

Nonprogressive and self-limiting.

Premature Adrenarche

DEFINITION

Early appearance of sexual hair without other signs of sexual development.
- < 8 years in girls
- < 9 years in boys

ETIOLOGY

Early maturation of adrenal androgen.

DIAGNOSIS
- Androgen normal for pubertal stage but elevated for chronologic age.
- Adrenal tumor needs to be excluded.

TREATMENT

Self-limiting.

Delayed Puberty

DEFINITION

Absence of pubertal development by 14 years in girls and 15 years in boys.

EPIDEMIOLOGY

More common in boys.

ETIOLOGY

Female
- Constitutional
- Primary ovarian failure
- Turner's syndrome
- Hypogonadotropic hypogonadism
- Kallmann's syndrome
- Hypopituitarism
- Prader–Willi syndrome

Male
- Constitutional
- Primary testicular failure
- Klinefelter's syndrome
- Hypogonadotropic hypogonadism
- Kallmann's syndrome
- Hypopituitarism
- Prader–Willi syndrome

Kallman Syndrome
X-linked hypogonadotropic hypogonadism affecting males and females, associated with anosmia, cleft lip/palate, and other midline defects.

- According to the Tanner English Series, most females begin menstruation between the ages of 9 and 16 years old (average age, 13.5 years old).
- Menarche occurs about 2 to 3 years after the initiation of puberty.
- Periods become regular after 2 to 2.5 years after menarche.
- The length of a cycle is between 21 to 45 days (average is 28 days).
- The length of flow is 2 to 7 days (average is 3 to 5 days).
- Blood loss is on average 40 mL (range, 25 to 70 mL).

Amenorrhea

PRIMARY AMENORRHEA

No menstrual flow by age 16.

Etiology

- Chromosomal
    - Turner's syndrome
    - Triple X syndrome
- Testicular feminization syndrome
- True hermaphroditism
- Congenital
- Imperforate hymen
- Primary ovarian failure

Turner's syndrome is the most common cause of primary amenorrhea.

Differential Diagnosis

- Pregnancy, hypothyroidism, hyperprolactinemia.
- Normal/low FSH:
    - Consider hypogonadotropic hypogonadism including hypothalamic causes like stress, weight loss, obesity, athletics, familial causes, or drugs.
    - Also consider CNS tumors, chronic disease, and other endocrinopathies including thyroid disorders.
- High FSH: Consider gonadal dysgenesis, autoimmune oophoritis, or other causes of ovarian failure.

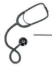

The most common causes of secondary amenorrhea include pregnancy, stress, and polycystic ovary disease.

SECONDARY AMENORRHEA

Absence of vaginal bleeding for > 3 months after menstrual cycles have already been established.

Differential Diagnosis

- Normal/low FSH:
    - Consider hypothalamic amenorrhea related to stress, weight loss, an eating disorder, competitive athletics, phenothiazine use, or substance abuse.
    - Also consider chronic disease, CNS tumor (i.e., prolactinoma), pituitary infiltration or infarction as in postpartum hemorrhage or sickle cell disease, and Asherman's syndrome (following endometrial currettage).
- High FSH:
    - Consider gonadal dysgenesis as in mosaic Turner's syndrome or autoimmune oophoritis.

Typical Scenario

A 16-year-old female adolescent had the onset of breast development at the age of 12 years and menses at age 14. She has not had menses for 2 months. She is active in sports. Physical exam is normal. *Think:* Rule out pregnancy, then consider the sports contribution to her secondary amenorrhea.

HIGH-YIELD FACTS

Endocrine Disease

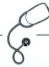

Dysmenorrhea

DEFINITION

Painful menstruation.

PRIMARY DYSMENORRHEA

Absence of any specific pelvic pathologic condition.

Etiology

Excessive amounts of prostaglandins F_2 and E_2, which cause uterine contractions, tissue hypoxia and ischemia, and increased sensitization of pain receptors.

Treatment

Recommend prostaglandin inhibitors for dysmenorrhea at the onset of flow or pain.

SECONDARY DYSMENORRHEA

Etiology

- Underlying structural abnormality of the vagina, cervix, or uterus:
  - Congenital anomalies
  - Pelvic adhesions
  - Endometriosis
- Foreign body such as an intrauterine device
- Endometritis: infection, especially secondary to sexually transmitted diseases (STDs)
- Complications of pregnancy such as ectopic pregnancy

TESTICULAR FEMINIZATION

DEFINITION
- Androgen insensitivity syndrome.
- XY male with testes appears as unambiguous female.

SIGNS AND SYMPTOMS
- Primary amenorrhea
- Presence of testes in inguinal hernia

TRUE HERMAPHRODITISM

DEFINITION

Presence of both ovarian follicles and seminiferous tubules in same patient with 46,XX karyotype.

ETIOLOGY

Abnormal gonadal differentiation.

SIGNS AND SYMPTOMS
- Ambiguous genitalia—significant masculinization (raised as male)
- Increased risk of malignant transformation of gonadal tissue

- 46,XX karyotype
- Normal 17-OH progesterone

PSEUDOHERMAPHRODITISM

Female

DEFINITION

Normal gonads and uterus (both gonads are ovaries) with virilization of external genitalia in a patient with a 46,XX karyotype.

ETIOLOGY

CAH (21-hydroxylase deficiency).

SIGNS AND SYMPTOMS

- Ambiguous genitalia
- Virilization of external genitalia
- Clitoral hypertrophy
- Labioscrotal fusion

Male

DEFINITION

- 46,XY male
- Normal testes (both gonads are testes)
- Undervirilization of external genitalia

ETIOLOGY

- Androgen insensitivity
- Enzyme defects in testosterone synthesis

SIGNS AND SYMPTOMS

- Small phallus
- Hypospadias
- Undescended testes

Neurologic Disease

Seizures are relatively common in the pediatric age group, occurring in 3–5% of children by 15 years of age. Most have either a single seizure or multiple seizures over many years.

DEFINITION

Abnormal rhythmic synchronous discharges of large collections central nervous system (CNS) neurons with electroencephalographic (EEG) or clinical manifestations.

ETIOLOGY

Multiple etiologies have been identified for seizures:

- Fever
- Acquired cortical defects (stroke, neoplasm, infection, trauma)
- Inborn errors of metabolism
- Congenital brain malformations
- Neurocutaneous syndromes
- Neurodegenerative diseases
- Toxins/drugs
- Electrolyte disturbances
- Idiopathic (epilepsy)

TYPES OF SEIZURES

See Table 17-1.

Partial (Focal) Seizures

1. Simple partial seizures:
   - Average duration is 10 to 20 seconds.
   - Consciousness is not altered.
   - Movements are characterized by asynchronous clonic or tonic movements.
   - Tend to involve the face, neck, and extremities.
   - Patients may complain of preictal aura, which is characteristic for the brain region involved in the seizure (i.e., visual aura, auditory aura, etc.).
2. Complex partial seizures:
   - Average duration is 1 to 2 minutes.
   - Hallmark feature is *alteration* or loss of consciousness.

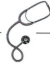

The diagnosis of epilepsy requires two or more unprovoked seizures.

In most children with seizures, an underlying cause cannot be determined and a diagnosis of idiopathic epilepsy is given.

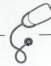

The first step in evaluating any seizure disorder is determining the type of seizure.

Motor activity is the most common symptom of simple partial seizures.

The presence of an aura always indicates a focal onset of the seizure. Physiologically, an aura is simply the earliest conscious manifestation of a seizure.

Automatisms are a common symptom of complex partial seizures.

Typical Scenario

While examining an 8-year-old girl in your office, the child suddenly develops a blank stare and flickering eyelids. Twenty seconds later she returns to normal and acts as if nothing out of the ordinary has occurred. *Think:* Absence seizure.

TABLE 17-1. Outline of the international classification of epileptic seizures.

I. Partial seizures (seizures with focal onset)
   A. Simple partial seizures (consciousness unimpaired)
      1. With motor signs
      2. With somatosensory of special sensory symptoms
      3. With autonomic symptoms or signs
      4. With psychic symptoms (higher cerebral functions)
   B. Complex partial seizures (consciousness impaired)
      1. Starting as simple partial seizures
         (a) Without automatisms
         (b) With automatisms
      2. With impairment of consciousness at onset
         (a) Without automatisms
         (b) With automatisms
   C. Partial seizures evolving into secondary generalized seizures
II. Generalized seizures
   A. Absence seizures: Brief lapse in awareness without postictal impairment (atypical absence seizures may have the following: mild clonic, atonic, tonic, automatism, or autonomic components)
   B. Myoclonic seizures: Brief, repetitive, symmetric muscle contractions (loss of tone)
   C. Clonic seizures: Rhythmic jerking; flexor spasm of extremities
   D. Tonic seizures: Sustained muscle contraction
   E. Tonic–clonic seizures
   F. Atonic seizures: Abrupt loss of muscle tone
III. Unclassified epileptic seizures

Reproduced, with permission, from Committee on Classification and Terminology of the International League Against Epilepsy. *Epilepsia* 1996;38(11):1051–1059.

- Automatisms are seen in 50–75% of cases (psychic, sensory, or motor phenomena carried out while unconscious and not recalled postictally).
- May begin as a simple partial seizure and progress until consciousness is affected.

Generalized Seizures
1. Typical absence seizures (formerly "petit mal"):
   - Characterized by sudden cessation of motor activity or speech.
   - May experience countless seizures daily.
   - More common in girls.
   - Never occur before age 5 (atypical absence can).
   - Duration is rarely longer than 30 seconds.
   - There is no postictal state.
   - Childhood absence epilepsy is accompanied by characteristic 3-Hz spike and wave.
2. Generalized tonic–clonic seizures (GTCs, formerly "grand mal"):
   - Extremely common and may follow a partial seizure with focal onset.
   - Patients suddenly lose consciousness, their eyes roll back, and their entire musculature undergoes tonic contractions, arresting breathing.
   - Gradually, the hyperextension gives way to a series of rapid clonic jerks.
   - Finally, a period of flaccid relaxation occurs, during which sphincter control is often lost (incontinence).
   - Prodromal symptoms (not aura) often precede the attack by several hours and include mood change, apprehension, insomnia, or loss of appetite.

Other seizures type listed in Table 17-1.

Simple Febrile Seizure

- The most common seizure disorder during childhood: occur in 2–5% of children 6 months to 6 years of age.
- Present as a brief tonic–clonic seizure associated with a fever.
- Risk of recurrence is 30% after first episode and 50% after second episode.
- There are no long-term sequelae, and children will outgrow by age 6.
- Increased risk of epilepsy (2% as opposed to 1% in the general population).
- An autosomal dominant inheritance pattern is demonstrated in some families (19p and 8q13–21).

Neonatal Seizure

- Metabolic, toxic, and infectious diseases are commonly present during the neonatal period, placing the child at an increased risk for seizures.
- Myelination and axonal formation are not complete at birth; thus, generalized tonic–clonic seizures will not be seen in the first month of life.
- May manifest as tonic, myoclonic, clonic, or subtle (prolonged non-nutritive sucking, nystagmus, color change, autonomic instability).
- EEG may show burst suppression (alternating high and very low voltages), low-voltage invariance, diffuse or focal background slowing, and focal or multifocal spikes.
- Neonatal seizures are typically treated with phenobarbital, fosphenytoin (oral form has variable absorption), or benzodiazepines.
- Benign neonatal familial convulsions is a brief self-limited autosomal-dominant condition with generalized seizures beginning in the first week of life and subsiding within 6 weeks. There is a normal interictal EEG. There is a 10–15% chance of future epilepsy, but otherwise carries an excellent prognosis. Always elicit a family history in neonatal seizures.

Infantile Spasm

- Begin between ages 4 and 8 months and present as short-lived, symmetric contractions of the neck, trunk, and extremities.
- Symptomatic type is most commonly seen with CNS malformations, brain injury, tuberous sclerosis, or inborn errors of metabolism and typically has a poor outcome.
- Cryptogenic type has a better prognosis and children typically have an uneventful birth history and reach developmental milestones before the onset of the seizures.
- Treated with adrenocorticotropic hormone (ACTH) in the United States.

Epilepsy

Definition

- A history of two or more unprovoked seizures.
- After a nebulous period (on the order of 5–10 years) of seizure freedom without the aid of antiepileptic medications or devices, the epilepsy can be considered to have resolved, particularly if the patient fits an epilepsy syndrome that is known typically to resolve.

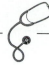

If you are present during a tonic–clonic seizure:

- Keep track of the duration.
- Place the patient between prone and lateral decubitus to allow the tongue to fall forward.
- Hyperextend the neck and jaw to enhance breathing.
- Loosen any tight clothing or jewelry around the neck.
- ***Do not try to force open the mouth or teeth!***

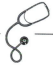

A febrile seizure lasting > 15 minutes suggests an organic cause such as meningitis or toxin exposure.

Etiologies of neonatal seizure:

- Hypoxic–ischemic encephalopathy (35–42%)
- Intracranial hemorrhage/infarction (15–20%)
- CNS infection (12–17%)
- Metabolic and inborn errors of metabolism (8–25%)
- CNS malformation (5%)

Unprovoked seizure: unrelated to current acute CNS insult such as infection, increased intracranial pressure (ICP), trauma, toxin, etc.

Evaluate patients following their first seizure (for mass lesion, etc.) prior to diagnosing and treating epilepsy.

EPIDEMIOLOGY

Epilepsy occurs in 0.5–1% of the population and begins in childhood in 60% of the cases.

SIGNS AND SYMPTOMS

- Vary depending on the seizure pattern. See above discussion of types of seizures.
- A seizure is defined electrographically as a hypersynchronous, hyper-rhythmic, high-amplitude signal that evolves in both frequency and space.
- An aura is a stereotyped symptom set that immediately precedes the onset of a clinical seizure and does not affect consciousness.
- Physiologically, the aura is probably simply the true beginning of the seizure, and as such its character can be quite useful for localizing seizure onset.
- A seizure prodrome is a set of symptoms, much less stereotyped than an aura, that precede seizures by hours to days. Symptoms such as headache, mood changes, and nausea are reported by over 50% of patients in some series.

TREATMENT

Therapy is directed at preventing the attacks. See Table 17-2 for current pharmacologic treatments for epilepsy.

COMMON EPILEPSY SYNDROMES

See Table 17-3 for localizing/lateralizing seizure semiologies.

- **Localization-related epilepsy:** Seizures secondary to a focal CNS lesion, not necessarily visible on imaging, best candidates for epilepsy surgery. Common examples include masses (particularly cortical tubers of tuberous sclerosis [TS]), cortical dysplasia, postencephalitic gliosis, and arteriovenous malformations (AVMs).
- **Benign focal epilesy of childhood (BFEC):** Includes benign rolandic epilepsy (BECTS), onset 1.5 to 13 years, peak at 7 to 8; infrequent par-

TABLE 17-2. Epilepsy drugs.

Drug	Simple Partial	Complex Partial	Tonic–Clonic	Absence	Status Epilepticus
Phenytoin	X	X	X		X
Carbamazepine	X	X	X		
Lamotrigine	X	X	X		
Gabapentin	X	X	X		
Topiramate	X	X			
Phenobarbital			X		X (infants)
Valproate			X	X	X (IV form)
Ethosuxamide				X	
Diazepam					X (often lorazepam)

X, clinical use.

TABLE 17-3. Localizing/lateralizing seizure semiologies.

Clinical Event	Lateralization	Localization
Ipsilateral indicates phenomenon is directed toward the seizing hemisphere.		
Head turn		
Early nonforced	Ipsilateral	Temporal
Forced		
Early forced		Frontal (less likely to generalize)
Late forced	Contralateral	Temporal (more likely to generalize)
Ocular version	Contralateral	Occipital
Focal clonus	Contralateral	Frontal = temporal
Dystonic limb	Contralateral	Temporal > frontal
Unilateral tonic limb	Contralateral	
M2e fencing	Contralateral	Frontal > temporal
Figure 4	Contralateral	
Ictal paresis	Contralateral	
Todd's (postictal) paresis	Contralateral	
Unilateral blinking	Ipsilateral	
Unilateral automatism	Ipsilateral	
Postictal nose rubbing	Ipsilateral (to hand used)	Temporal > frontal
Postictal cough		Temporal
Bipedal automatism		Frontal > temporal
Hypermotoric state		Supplementary motor area
Ictal spitting	Right	Temporal
Automatism with preserved responsiveness	Right	Temporal
Gelastic		Hypothalamic, mesial temporal
Ictal vomiting/retching	Right	Temporal
Ictal urinary urgency	Nondominant	Temporal
Loud vocalization		Frontal > temporal
Ictal speech arrest		Temporal
Postictal aphasia	Dominant	

tial seizures; arising out of sleep is usual but not required; unilateral face/arm, motor/sensory symptoms most common; tendency to secondary generalization in younger age groups; EEG shows interictal focal sharp waves activated by sleep and sometimes generalized spike and wave; good response to antiepileptic drugs (AEDs); resolution by age 16.

Epilepsy History

- Age, sex, handedness
- Seizure semiology (what the seizures look like, details about right/left). If more than one type, the pattern of progression (if any)
- Seizure duration/history of status epilepticus
- Postictal lethargy or focal neurologic deficits
- Current frequency/tendency to cluster
- Age at onset
- Date of last seizure
- Longest seizure-free interval
- Known precipitants (don't forget to ask if the seizures typically arise out of sleep)
- History of head trauma, difficult birth, intrauterine infection, hypoxic/ischemic insults, meningoencephalitis or other CNS disease
- Developmental history (delay strongly correlated with poorer prognoses)
- Family history of epilepsy, febrile seizures
- Psychiatric history
- Current AEDs
- AED history (maximum doses, efficacy, reason for stopping)
- Previous EEG, magnetic resonance imaging (MRI) findings

- **West syndrome:** Triad of infantile spasms, arrest of development, and hypsarrhythmia (generalized, high-voltage, chaotic pattern) on EEG, onset usually 4 to 7 months, up to 1 year, boys more commonly affected, generally poor prognosis. Differential includes TS (largest group), CNS malformation, intrauterine infection, inborn metabolic disorders, and idiopathic. Idiopathic group fares the best. Treatment in the United States is restricted to daily intramuscular (IM) ACTH.

- **Juvenile myoclonic epilepsy (JME):** Begins around puberty; repetitive myoclonic jerks, particularly in the morning; GTCs and abscence seizures appear later; photosensitivity is common; irregular generalized polyspike and wave on EEG; AED response is good; no spontaneous resolution.

- **Childhood absence epilepsy (CAE, pyknolepsy):** Peak incidence 6 to 7 years, strong genetic predisposition, inheritance unclear, girls more frequently affected, multiple absence seizures per day; EEG shows bilateral 3-Hz spike and wave; GTCs often develop in adolescence; spontaneous resolution is the rule, however.

- **Juvenile absence epilepsy (JAE):** Similar to CAE except beginning in adolescence, seizure frequency lower, sexes affected equally, EEG spike and wave often faster than 3 Hz.

- **Lennox–Gastaut syndrome:** Onset from 1 to 8 years, tonic, atonic, and atypical absence (prolonged) seizure types define the syndrome, but GTCs, myoclonic, and partial seizures are also commonly seen. Developmental delay/regression is usually present. Seizures are frequent and resistant to treatment with AEDs. EEG shows abnormal background, generalized slow spike and wave, and multifocal spikes. Poor prognosis.

- **Landau–Kleffner syndrome (acquired epileptic aphasia):** Progressive loss of spontaneous speech beginning in early to mid childhood; interictal EEG may be normal or show multifocal spikes, spike wave abnormalities. Nonconvulsive status epilepticus during slow-wave sleep consisting of continuous 1.5- to 5-Hz spike and wave bilaterally on EEG. Clinical seizures, if present, are GTCs or partial motor. Resolution by age 15 but long-term cognitive/developmental sequelae in more than 50%. May respond to high-dose benzodiazepines prior to bed.

- **Progressive myoclonic epilepsies:** A group of diseases including Unverricht–Lundborg disease, myoclonic epilepsy with ragged-red fibers (MERRF), Lafora's disease, neuronal ceroid lipofuscinosis, and sialidosis/mucolipidosis that as a group begin late childhood to adolescence, and entail progressive neurologic deterioration with myoclonic seizures, dementia, and ataxia. Death within 10 years of onset is common, but survival to old age occurs.

- **Mesial temporal sclerosis:** Gliotic scarring and atrophy of the hippocampal formation creating a seizure focus. Etiology is debated, but remote excitotoxic damage from multiple recurrent or prolonged seizures is the reigning theory. Abnormality is often apparent on high-resolution MRI. Curative resection is often possible.

RETT SYNDROME

DEFINITION

A neurodegenerative disorder of unknown cause.

EPIDEMIOLOGY

- Occurs almost exclusively in females; thought to be X-linked recessive and lethal to males
- Prevalence of 1:15,000 to 1:22,000

SIGNS AND SYMPTOMS

- Normal development until 12 to 18 months, before undergoing a period of regression of language and motor milestones.
- Ataxia, hand-wringing, reduced brain weight, and episodes of hyperventilation are typical.

PROGNOSIS

- After the initial period of regression, the disease appears to plateau.
- Death occurs during adolescence or the third decade of life.

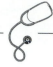

The hallmark of Rett syndrome is repetitive hand-wringing and resultant loss of use of the hands.

STURGE–WEBER SYNDROME

EPIDEMIOLOGY

Occurs sporadically in 1:50,000.

ETIOLOGY

Abnormal development of the meningeal vasculature resulting in hemispheric vascular steal phenomenon and resultant hemiatrophy. Facial capillary hemangioma usually accompanies.

SIGNS AND SYMPTOMS

A constellation of symptoms including a facial nevus, seizures, hemiparesis, intracranial calcifications, mental retardation, and vascular malformations in the eye.

If you see "port-wine stain," *think:* Sturge–Weber syndrome.

STATUS EPILEPTICUS

DEFINITION

A continuous seizure or multiple seizures lasting for > 30 minutes without regaining consciousness.

ETIOLOGY

Febrile seizures, idiopathic status epilepticus, and symptomatic status epilepticus.

PATHOPHYSIOLOGY

Prolonged neural firing may result in neuronal cell death, called excitotoxicity.

TREATMENT

Initial treatment includes assessment of the respiratory and cardiovascular systems.

In children under 3 years, febrile seizures are the most likely etiology of status epilepticus.

Status Protocol
1. Airway, breathing, circulation (ABCs); give O_2
2. Vitals, particularly blood pressure (BP)
3. Intravenous (IV) access
4. Labs: glucose, sodium (Na), potassium (K), calcium (Ca), magnesium (Mg), phosphorus (P), blood urea nitrogen (BUN), creatinine (Cr), ammonia (NH_3), aspartate transaminase (AST), alanine transaminase (ALT), AED levels, tox screen, blood cultures, complete blood count (CBC)
5. If seizing for > 5 minutes: lorazepam 0.1 mg/kg IV
6. If lorazepam fails, fosphenytoin 20 mg/kg IV (doses of fosphenytoin are in "phenytoin equivalents" by convention)

Neonatal status that is refractory to the usual measures may respond to pyridoxine. This is seen in pyridoxine dependency (due to diminished glutamate decarboxylase activity, a rare autosomal recessive condition) or pyridoxine deficiency in children born to mothers on isoniazid.

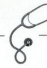

Since obstructive sleep apnea causes hypoxia, it may be associated with polycythemia vera, growth failure, and serious cardiorespiratory pathophysiology.

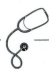

Sleep deprivation causes attention deficit, hyperactivity, and behavior disturbances in children — often mistaken for attention deficit–hyperactivity disorder (ADHD).

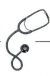

Coma can be caused by only:
- Diffuse bilateral cortical disease
- Bilateral thalamic lesions
- Lesions of the medullary reticular-activating system or its ascending projections. Ventral pontine lesions can lead to the locked-in syndrome, which is not coma.

7. If fosphenytoin fails, give a second dose of 5 mg/kg IV
8. If second fosphenytoin fails, either:
   - Load with phenobarbital 20 mg/kg IV or
   - Load with midazolam 0.1 mg/kg IV and start drip at 2 µg/kg/min and titrate to effect

SLEEP DISORDERS

Obstructive Sleep Apnea

- Occurs in 1% of children, most often between ages 2 and 5.
- Characterized by chronic partial airway obstruction with intermittent episodes of complete obstruction during sleep.
- Snoring is the most common symptom, occurring in 8–10%.

Night Terrors

- Occur in 1–3% of the population, primarily in boys between 5 and 7 years old.
- Transient, sudden-onset episodes of terror in which the child cannot be consoled and is unaware of the surroundings.
- There is total amnesia following the episodes.
- Often, incontinence and diaphoresis.
- Occurs in stage 4 (deep) sleep.

Somnambulance (Sleepwalking)

Complex motor acts that occur during the first third of the night but not during rapid eye movement (REM) sleep.

Insomnia

- Affects 10–20% of adolescents.
- Depression is a common cause and should be ruled out.

COMA

- Consciousness refers to the state of awareness of self and environment.
- Pediatric evaluation of consciousness is dependent on both age and developmental level.

DEFINITION

Refers to a pathologic cause of loss of normal consciousness.

PATHOPHYSIOLOGY

Consciousness is the result of communication between the cerebral cortex and the ascending reticular-activating system.

ETIOLOGY

- Structural causes include trauma, vascular conditions, and mass lesions.
- Metabolic and toxic causes include hypoxic–ischemic injury, toxins, infectious causes, and seizures.

EVALUATION

- ABCs must be initially assessed.
- Supply glucose via IV line so that the brain has an adequate energy supply.

TABLE 17-4. Glasgow Coma Scale (GCS).

Eye Opening (Total Points: 4)

Spontaneous	4
To Voice	3
To Pain	2
None	1

Verbal Response (Total Points: 5)

Infants and Young Children		*Older Children*	
Appropriate words; smiles, fixes, and follows	5	Oriented	5
Consolable crying	4	Confused	4
Persistently irritable	3	Inappropriate	3
Restless, agitated	2	Incomprehensible	2
None	1	None	1

Motor Response (Total Points: 6)

Obeys	6
Localizes pain	5
Withdraws	4
Flexion	3
Extension	2
None	1

Note minimum score is 3, not 0.

- Attempt to determine the underlying cause of the impaired consciousness through a thorough history and physical/neurologic exam.
- Treat underlying cause (toxin antidote, reduce ICP, antibiotics, etc.)

PROGNOSIS

- Overall, children tend to do better than adults.
- Several measurement scales have been published attempting to predict outcome. The most widely accepted is the Glasgow Coma Scale (see Table 17-4).
- Another scale that you should know exists is the Pediatric Cerebral Performance Category Scale, which, unlike the Glasgow, was specifically designed for pediatric patients.

CNS INFECTION

- May be caused by virtually any microbe
- In general incidence: viral > bacterial > fungal and parasitic

SIGNS AND SYMPTOMS

- Headache, nausea, vomiting, anorexia, restlessness, and irritability are common nonspecific findings.
- Photophobia, nuchal rigidity, stupor, coma, seizures, and focal neurologic deficits are more specific for CNS infection.

MENINGITIS

- A diffuse CNS infection primarily affecting the meninges.
- Typically caused by infection, but both chemical and neoplastic spread may also cause inflammation.

Herniation syndromes that may result in coma:
- Ipsilateral oculomotor dysfunction, *Think:* Uncal herniation.
- Cheyne–Stokes respirations. *Think:* Transtentorial (central) herniation.

Prognosis depends on the etiology of the insult and the rapid initiation of treatment!

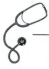

Emergent Treatment of Increased ICP:
1. Elevate head of bed to 30 degrees.
2. Intubate and hyperventilate (20 breaths/min). This will provide relief for about 30 minutes; onset is immediate.
3. Osmotic diuresis with mannitol (1 g/kg) will provide relief with q6h doses for several days; onset in 1 hour.
4. Emergent neurosurgical consult for extraventricular drain (EVD) or craniectomy.
5. High BP needed to maintain cerebral perfusion pressure; if BP falls, consider pressor support.

Emergent Treatment of Increased ICP:

6. Watch for signs of herniation; head computed tomography (CT) if in doubt.

7. Cushing triad (hypertension, bradycardia, bradypnea) may develop; recognize and manage conservatively.

8. Consider AED load with phenobarbital or fosphenytoin for seizure prophylaxis. Phenobarbital may also decrease cerebral metabolic demand.

9. Manage pain

- Can be classified as pyogenic (bacterial), aseptic (viral), or chronic (can be either).
- Diagnosis is made via cerebrospinal fluid (CSF) analysis following a lumbar puncture (LP) (be certain to rule out increased cranial pressure before getting LP) (see Table 17-5).

Bacterial Meningitis

- See Table 17-6 for common meningitis-causing bacteria.
- Associated with high rate of complications and chronic morbidity.
- Most often results from hematogenous spread from a distant site of infection.
- Blood vessels become inflamed and occluded, leading to cerebral infarcts.
- Patients show typical signs of inflammation as well as meningeal signs.

Viral Meningitis

- Enterovirus, echovirus, coxsackievirus, and nonparalytic poliovirus comprise 80% of cases.
- Other classic causes are herpes simplex virus type 1 (HSV-1), Epstein–Barr virus (EBV), mumps, influenza, and adenoviruses.
- Clinical course is milder than that of bacterial meningitis.
- Patients show typical viral-type infectious signs (fever, malaise, myalgia, nausea, rash) as well as meningeal signs.
- Typically is a self-limited process, and treatment is supportive.

Fungal Meningitis

- Although relatively uncommon, the classic organism is *Cryptococcus*.
- Encountered primarily in the immunocompromised patient.
- May be rapidly fatal (as quickly as 2 weeks) or evolve over months to years.
- Tends to cause direct lymphatic obstruction, leading to hydrocephalus.

TABLE 17-5. Cerebrospinal fluid (CSF) findings in meningitis.

	Normal Levels	Bacterial	Viral	Fungal
Pressure (mm Hg)	50–80	Usually elevated 100–300	Normal or slightly elevated 80–150	Usually elevated
Leukocytes (mm³)	< 5	> 1,000	100–500	10–500
% Neutrophils	0	> 50	< 20	Varies
Protein (mg/dL)	20–45	100–500	50–200	25–500
Glucose (mg/dL)	> 50 or 75% serum glucose	Decreased < 40 or 66% serum	Generally normal	< 50 Continues to decline if untreated
Lab cultures		■ Gram stain of CSF	■ Hard to detect ■ PCR of CSF may show HSV or enteroviruses	■ Budding yeast may be seen ■ Cryptococcal antigen may be positive in serum and CSF

PCR, polymerase chain reaction; HSV, herpes simplex virus.

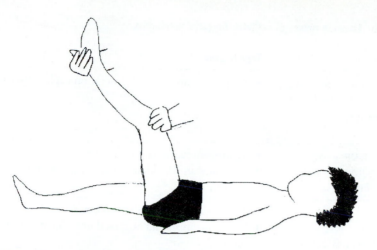

FIGURE 17-1. Kernig's sign. Flex patient's leg at both hip and knee, and then straighten knee. Pain on extension is a positive sign.

Meningitis is associated with the following:
Kernig's sign: Flex patient's leg at both hip and knee, and then straighten knee. Pain on extension is a positive sign (see Figure 17-1).
Brudzinski's sign: Involuntary flexion of the hips and knees with passive flexion of the neck while lying down (see Figure 17-2).

ENCEPHALITIS

DEFINITION

- A disease process in the brain primarily affecting the brain parenchyma.
- Typically is caused by infection, but both chemical and neoplastic spread may also cause inflammation.
- Because patients often have symptoms of both meningitis and encephalitis, the term *meningoencephalitis* is often applied.

ETIOLOGY

Chronic Bacterial Meningoencephalitis

1. **Tuberculosis and mycobacterioses**
   - Patients have generalized complaints of headache, malaise, and confusion.
   - Vomiting is common.
   - Serious complications include arachnoid fibrosis, leading to hydrocephalus, and arterial occlusion, leading to infarcts.
   - *Mycobacterium avium-intracellulare* is common in acquired immune deficiency syndrome (AIDS) patients.

Take some time to familiarize yourself with Tables 17-5 and 17-6: *You will be asked this!*

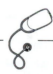

Treat all acute cases of meningitis as if they are bacterial until cultures return.

Nuchal rigidity. *Think:* Meningitis.

Acyclovir is the treatment of choice for herpetic meningitis.

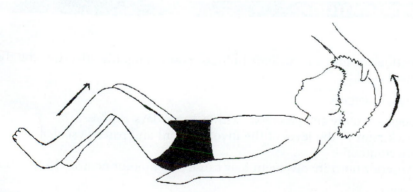

FIGURE 17-2. Brudzinski sign. Involuntary flexion of the hips and knees with passive flexion of the neck while supine.

TABLE 17-6. Common causes of pediatric bacterial meningitis.

Age	Bacteria	Treatment
Neonates (< 1 month)	Group B streptococcus Gram-negative enteric bacilli *Listeria monocytogenes* *Escherichia coli*	■ Ampicillin and a third-generation cephalosporin
Infants (1–24 months)	*Streptococcus pneumoniae* *Neisseria meningitidis* *Haemophilus influenzae* type B	■ Third-generation cephalosporin ■ Vancomycin should be added until susceptibility is known
Children (> 24 months)	*S. pneumoniae* *N. meningitidis* *H. influenzae* type B	■ Third-generation cephalosporin ■ Vancomycin should be added until susceptibility is known

The transmission rate of syphilis from infected mother to infant is nearly 100%. Treat infant with IV penicillin G.

Congenital syphilis may manifest around age 2 with **Hutchingson's triad:**
- Interstitial keratitis
- Peg-shaped incisors
- Deafness (cranial nerve [CN] VIII)

Argyll–Robertson pupil is discrepancy in pupil size seen in neurosyphilis. Pupil reacts poorly to light but accommodation is normal.

2. **Neurosyphilis (tabes dorsalis)**
- Causative organism is *Treponema pallidum*.
- Tertiary syphilis (late-stage syphilis) manifests with neurologic, cardiovascular, and granulomatous lesions.
- Congenital syphilis presents with a maculopapular rash, lymphadenopathy, and mucopurulent rhinitis.
- Routine prenatal screening for syphilis is now mandatory in most states to prevent congenital syphilis.

Viral Meningoencephalitis
1. **Herpes simplex virus**
- HSV-1 produces alterations in mood, memory, and behavior.
- HSV-2 is more commonly the cause of meningoencephalitis and is the congenitally acquired form, transmitted to 50% of babies born to a mother with active vaginal lesions.
2. **Rabies**
- Causes severe encephalitis, coma, and death due to respiratory failure.
- Transmitted via bite from an infected animal, usually associated with dogs or bats.
- The virus travels up the peripheral nerves from the bite site and enters the brain.
- Nonspecific symptoms (fever, malaise) and paresthesia around the bite site are pathopneumonic.

TRANSVERSE MYELITIS

DEFINITION
An infectious or immune-mediated illness most commonly affecting the thoracic spinal cord.

SIGNS AND SYMPTOMS
- Begins acutely and progresses within 1 to 2 days.
- Back pain at the level of the involved cord and paresthesias of the legs are common.
- Anterior horn involvement may cause lower motor neuron dysfunction.

PROGNOSIS
Recovery can take months to occur, if it occurs at all.

DEFINITION

An acute spastic illness caused by the neurotoxin produced by *Clostridium tetani*.

SIGNS AND SYMPTOMS

- Trismus (masseter muscle spasm) is the characteristic sign.
- Risus caninus, a grin caused by facial spasm is also classic.
- Once the paralysis extends to the trunk and thigh, the patient may exhibit an arched posture in which only the head and heels touch the ground.
- Late stages manifest with recurrent seizures consisting of sudden severe tonic contractions of the muscles with fist clenching, flexion and adduction of the upper limb, and extension of the lower limb.
- Incubation period varies from 2 to 14 days.

DIAGNOSIS

- Diagnosis is typically made clinically.
- Lab studies are usually normal.
- Gram stain is positive in only one third of cases.

TREATMENT

- Rapid administration of human tetanus immune globulin.
- IV penicillin G or metronidazole.
- Surgical excision and debridement of the wound.
- Muscle relaxants such as diazepam should be used to promote relaxation and seizure control.

PROGNOSIS

- Mortality rate: 5–35%.
- Neonatal tetanus mortality ranges from 10 to 75%, depending on quality of care received.

DEFINITION

A generalized disorder of the brain.

TYPES

Mitochondrial Encephalopathy

A group of disorders that can be caused by mutations in either nuclear or mitochondrial DNA, resulting in a variety of symptoms:

1. **Mitochondrial encephalopathy, lactic acidosis, and stroke-like episodes (MELAS):**
   - Patients present before age 15 with hemianopsia or cortical blindness and typically are of short stature.
   - Children are normal for the first several years and then gradually develop motor and cognitive deficiencies and die before age 20.
   - Muscle biopsy is diagnostic.
2. **Myoclonic epilepsy with ragged-red fibers (MERRF):**
   - Onset may be in childhood or adult life.
   - Children are normal for the first several years and then develop progressive epilepsy, cerebellar ataxia, and dysarthria.

Numerous viruses as well as the rabies vaccination and smallpox vaccination have been linked to transverse myelitis.

Typical Scenario

A 1-week-old child born to an immunocompromised mother presents with difficulty feeding, trismus, and other rigid muscles. *Think:* Generalized tetanus.

Tetanus seizures can be triggered by minor stimuli, such as a flashing light. Patients should be sedated, intubated, and put in a dark room in severe cases.

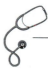

Tetanus is an entirely preventable disease via immunization.

MELAS and MERRF are caused by point mutations in transfer RNA (tRNA) in mitochondrial DNA.
MELAS = leucine
MERRF = lycine

MERRF is often confused with Friedreich's ataxia.

HIGH-YIELD FACTS

Neurologic Disease

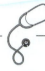

3. **Reye's syndrome:**
   - Characterized by microvesicular steatosis and aberrant mitochondrial metabolism.
   - Sporadic syndrome can occur with varicella-zoster or influenza B infection and ingestion of aspirin.
   - Recurrent Reye's-like syndrome is seen in children with genetic defects of fatty acid oxidation.

Hepatic Encephalopathy

- In children is most commonly related to fulminant viral hepatitis (50–75%).
- Hallmark feature is mental status change.
- The most likely pathophysiology is related to the buildup of ammonia due to impaired hepatic function.
- Increased levels of gamma-aminobutyric acid (GABA) may also play a role.
- Hepatic encephalopathy is reversible with treatment, and most therapies are aimed at lowering the ammonia level (decrease dietary protein, stop gastrointestinal [GI] bleed, treat constipation).
- Acute cerebral edema is treated with fluid restriction and the use of hyperosmolar agents (mannitol).
- Fulminant hepatic failure has a mortality of 75%.
- Patients who recover typically have no long-term sequelae.

Human Immunodeficiency Virus (HIV)/AIDS Encephalopathy

- There is a 40–90% incidence of CNS involvement in perinatally infected children.
- Commonly present with progressive encephalopathy, leading to failure to meet developmental milestones, impaired brain growth, and symmetrical motor dysfunction.
- Imaging techniques reveal cerebral atrophy in 85% of children and ventricular enlargement.
- Basal ganglia calcifications may be present.
- Opportunistic infections such as toxoplasmosis typically occur later in adolescence.
- Diagnosis is via immunoglobulin G (IgG) antibody to HIV for patients > 18 months and a confirmatory test.
- Polymerase chain reaction (PCR) analysis of HIV DNA or RNA is used to detect HIV infection in infants < 18 months.

Lead Encephalopathy

- There is no direct correlation to the level of lead and clinical manifestations.
- Vomiting, abdominal pain, seizures, papilledema, and impaired consciousness are common.
- Peripheral neuropathy, while common in adults, is rarely seen in children unless they also have sickle cell anemia.
- Pica is common in these children (e.g., eating paint chips).
- Diagnosis is made primarily through history and also via blood lead testing.
- Treatment consists of removing the source of lead and chelation therapy.

Sydenham's Chorea

Postinfectious chorea appearing several months after a group A streptococcal infection with subsequent rheumatic fever:

- Is rare under the age of 3 and occurs more commonly in girls
- Resolves after 1 to 6 months
- Is thought to be due to autoantibodies directed at the neurons in the basal ganglia.
- Treatment includes treatment of the primary infection, dopamine-blocking agents for the chorea, and prophylactic penicillin to prevent future episodes.
- Elevated antistreptolysin-O and/or deoxyribunuclease (DNase) B titers may be seen.

Adrenoleukodystrophy

A progressive disease, characterized by demyelination of the CNS and peripheral nerves and adrenal insufficiency:

- The defect is in the ability to catabolize long-chain fatty acids (LCFAs), and high levels of very-long-chain fatty acids (VLCFAs) can be detected in serum.
- X-linked form presents in early school years, progresses rapidly, and is fatal.
- Another form of the disease presents in adulthood and has a better prognosis.

Tourette's Syndrome

A lifelong condition affecting 1:2,000 that presents during childhood with motor tics, vocal tics, obsessive–compulsive behavior, and ADHD.

- Symptoms are enhanced by stress and anxiety.
- Treatment should be initiated when tics interfere with child's developmental learning.

Methylphenidate may unmask Tourette's syndrome, but does not cause it.

CEREBRAL PALSY (CP)

DEFINITION

- A nonprogressive disorder of movement resulting from damage to the brain prior to or surrounding birth.
- Most cases occur in the absence of identifiable causes.

ETIOLOGY

- Prematurity with intraventricular hemorrhage
- Birth or other asphyxia
- Intrauterine growth retardation (IUGR)
- Early infection
- Head trauma

SIGNS AND SYMPTOMS

Prenatal and Perinatal History

- Delayed motor, language, or social skills
- Not losing skills previously acquired
- Feeding difficulties

EXAMINATION

- Hypertonia
- Hyperreflexia

CP is a static disorder, meaning that it does not result in the loss of previously acquired milestones.

- Posture and movement may be spastic, ataxic, choreoathetoid, and dystonic
- Abnormal primitive reflexes
- Abnormal gait
- Impaired growth of affected extremity

Associated Problems
- Seizure disorder
- Mental retardation
- Developmental disorders

TREATMENT

- Multidisciplinary approach with goals of maximizing function and minimizing impairment.
- Team includes general pediatrician, physiotherapist, occupational therapist, language therapist, neurologist, and social and educational support services.

Extensor plantar response (presence of Babinski sign) can be present up to 1 year of age, but should be present symmetrically.

MENTAL RETARDATION (MR)

DEFINITION

- Subaverage intellectual functioning in association with deficits in adaptive behavior prior to 18 years of age
- Intelligence quotient (IQ) or developmental quotient (DQ) < 70

EPIDEMIOLOGY

- Affects 0.8% of the population in the United States, varying significantly by region.
- Approximately 85% are mild cases.
- Males are affected twice as often as females.

SIGNS AND SYMPTOMS

- Significant delay in reaching developmental milestones.
- Delayed speech and language skills in toddlers with less severe MR.
- The child will continue to learn new skills.

Diagnosis

Classification is based on IQ:
- Mild: IQ 55–70, 1–2% of cases
- Moderate: IQ 40–55, 3–5% of cases
- Severe: IQ 25–40, 10% of cases
- Profound: IQ < 25, 85% of cases

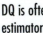

DQ is often used as a rough estimator of IQ in infants and younger children. It is simply the mental age (estimated from historical milestones and exam) divided by the chronologic age.

The IQ is scaled such that the mean is 100 and the standard deviation (SD) is 15. So MR is simply defined as an IQ two SDs below the mean.

LEARNING DISABILITY (LD)

- Significant discrepancy between a person's intellectual ability and academic acheivement.
- Often learn best in unconventional ways.
- Often restricted to a particular realm such as reading or mathematics with correspondingly discrepant scores on standardized measures of intelligence or academic achievement.
- Significant improvement with approriate interventions.

Earlier classification:
Moron: IQ 51–75
Imbecile: IQ 26–50
Idiot: IQ ≤ 25

This is no longer considered politically correct.

Inability to coordinate muscle activities.

TYPES

Acute Cerebellar Ataxia

- A diagnosis of exclusion occurring in children 1 to 3 years old.
- Often follows virus by 2 to 3 weeks; thought to be autoimmune response to virus on cerebellum.
- Sudden onset of severe truncal ataxia; often, the child cannot stand or sit.
- Horizontal nystagmus in 50%.
- Complete recovery typically occurs within 2 months.

Freidreich's Ataxia

- Autosomal recessive mutation (usually a triplet expansion) in the X25 gene on chromosome 9 encoding the mitochondrial protein Frataxin.
- Degeneration of the dorsal columns and rootlets, spinocerebellar tracts, and to a lesser extent the pyramidal tracts and cerebellar hemispheres.
- Onset before age 10.
- Slow progressive ataxia involving the lower limbs greater than the upper limbs.
- Profound hypotonia.
- Peripheral nerve sensory deficits.
- Romberg test is positive; deep tendon reflexes diminished to absent.
- Associated abnormalities include skeletal abnormalities, cardiomyopathy, and optic atrophy.

MERRF is often confused with Friedreich's ataxia.

Ataxia–Telangiectasia

- Autosomal recessive.
- The most common degenerative ataxia.
- Ataxia beginning at age 2 progresses to inability to walk by adolescence.
- Oculomotor apraxia is a common finding.
- Telangiectasia becomes evident in the teenage years and is most prominent on the bridge of nose, conjunctiva, and exposed surfaces of the extremities.
- Have a 50- to 100-fold greater chance of brain tumors and lymphoid tumors.

PERIPHERAL NEUROPATHIES

Injuries to the peripheral nerves may be either:
- Demyelinating (injury to Schwann cells)
- Degenerating (injury to the nerve or axon)

TYPES

Guillain–Barré Syndrome

- A postinfection demyelinating neuropathy affecting predominantly the motor neurons.
- Classically, it occurs 10 days following *Campylobacter jejuni* or *Mycoplasma pneumoniae* infection.
- Weakness begins in the legs and progresses upward to the trunk, arms, then bulbar muscles.
- Treatment includes close monitoring for respiratory weakness and intravenous immune globulin (IVIG) or plasmapheresis in more severe cases.

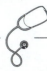

Botulism

- Botulinum toxin is disseminated through the blood and, due to the rich vascular network in the bulbar region, symmetric flaccid paralysis of the cranial nerves is the typical manifestation.
- Infant botulism: The first sign is usually absence of defecation.
- Most dreaded complication is respiratory paralysis, and approximately 50% of patients are intubated.
- Prognosis is good in noncomplicated cases.
- Antibiotics and blocking antibodies have not been shown to affect the course of the disease.
- Electromyogram (EMG) with high frequency (20–50 Hz) reverses the presynaptic blockade and produces an incremental response.

Myasthenia Gravis

- Decrease in postsynaptic acetylcholine receptors due to autoimmune degradation, resulting in rapid fatigability of muscles.
- Ptosis and extraocular eye weakness are the earliest and most diagnostic symptoms.
- Onset usually after age 10, as early as 6 months. Prepubertal male bias, postpubertal female bias.
- Diagnosis is made by EMG with repetitive stimulation, edrophonium (Tensilon) test (acetylcholinesterase inhibitor). Acetylcholine receptor-binding or -blocking antibodies are detected in the seropositive forms and are an indication for thymectomy.
- Cholinesterase drugs are the mainstay of treatment, with oral steroids used as needed for immune suppression.
- Prognosis varies, with some children undergoing spontaneous remission, while in others the disease persists into adulthood.

Transitory Neonatal Myasthenia

- Passive transfer of antibodies from myasthenic mothers (10–15% incidence).
- Self-limited disease consisting of generalized weakness and hypotonia for 1 week to 2 months.
- Supportive care usually suffices. Neostigmine or exchange transfusion can be used in more severe cases.

Familial Infantile Myasthenia

- Collection of autosomal recessive seronegative disorders of the neuromuscular junction. Most defects are postsynaptic, but presynaptic forms are described.
- Onset can be neonatal. Diagnosis by EMG with repetive stimulation, response to edrophonium, specialized testing for identification of the specific defect.
- Long-term treatment with neostigmine or pyridostigmine (acetylcholinesterase inhibitors). Thymectomy and immunosuppression are of no benefit.

Electrolyte Imbalances

- See Table 17-7 for common electrolyte imbalances affecting the nervous system.

TABLE 17-7. Electrolyte disturbances and the nervous system.

Disturbance	Manifestation	Common Causes
Hyponatremia	■ Rapid onset: brain swelling, lethargy, coma, and seizures ■ Slow onset: usually asymptomatic	■ Typically impaired renal water excretion in the presence of normal water intake
Hypernatremia	■ Intracranial bleeding is common in children (dehydrated brain shrinks and can tear bridging veins)	■ Most common cause is dehydration or inadequate intake of water ■ Rare
Hypokalemia	■ Neuromuscular: weakness, paralysis, rhabdomyolysis ■ Gastrointestinal: constipation, ileus ■ Nephrogenic diabetes insipidus ■ ECG changes: prominent U-waves, T-wave flattening ■ Arrhythmias	■ Uptake into cells ■ Renal loss ■ Severe diarrhea, laxative abuse ■ Magnesium depletion is an important and often overlooked cause

Hyperkalemia	■ Severe cases are a medical emergency!
	■ Neuromuscular: weakness, ascending paralysis, respiratory failure
	■ Progressive ECG changes with increasing potassium:
	  ■ Peaked T-waves
	  ■ Flattened P-waves
	  ■ Long PR interval
	  ■ Idioventricular rhythm
	  ■ Wide QRS and deep S-waves
	  ■ Sine wave pattern and ventricular fibrillation
		■ Shift out of cells
		■ Aldosterone deficiency/unresponsiveness
		■ Renal failure

HEADACHES

Migraine

The most important and common type of headache in the pediatric population.

DEFINITION

A recurrent headache with symptom-free intervals and at least three of the following:
- Abdominal pain
- Nausea and/or vomiting
- Throbbing headache
- Unifocal location
- Associated aura
- Relieved by sleep
- Family history of migraines

CLASSIFICATION

Migraines may be classified into the following subgroups:

Common Migraine
- The most prevalent type of migraine in children.
- Intense nausea and vomiting are classic.

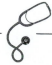

Common migraines may present with vomiting, abdominal pain, and fever, and should be included in the differential of increased ICP diseases.

- Aura is absent.
- Family history is present in 90%, most often on the maternal side.

Classic Migraine
- An aura precedes the headache by 30 minutes and nearly always disappears before the headache begins.
- The auras most often manifest as paresthesias and rarely as visual disturbances such as flashing lights.

Complicated Migraine
- Neurologic signs develop during a headache and persist after the resolution of the headache.

TREATMENT
- Often, migraines occur in response to specific triggers, such as psychological stress, strenuous exercise, sleep deprivation, or moving vehicles, and minimizing these factors may have great therapeutic effect.
- Acute treatment with dark, quiet environment, sleep, and nonsteroidal anti-inflammatory drugs (NSAIDs). Caffeine, triptans, ergots (older children), and antiemetics are other measures that can be tried.
- Treatment should be instituted as early as possible in an attack.
- Prophylaxis begins by establishing a regular sleep schedule and ensuring adequate daily sleep, not skipping meals, and eliminating methylxanthines (caffeine, chocolate) from the diet.
- Daily prophylactic treatment with valproic acid, a tricyclic antidepressant (TCA), β blocker, calcium channel blocker, or topiramate may be indicated.

> Prophylaxis should be offered to children with two or more migraines per month that interfere with activities such as school or recreation.

Cluster Headache
- Brief, severe, unilateral stabbing headaches that occur multiple times daily over a period of several weeks and tend to be seasonal
- Conjunctival injection, tearing, rhinorrhea
- Prophylaxis with lithium or calcium channel blocker
- Acute treatment with oxygen or steroids

Tension Headache

Tension or stress headaches are rare in children prior to puberty and are often difficult to differentiate from migraines.

PRESENTATION
- Most often occur with a stressful situation, such as an exam.
- Described as "hurting" but not "throbbing."
- Most often occur in the frontal region.
- Unlike migraines and increased cranial pressure, tension headaches are not associated with nausea and vomiting.

DIAGNOSIS
- Diagnosis of exclusion.
- EEG or CT is not necessary.
- A poor self-image, fear of failure, and low self-esteem are common factors.

TREATMENT
Steps should be taken to minimize anxiety and stress:
- Mild analgesics often are ample.

- Other options include counseling and hypnosis.
- Sedatives or antidepressants are rarely necessary.

Increased Intracranial Pressure (ICP)

Headache due to tension of the blood vessels or dura may be the first symptom of an increase in cranial pressure.

SYMPTOMS

- In the first 3 years of life, the first indication may be an abnormal increase in head circumference.
- A diffuse headache that often is most prominent in the frontal or occipital regions.
- Coughing or Valsalva's maneuver tends to make the pain worse by increasing ICP further.
- At high pressures, vomiting, lethargy, and mood changes are common.
- CN VI traction may result in vision changes and diplopia.

ETIOLOGY

Common causes include posterior fossa brain tumors (and other brain tumors), obstructive hydrocephalus, hemorrhage, meningitis, abscesses, and chronic lead poisoning.

DIAGNOSIS

- Thorough history and physical exam are vital.
- Papilledema and nuchal rigidity are helpful signs.
- Obtain CBC, erythrocyte sedimentation rate (ESR), and CT/MRI to narrow the differential.
- If CT/MRI is negative, consider lumbar puncture (LP).

TREATMENT

- Varies with particular diagnosis, and should be directed at the underlying etiology
- Techniques to lower ICP acutely are as follows:
  1. Intubation and subsequent hyperventilation results in cerebral vasoconstriction, effective for about 30 minutes.
  2. Elevating the head 15 to 30 degrees facilitates venous return.
  3. Hyperosmolar agents such as mannitol facilitate a fluid shift from the brain to the intravascular compartment.
  4. Extraventricular drain provides temporarary relief and can provide continuous monitoring of ICP.

ANEURYSMS

- Most aneurysms in childhood are related to focal congenital weakness of the elastic and muscular layers in the cerebral arteries.
- Saccular aneurysms are the most common type.
- More likely to rupture in patients < 2 years of age or > 10 years
- Early warning signs are headaches or localized cranial nerve compression.
- More common in males 2:1.
- Familial occurrence is common.

PRESENTATION

- The most common presentation is with a subarachnoid hemorrhage.
- Early warning signs include headache and focal neurologic deficits due to localized nerve compression.

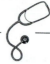

Normal ICP
- Newborns: 6 mm Hg
- Children: 6–13 mm Hg
- Adolescents/adults: 0–15 mm Hg

Any time you see papilledema, *think:* Increased ICP.

A classic textbook finding due to compression of the brain stem is **Cushing's triad:**
1. Decreased respiratory rate
2. Decreased heart rate
3. Increased BP (actually seen in 20–30%)

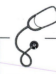

MRI is the best test for a posterior fossa tumor.

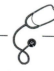

Never perform an LP if papilledema is present.

ETIOLOGY

Most often are related to a congenital disease:
- Ehlers–Danlos syndrome
- AVMs
- Coarctation of the aorta
- Polycystic kidney disease (likely develop secondary to hypertension in this condition); called *berry aneuryms*

Acquired aneurysms are most often related to bacterial endocarditis:
- Embolization of bacteria results in mycotic aneurysms in the cerebral vasculature.
- Twenty-five percent present with bleeding, such as a subarachnoid or intraparenchymal hemorrhage.

DIAGNOSIS

- Angiography is the gold standard for aneurysms in both children and adults.
- MR angiography may also be used and is becoming more reliable.

TREATMENT

If ruptured, surgical clipping or endovascular coiling within 2 days of hemorrhage is the treatment of choice as the risk of rebleeding is significant.

Subarachnoid hemorrhage can present as subacute or repeated headaches.

Relatively more children have aneurysms in the vertebrobasilar circulation (23%) compared to adults (12%).

ARTERIOVENOUS MALFORMATIONS (AVMs)

True AVMs consist of an admixture of both arteries and veins and can vary greatly in size from several millimeters to several centimeters. The larger ones create a significant atrioventricular (AV) shunt and considerable damage if they rupture.

PRESENTATION

- Small unruptured malformations present with headache or seizures.
- Larger malformations may present with progressive neurologic deficit.
- Hemorrhage is more often than not the initial finding, either with a subarachnoid hemorrhage or a smaller leak.

DIAGNOSIS

- Angiography is the test of choice and is required to direct the future therapy.
- MRI or CT with contrast can demonstrate an AV malformation but provide less information than angiography.

COMMON AVM VARIANTS

Vein of Galen Malformations
- Consists of a large shunt between the cerebral arteries and the vein of Galen.
- Typically present during infancy with high-output congestive heart failure (CHF) and failure to thrive.
- Mortality is 50%.
- Treatment is difficult, but surgery is currently the standard.

Cavernous Hemangiomas
- Low-flow AVM with tendency to leak but not cause large-scale intracerebral hemorrhage.
- Seizure is the most common presentation.
- "Popcorn" appearance on MRI.
- Surgical resection is indicated if symptomatic.

Venous Angiomas

- Rarely symptomatic (seizures are the most common presenting sign).
- Surgery is not indicated unless complications arise.

TREATMENT

- Treatment consists of surgical resection or embolization.
- Focused gamma knife radiation has some benefit in smaller lesions.

STROKE

EPIDEMIOLOGY

Hemiplegia in children secondary to vascular disorders occurs with an incidence of 1 to 3:100,000 per year.

ETIOLOGY

- The cause of stroke is established in ~75% of children.
- Pediatric causes of stroke differ from those in the adult population.
- Types of stroke include:
  - Arterial and venous thrombosis
  - Intracranial hemorrhage
  - Arterial embolism
  - A variety of other conditions

CLINICALLY RELEVANT TYPES OF STROKE

Arterial Thrombosis/Embolism

- Thrombosis of the internal carotid artery may occur due to blunt trauma of the posterior pharynx, often due to a fall with an object such as a pencil in the child's mouth.
  - Results in a tear in the intima and subsequent dissection.
  - Cerebral symptoms such as a progressive hemiplegia, lethargy, or aphasia result from the shedding of small emboli into the carotid circulation.
  - Seizures are the most common presenting symptom.
- A retropharyngeal abscess presents with a similar presentation, except inflammation of the intima is the etiology.
- Cardiac abnormalities such as arrhythmias, myxoma, paradoxical emboli through a patent foramen ovale, and septic emboli from bacterial endocarditis.

Venous Thrombosis

- May be subdivided into septic and nonseptic causes.
- Septic causes include bacterial meningitis, otitis media, and mastoiditis.
- Aseptic causes are numerous and include severe dehydration, hypercoagulable states, and congenital heart disease.
- Neonates present with diffuse neurologic signs and seizures.
- In children, focal neurologic signs are more common.

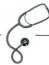

Gamma knife radiation typically takes up to 2 years to see resolution of the AV malformation, during which time the patient is at risk for hemorrhage; thus, surgery is the treatment of choice.

Cardiac abnormalities are the most common cause of thromboembolic stroke in children.

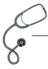

History and physical exam are critical to search for the etiology.

A typical workup for a stroke syndrome will include head CT or MRI scan, followed by an angiogram (if the CT/MRI is nondiagnostic), and a cardiac echo to exclude cardiac causes.

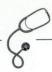

Low-molecular-weight heparin has been shown to be safe, effective, and well tolerated in children.

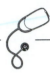

The extent of brain damage directly attributable to impact is the most important prognostic factor.

See Table 17-8 for a comparison of subdural and epidural hematomas.

Subdural Hematoma

EPIDEMIOLOGY

The most frequent focal brain injury in sports and the most common form of sports-related intracranial hemorrhage. Seen most often in infants, with a peak at 6 months.

ETIOLOGY

- Occurs when a bridging vein is torn between the dura and the brain.
- Skull fracture is seen in 30%.
- Typically frontoparietal location.
- Seventy-five percent are bilateral.

SIGNS AND SYMPTOMS

- Seizures in 60–90%
- Retinal and preretinal hemorrhages common
- Increased ICP (irritability, lethargy, vomiting, papilledema, headache)

DIAGNOSIS

Gold standard is CT scan.

Epidural Hematoma

EPIDEMIOLOGY

Seen most often in children > 2 years of age.

TABLE 17-8. Features of acute epidural and subdural hematomas.

	Epidural	Subdural
Supratentorial		
Frequency	Less common	More common
Skull fracture	70%	30%
Source of hemorrhage	Arterial or venous	Venous
Age	> 2 years	< 2 years
Location	Temporoparietal	Frontoparietal
Seizures	< 25%	75%
Mortality	High	Low
Morbidity	Low	High
Infratentorial		
Frequency	More common	Less common
Skull fracture	Almost always	Frequent
Source of hemorrhage	Venous	Venous

ETIOLOGY

- Most commonly results from a fracture in the temporal bone, lacerating the middle meningeal artery.
- Skull fracture is seen in 70%.
- Nearly always unilateral.

SIGNS AND SYMPTOMS

- Classic progression involves an initial loss of consciousness, followed by a lucid interval, and then abrupt deterioration and death (not as helpful in younger children).
- Seizures in < 25%.
- Retinal and preretinal hemorrhages are not common.
- Increased ICP is seen (irritability, lethargy, vomiting, papilledema, headache).

DIAGNOSIS

Gold standard is CT scan.

TREATMENT

Epidural hematomas may progress rapidly, and immediate neurosurgical treatment is indicated.

Coup/Contrecoup Injuries

Cerebral contusion injury mainly occurs when the head is subjected to a sudden acceleration or deceleration.

Coup Injuries
- Located directly at the point of impact
- More common in acceleration injuries such as being hit with a baseball bat

Contrecoup Injuries
- Located opposite (180 degrees) from the point of impact
- More common in deceleration injuries, such as striking one's head on the pavement after a fall

Diffuse Axonal Injury

EPIDEMIOLOGY

- Occurs in 50% of severe head injury cases.
- Causes 35% of all head injury deaths.
- Survivors often have substantial long-term cognitive and behavioral morbidity.

ETIOLOGY

- Impact results in diffuse white matter damage to the brain.
- A result of shearing forces within the brain secondary to differential movement of brain regions due to their different densities

LOCATION

- Most often occur at the cortical/white matter junction of the frontal and parietal lobes.
- The corpus callosum, brain stem, and basal ganglia are the other common locations of damage.

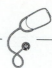

Subdural hematomas appear crescent shaped (concave) on CT and will not cross the midline, but will cross ipsilateral suture lines.

Lucid interval. *Think:* Epidural hematoma.

Epidural hematomas appear lens shaped (convex) on CT and will not cross the midline or other cranial sutures.

Old contusions develop an orange color secondary to hemosiderin deposition and are referred to as *plaques jaunes* by pathologists.

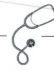

Contrecoup injuries tend to be more severe than coup injuries.

IMAGING

CT scan is usually unremarkable, with only 10% showing abnormalities.

HYDROCEPHALUS

PHYSIOLOGY

- CSF is made by the choroid plexus in the walls of the lateral, third, and fourth ventricles.
- CSF flows in the following direction: lateral ventricles → foramen of Monro → third ventricle → cerebral aqueduct → fourth ventricle → foramena of Magendie and Luschka → subarachnoid space of spinal cord and brain → arachnoid villi.
- CSF is absorbed primarily by the arachnoid villi through tight junctions.

ETIOLOGY

Obstructive (Noncommunicating) Hydrocephalus
- Most commonly due to stenosis or narrowing of the aqueduct of Sylvius.
- An obstruction in the fourth ventricle is a common cause in children, including posterior fossa brain tumors, Arnold–Chiari malformations (type II), and the Dandy–Walker syndrome.

Nonobstructive (Communicating) Hydrocephalus
- Most commonly follows a subarachnoid hemorrhage.
- Blood in the subarachnoid spaces may obliterate the cisterns or arachnoid villi and obstruct CSF flow.
- Meningitis and intrauterine infections are two other common causes.

Ex Vacuo
Hydrocephalus resulting from decreased brain parenchyma.

CLINICAL MANIFESTATIONS

Infants
- Accelerated rate of enlargement of the head is most prominent sign.
- Bulging anterior fontanelle (fontanelles can provide some pressure relief in infants, delaying symptoms of increased ICP).
- Upper motor neuron signs such as a positive Babinski and brisk reflexes are common findings due to stretching of the descending cortical spinal tract.
- Increased ICP signs (lethargy, vomiting, headache, etc.) may be present.
- Ocular bobbing

Children and Adolescents
- Signs are more subtle because the cranial sutures are partially closed.
- Increased ICP signs may be present.
- A gradual change in school performance may be the first clue to a slowly obstructing lesion.

DIAGNOSIS
- As always, a detailed history and physical exam is key to discovering the underlying etiology.
- Ultrasound and head CT/MRI are the most important studies to identify the cause of hydrocephalus.
- Familial cases of aqueductal stenosis have been reported and have an X-linked pattern of inheritance.

- Neurofibromatosis and meningitis have also been linked to aqueductal stenosis.
- A cranial bruit is often present with vein of Galen malformations.

TREATMENT

- Medical management with acetazolamide (may decrease CSF production) and furosemide may provide temporary relief.
- Placement of an extraventricular drain (EVD) or ventriculoperitoneal shunt (VPS), if the etiology is permanent, may be required.

NEOPLASMS

Pediatric Brain Tumors

EPIDEMIOLOGY

- Two thirds of intracranial tumors are located in the posterior fossa.
- Glial cell tumors are the most common tumors in childhood and consist of astrocytomas and ependymomas.
- Medulloblastoma is a primitive neuroectodermal tumor (PNET) common only in childhood.

CLINICAL MANIFESTATIONS

- Generally present with either signs and symptoms of increased ICP or with focal neurologic signs.
- Alterations in personality are often the first symptoms of a brain tumor.
- Nystagmus is the classic finding in posterior fossa tumors.
- Tumors in the posterior fossa tend to result in hydrocephalus secondary to CSF flow obstruction.

INFRATENTORIAL TUMORS

Cerebellar Astrocytoma

- The most common posterior fossa tumor of childhood.
- Histologically shows fibrillary astrocytes with dense cytoplasmic inclusions called Rosenthal fibers.
- Good prognosis, 5-year survival > 90%.
- Treatment is surgical resection.

Medulloblastoma (PNET)

- The second most common posterior fossa tumor and the most prevalent brain tumor in children under the age of 7 years.
- Tends to invade the fourth ventricle and spread along CSF pathways.
- Histologic analysis shows deeply staining nuclei with scant cytoplasm arranged in pseudorosettes.
- "Drop metastases" occur in medulloblastoma, seeding the spinal cord from the fourth ventricle.
- Treatment consists of surgical resection followed by irradiation.
- Prognosis is dependent on size and dissemination of the tumor, but most studies show 5-year survival rates of > 80%.

Craniopharyngioma

- One of the most common supratentorial brain tumors of childhood.
- Short stature or other endocrine associated problems are common initial signs.
- Typically slow growing and benign.

Glioblastoma multiforme (GBM) is a high-grade glioma common in adults but rare in children.

Rosenthal fibers are also seen in Alexander's disease, a progressive leukodystrophy with mental retardation, spasticity, and megalencephaly.

HIGH-YIELD FACTS

Neurologic Disease

- The tumor may be confined to the sella turcica or extend through the diaphragma sellae and compress the optic nerve or, rarely, obstruct CSF flow.
- Due to location, surgical resection is often subtotal.

DIAGNOSIS

- Ninety percent of craniopharyngiomas show calcification on CT scan; MRI provides better images of surrounding structures.
- Baseline endocrine studies and visual fields should be done prior to surgery.

Neurofibromatosis (NF)

EPIDEMIOLOGY

Both types display autosomal recessive inheritance patterns.
- **Type 1:** The most prevalent type (~90%) with an incidence of 1:4,000 (chromosome 17)
- **Type 2:** Account for 10% of all cases of NF, with an incidence of 1:50,000 (chromosome 22)

CLINICAL MANIFESTATIONS

Type 1

- Diagnosis is made by the presence of two or more of the following:
  - Six or more café-au-lait macules (must be > 5 mm prepuberty, > 15 mm postpuberty)
  - Axillary or inguinal freckling
  - Two or more iris Lisch nodules (melanocytic hamartomas)
  - Two or more neurofibromas
  - A characteristic osseous lesion (sphenoid dysplasia, thinning of long bone cortex)
  - Optic glioma
  - A first-degree relative with confirmed NF-1
- Learning disabilities, abnormal speech development, and seizures are common.
- Patients are at a higher risk for other tumors of the CNS such as meningiomas and astrocytomas (but not as significantly as in NF-2)

Type 2

- Diagnosis is made when one of the following is present:
  - Bilateral CN VIII masses
  - A parent or sibling with the disease and either a neurofibroma, meningioma, glioma, or schwannoma
- Café-au-lait spots and skin neurofibromas are not common findings.
- Patients are at significantly higher risk for CNS tumors than in NF-1 and typically have multiple tumors.

TREATMENT

Treatment is mainly aimed at preventing future complications and early detection of malignancies.

Tuberous Sclerosis

EPIDEMIOLOGY

- Inherited as an autosomal dominant trait, with a frequency of 1:6,000.
- Fifty percent are new mutations.

About 50% of NF-1 results from new mutations. Parents should be carefully screened before counseling on the risk to future children.

NF-1: café-au-lait spots, childhood onset
NF-2: bilateral acoustic neuromas, teenage onset, multiple CNS tumors

Café-au-lait is French for "coffee with milk," which is the color of these lesions.

Prenatal diagnosis and genetic confirmation of diagnosis is available in familial cases of both NF-1 and NF-2, but not new mutations.

PATHOLOGY

- Characteristic brain lesions consist of tubers, which are located in the convolutions of the cerebrum, where they undergo calcification and project into the ventricles.
- There are two recognized genes: TSC1 on chromosome 9, encoding a protein called hamartin; and TSC2 on chromosome 16, encoding a protein called tuberin.
- Two additional genes, TSC3 on chromosome 12 and TSC4 on chromosome 11, are identified as additional putative loci causing the disease.
- Tubers may obstruct the foramen of Monro, leading to hydrocephalus.

CLINICAL MANIFESTATIONS

- "Ash leaf" skin lesions (hypopigmented regions) are seen in 90% and are best viewed under a Wood's lamp (violet/ultraviolet light source).
- CT scan shows calcified hamartomas (tubers) in the periventricular region.
- Seizures and infantile spasms are common.
- Adenoma sebaceum—small, raised papules resembling acne that develop on the face between 4 and 6 years of age—actually are small hamartomas.
- A Shagreen patch (rough, raised lesion with an orange-peel consistency in the lumbar region) is also a classic finding; typically does not develop until adolescence.
- Fifty percent of children also have rhabdomyomas of the heart, which may lead to CHF or arrhythmias.
- Hamartomas of the kidneys and the lungs are also frequently present.

DIAGNOSIS

- A high index of suspicion is needed, but all children presenting with infantile spasms should be carefully assessed for skin and retinal lesions.
- CT or MRI will confirm the diagnosis.
- Genetic testing is available for mutations in TSC1 and TSC2.

Neuroblastoma (NB)

EPIDEMIOLOGY

- A common tumor of neural crest origin, representing the most common neoplasm in infants and 8% of all childhood malignancies.
- Ninety percent are diagnosed before age 5, with a peak at 2 years.

PATHOGENESIS

NB is a small, round blue cell tumor with varying degrees of neuronal differentiation.

CLINICAL PRESENTATION

- The tumor may arise at any site of sympathetic nervous tissue.
- The abdomen, adrenals, and retroperitoneal sympathetic ganglia are the most common sites.
- Thirty percent arise in the cervical or thoracic region and may present with Horner's syndrome.
- Opsoclonus–myoclonus—"dancing eyes, dancing feet"—is the telltale symptom of this disease.

DIAGNOSIS

- Typically, a mass is seen on CT or MRI.
- Ninety-five percent of cases have elevated tumor markers, most often homovanillic acid (HVA) and vanillylmandelic acid (VMA) in the urine.

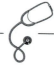

In general, the younger that a child presents with signs and symptoms, the greater the likelihood of mental retardation.

Tuberous sclerosis is the most common cause of infantile spasms, an ominous seizure pattern in infants.

Hamartoma: a tumor-like overgrowth of tissue normally found in the area surrounding it.

Infants tend to have localized NB in the cervical or thoracic region, whereas older children tend to have disseminated abdominal disease.

- MIBG (metaiodobenzylguanidine) radioisotope scan for detecting small primaries and metastases.
- Stage 4s—infantile form, self-limited with good prognosis.

von Hippel–Lindau Disease

DEFINITION

A neurocutaneous syndrome affecting many organs, including the cerebellum, spinal cord, medulla, retina, kidneys, pancreas, and epididymis.

SIGNS AND SYMPTOMS

The major neurologic manifestations are:
- **Cerebellar hemagioblastomas:** present in early adult life with signs of increased ICP
- **Retinal angiomata:** small masses of thin-walled capillaries in the peripheral retina

Renal carcinoma is the most common cause of death associated with von Hippel–Lindau disease.

Neurologic Disease

CONGENITAL MALFORMATIONS

Agenesis of the Corpus Callosum

- Associated with numerous syndromes and several inborn errors of metabolism, including patients with lissencephaly, Dandy–Walker syndrome, Arnold–Chiari type 2 malformations, and Aicardie syndrome.
- Imaging techniques reveal that the lateral ventricles are shifted laterally.
- Normal intelligence is not unusual, and often only mild clinical signs are seen.
- The severity of the disease varies greatly, from only mild deficits to marked retardation and severe epilepsy.

Syringomyelia

- A slowly progressive cavity formation within the brain or spinal cord, most often in the cervical or lumbar regions.
- Thought to arise from incomplete closure of the neural tube during the fourth week of gestation.
- MRI is the test of choice for diagnosis.
- Often develops post-traumatically in the setting of an undiagnosed Chiari I malformation or tethered cord.
- Symptoms include bilateral impaired pain and temperature sensation due to decussation of these fibers near the central canal.

Typical Scenario

A teenage girl has a headache and a cape-like distribution of pain and temperature sensory loss that developed after a minor motor vehicle accident. *Think:* Cervical syringomyelia with undiagnosed Chiari I.

Dandy–Walker Malformation

- Results from a developmental failure of the roof of the fourth ventricle to form, resulting in a cystic expansion into the posterior fossa.
- Ninety percent of patients have hydrocephalus.
- Agenesis of the cerebellar vermis and corpus callosum is also common.
- Infants present with a rapid increase in head size.
- Management is via shunting of the cystic cavity to prevent hydrocephalus.

Arnold–Chiari Malformations

- Four variations exist (see Figure 17-3), with type 2 being the most common, in which the cerebellum and medulla are shifted caudally, resulting in crowding of the upper spinal column.
- Type 2 is also associated with meningomyelocele in > 95% of cases.
- Syringomyelia is associated in 70% of type 1, and 20–50% overall.
- Management includes close observation with serial MRIs and surgery as required.

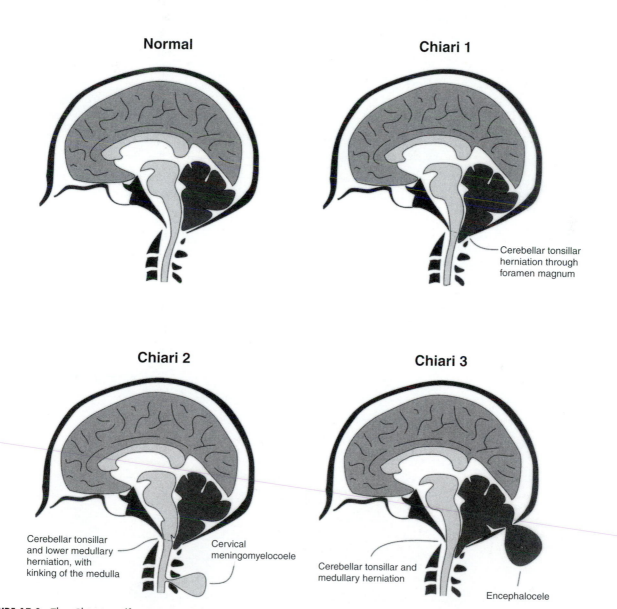

Normal

Chiari 1

Cerebellar tonsillar herniation through foramen magnum

Chiari 2

Cerebellar tonsillar and lower medullary herniation, with kinking of the medulla

Cervical meningomyelocoele

Chiari 3

Cerebellar tonsillar and medullary herniation

Encephalocele

FIGURE 17-3. The Chiari malformations. Schematic representations of the Chiari malformations. Commonly associated hydrocephalus and syringomyelia not depicted. (Artwork by S. Matthew Stead.)

Special Organs—Eye, Ear, Nose

Amblyopia

DEFINITION

A decrease in visual acuity in one or both eyes caused by blurred retinal images, which leads to failure of the visual cortex to develop properly.

ETIOLOGY

- Strabismus
- Refractive errors
- Opacity in the visual path (e.g., cataract)

DIAGNOSIS

Diagnosis is made by visual acuity testing.

TREATMENT

- Removal of the pathology such as a cataract
- Prescription glasses to correct refractive errors
- Patching the good eye until the ambylopic eye has improved its vision

Strabismus

DEFINITION

Deviation or misalignment of the eye (see Figure 18-1).

DIAGNOSIS

- Corneal light reflex: The child looks directly into a light source and the doctor observes where the reflex lies in both eyes; if the light is off center in one pupil or asymmetric, then strabismus exists.

Amblyopia has been called "lazy eye."

Strabismus is the most common cause of amblyopia.

For the best results, amblyopia should be treated by age 4.

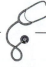

A deviated eye is described as being turned "eso" (inward), "exo" (outward), "hypo" (downward), or "hyper" (upward).

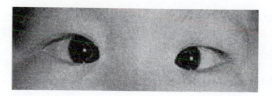

FIGURE 18-1. Child with strabismus.

- Cover–uncover test: The child stares at an object in the distance and the doctor covers one of the child's eyes; if there is movement of the uncovered eye once the other eye is covered, then strabismus exists.

TREATMENT

- Prescription glasses may help if the strabismus is secondary to refraction.
- Eye muscle surgery may be necessary.

Optic Neuritis

DEFINITION

Inflammation of the optic nerve.

ETIOLOGY

- Extension from an infection involving the teeth, sinuses, or meninges
- Side effect of treatment with vincristine or chloramphenicol
- Secondary to a toxin such as lead
- Associated with viral diseases such as measles, chickenpox, influenza, Guillain–Barré

SIGNS AND SYMPTOMS

- Loss of vision
- Pain with extraocular motion
- Pain to palpation of the globe

COMPLICATIONS

- Color deficits
- Motion perception deficits
- Brightness sense deficits

TREATMENT

A trial of intravenous (IV) steroids may decrease the length of time for symptoms but has no effect on the outcome.

In children, optic neuritis is rarely associated with multiple sclerosis.

Conjunctivitis

DEFINITION

Inflammation of the conjunctiva.

TYPES

Allergic

- Immunoglobulin E (IgE)-mediated reaction caused by triggers such as pollen or dust.
- Signs and symptoms include watery, itchy, red eyes with edema to the conjunctiva and lids.
- Treatment includes removal of the trigger, cold compresses, and antihistamines.

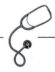

Adenovirus is the most common viral cause of conjunctivitis.

Viral

- Adenovirus and coxsackievirus are typical causes.
- Signs and symptoms include watery, red eyes with preauricular lymph nodes.
- Treatment includes supportive treatment with constant hand washing to prevent transmission.

Conjunctivitis with lymph nodes. *Think:* Viral etiology.

Bacterial

- *Haemophilus influenzae* and *Streptococcus pneumoniae* are typical causes.
- Signs and symptoms include a mucopurulent discharge, red eyes, and edema of the conjunctiva.
- Treat with topical antibiotics.

Episcleritis/Scleritis

DEFINITION

Inflammation of the episclera or sclera.

ETIOLOGY

High association with autoimmune diseases.

SIGNS AND SYMPTOMS

- Eye pain.
- Photophobia.
- Erythema.
- Perforation is associated only with scleritis.

TREATMENT

- Topical steroids
- Nonsteroidal anti-inflammatory drugs (NSAIDs)
- Surgery for thinning or perforated sclera

Episcleritis/scleritis is usually unilateral.

Blepharitis

DEFINITION

Inflammation of the eyelid margins.

ETIOLOGY

- *Staphylococcus aureus*
- *Staphylococcus epidermidis*
- Seborrheic
- A combination of the above

SIGNS AND SYMPTOMS

- Burning
- Itching
- Erythema
- Scaling
- Ulceration of the lid margin

TREATMENT

- Daily eyelid cleansing to remove scales
- Topical antibiotics

Dacryostenosis

DEFINITION

A congenital nasolacrimal duct obstruction.

EPIDEMIOLOGY

Occurs in 5% of infants; appears a few weeks after birth.

ETIOLOGY

Failure of the epithelial cells of tear duct to come apart.

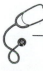

Dacryostenosis is the most common disorder of the lacrimal system.

SIGNS AND SYMPTOMS

- Chronic tearing.
- Erythema occurs secondary to rubbing the tears.

COMPLICATIONS

Dacrocystitis—inflammation of the nasolacrimal sac; this must be treated with topical or systemic antibiotic and warm compresses.

TREATMENT

- Digital massage of the lacrimal sac
- Eyelid cleansing
- Probing if still present after 1 year of age to rupture the membrane

Chalazion

DEFINITION

Inflammation of a meibomian gland leading to the formation of a granuloma.

SIGNS AND SYMPTOMS

- Firm nodule on the eyelid
- Nontender

TREATMENT

- Warm compresses
- Excision if necessary
- Most subside spontaneously over months

Hordeolum

TYPES

- **External hordeolum,** or stye, is an infection of the glands of Zeis or Moll.
- **Internal hordeolum** is infection of the meibomian gland.

ETIOLOGY

S. aureus.

SIGNS AND SYMPTOMS

- Localized swelling
- Tenderness
- Erythema

TREATMENT

- Warm compresses
- Topical antibiotics (e.g., erythromycin)
- Incision and drainage if there is no spontaneous rupture

Orbital Cellulitis

DEFINITION

Inflammation of the orbital tissues behind the septum.

ETIOLOGY

- Extension of a local infection including paranasal sinusitis, facial cellulitis, or dental abcess.
- Trauma.
- The most common organisms are *H. influenza, S. aureus,* and *S. pneumoniae.*

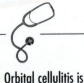

SIGNS AND SYMPTOMS

- Painful extraocular motion
- Proptosis
- Decreased vision
- Erythema
- Edema

COMPLICATIONS

- Loss of vision
- Meningitis
- Central nervous system (CNS) abscess

TREATMENT

Intravenous antibiotics.

Periorbital Cellulitis

DEFINITION

Inflammation of the eyelids and periorbital tissue anterior to the septum.

ETIOLOGY

- Extension of local infections including upper respiratory infection (URI), sinusitis, facial cellulitis, or eyelid infection
- Trauma

SIGNS AND SYMPTOMS

- Erythema
- Edema
- No pain with extraocular movements

COMPLICATIONS

Development of an orbital cellulitis.

TREATMENT

Oral or IV antibiotics (e.g., ceftriaxone).

Corneal Ulcer

ETIOLOGY

- Trauma (sand, contact lens, etc.) with secondary infection
- Bacterial—*Pseudomonas aeruginosa, Neisseria gonorrhoeae*
- Fungal—especially in contact lens users

SIGNS AND SYMPTOMS

- Corneal haze
- Pain
- Photophobia
- Tearing

COMPLICATIONS

- Perforation
- Scarring
- Blindness

DIAGNOSIS

- Slit-lamp exam
- Scraping of the cornea to identify infectious etiology

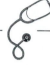

Periorbital cellulitis is preseptal.

The most common organisms causing both preorbital and orbital cellulitis: **SHIP**
S. aureus
H. influenzae
S. pneumoniae

TREATMENT

- Local antibiotics.
- In some cases, systemic treatment may be required.

Retinoblastoma

SIGNS AND SYMPTOMS

- Leukocoria—white pupillary reflex
- Strabismus
- Orbital inflammation
- Hyphema—blood layering anterior to the iris

DIAGNOSIS

- Direct visualization during eye exam.
- Computed tomography (CT) or ultrasound (US) can help confirm and evaluate spread

TREATMENT

- Chemotherapy
- Laser photocoagulation
- Cryotherapy
- Enucleation for unresponsive tumors

EAR

Otitis Media

DEFINITION

Inflammation of the middle ear.

EPIDEMIOLOGY

- The incidence of otitis media is higher in:
  - Boys
  - Daycare children
  - Children exposed to secondhand smoke
  - Non–breast-fed infants
  - Immunocompromised children
  - Children with craniofacial defects like cleft palate
  - Children with a strong family history for otitis media
- The incidence of infection is higher in children because of their eustachian tube anatomy:
  - Horizontal
  - Short in length
  - Decreased tone

ETIOLOGY

- *S. pneumoniae*
- *H. influenzae*
- *Moraxella catarrhalis*

COMPLICATIONS

- Hearing loss
- Perforation
- Mastoiditis
- Cholesteatoma—saclike epithelial structures

The most common cause of leukocoria is a cataract.

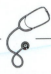

Retinoblastoma is the most common primary malignant intraocular tumor in children.

Family members of a patient with retinoblastoma should be checked because it may be hereditary.

- Facial nerve paralysis—the facial nerve may not be completely covered with bone in the middle ear; therefore, infection can spread to the nerve
- Labyrinthitis
- Abscess formation
- Tympanosclerosis—scarring of the tympanic membrane
- Meningitis

Acute Otitis Media

SIGNS AND SYMPTOMS

- Ear tugging
- Ear pain
- Fever
- Malaise
- Irritability
- Hearing loss
- Nausea and vomiting

DIAGNOSIS

- Diagnosis is made with a pneumatic otoscope—the tympanic membrane will have decreased mobility and will appear hyperemic and bulging with loss of landmarks.
- Tympanocentesis should be used as an adjunct in patients who are < 8 weeks old, are immunodeficient, have a complication, or were treated with multiple courses of antibiotics without improvement; the fluid is sent for culture and sensitivity.

TREATMENT

- Typically, the first-line antibiotic is amoxicillin. High dose can be used for cases most likely to be resistant.
- Antipyretics—ibuprofen and/or acetaminophen.

Recurrent Acute Otitis Media

DEFINITION

Three to four episodes of acute otitis media in 6 months or six episodes in a year.

TREATMENT

- Prophylactic antibiotics.
- Myringotomy and ventilating tubes should be considered.

Otitis Media with Effusion

SIGNS AND SYMPTOMS

- Hearing loss
- Dizziness
- No fever
- No ear pain

DIAGNOSIS

Pneumatic otoscope shows a retracted eardrum with loss of landmarks and air–fluid levels or bubbles.

TREATMENT

- If asymptomatic, a child is observed for 3 months to see if effusion resolves.

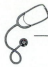

The most common overall complication of otitis media is hearing loss.

The most common intracranial complication of otitis media is meningitis.

Remember that younger children who are unable to communicate may have only nonspecific signs like nausea and vomiting with an acute illness such as acute otitis media.

A red eardrum in a crying child is normal; the most specific sign of acute otitis media is decreased mobility of the tympanic membrane.

Typical Scenario

A 4-year-old boy presents with what looks like herpetic vesicles in the ear canal and tympanic membrane. *Think:* Ramsay–Hunt syndrome. Syndrome includes ipsilateral facial nerve paralysis and loss of taste in the anterior two thirds of the tongue.

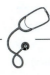

Malignant otitis externa is caused by *P. aeruginosa.*

- If symptomatic after 3 months of observation, treatment includes antibiotics and possibly myringotomy and insertion of tympanostomy tubes.

Otitis Externa

DEFINITION

- Inflammation of the external auditory canal
- Occurs when trauma introduces bacteria into an area that is excessively wet or dry

ETIOLOGY

- Bacterial—*Pseudomonas aeruginosa, S. aureus, Proteus mirabilis, Klebsiella pneumoniae*
- Viral—herpes
- Fungal—*Candida*

SIGNS AND SYMPTOMS

- Ear pain with movement of the pinna
- Pruritus of the ear canal
- Edema of the ear canal
- Otorrhea—usually white in color
- Palpable lymph nodes—peri- and preauricular

COMPLICATIONS

- Malignant otitis externa leads to hearing loss, vertigo, and facial nerve paralysis.
- Temporary hearing loss secondary to swelling.

DIAGNOSIS

Diagnosis is made by otoscopic examination.

TREATMENT

Topical antibiotics and steroids to reduce edema (e.g., Cortisporin ointment [hydrocortisone–polymyxin–neomycin–bacitracin]).

Mastoiditis

DEFINITION

Inflammation of the mastoid cells.

ACUTE MASTOIDITIS

- This condition is mostly seen in children after/with an acute otitis media (see Figure 18-2).
- It typically resolves with the treatment of the otitis.
- If resolution does not occur, it may lead to acute mastoiditis with periosteitis, acute mastoid osteitis, or chronic mastoiditis.

ACUTE MASTOIDITIS WITH PERIOSTEITIS

- Includes the involvement of the periosteum.
- Treatment includes myringotomy with ventilation tube placement and IV antibiotics.

ACUTE MASTOID OSTEITIS

- Occurs when there is destruction of the mastoid cells and empyema is present.
- The child will have a tender, swollen, red mastoid process with his/her ear displaced down and out.

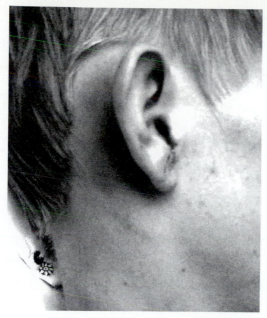

FIGURE 18-2. Child with mastoiditis secondary to otitis media. Note the erythema and swelling behind the ear, which makes the pinna protrude forward.

- Treatment includes IV antibiotics, and mastoidectomy may be necessary.

CHRONIC MASTOIDITIS

Involves treatment with antibiotics and possibly a mastoidectomy if osteitis is present.

Tinnitus

DEFINITION

- Ringing heard in the ear
- Commonly found in children who have middle ear disease or hearing loss

Vertigo

DEFINITION

Dizziness with the feeling that one's body is in motion.

SIGNS AND SYMPTOMS

- Difficulty walking straight or stumbling
- Spinning sensation

ETIOLOGY

May occur secondary to the following conditions:
- Otitis media
- Labyrinthitis
- Trauma
- Cholesteatoma
- Benign positional vertigo
- Ménière's disease
- CNS disease

Benign positional vertigo (BPV) will present with ataxia and horizontal nystagmus.

Ménière's triad includes vertigo, tinnitus, and hearing loss.

Minocycline and quinolones are not used in children because of side effects.

TABLE 18-1. Ototoxic drugs.	
Diuretics	**Furosemide** Ethacrynic acid
Antibiotics	**Aminoglycosides** Gentamicin, erythromycin Minocycline Quinolones
Chemotherapeutics	Cisplatin Vinblastine
Antimalarials	Quinine Chloroquine Mefloquine
Antiarrhythmics	Quinidine
Salicylates	Aspirin

TREATMENT

Address the underlying cause.

Ototoxic Drugs

See Table 18-1.

NOSE

Sinusitis

DEFINITION

Inflammation of the membranes covering the sinuses.

ETIOLOGY

- A child may be at increased risk for sinusitis if there is an obstruction or cilia impairment.
- S. *pneumoniae*.
- H. *influenzae*.
- M. *catarrhalis*.

SIGNS AND SYMPTOMS

- Headache
- Sinus tenderness to palpation
- Nasal discharge
- Halitosis
- Cough secondary to postnasal drip

COMPLICATIONS

- Cellulitis.
- Abscess formation.
- Osteomyelitis.
- Meningitis may occur through spread of the ethmoid, sphenoid, or frontal sinuses.

At birth, only the maxillary and ethmoid sinuses are present.

326

DIAGNOSIS

- Diagnosis is made by physical exam.
- If a test is required, a CT scan is preferred over plain films, which are not as sensitive.

TREATMENT

- Antibiotics (e.g., amoxicllin) for 14 to 21 days.
- If no improvement, a macrolide or amoxicillin–clavulanate may be used.
- Decongestants.
- Nasal saline drops.

Epistaxis

DEFINITION

Nosebleed.

ETIOLOGY

- The most common location for a nosebleed in children is the anterior septum.
- The most common cause is trauma secondary to a fingernail.
- Other causes may include foreign bodies, inflammation, or dry air.
- If a child has recurrent, severe epistaxis, other, more serious causes should be looked into such as thrombocytopenia, clotting deficiencies, and angiofibromas.

SIGNS AND SYMPTOMS

Bleeding may occur from one or both nostrils.

TREATMENT

- Compression for 10 minutes with head tilted forward.
- Cold compresses to the nose.
- Topical vasoconstrictors may allow visualization of the bleeding site.
- Cauterization using silver nitrite.
- Packing the nose.

Allergic Rhinitis

DEFINITION

An IgE-mediated response to an allergen causing an inflammation of the nasal mucous membranes.

SIGNS AND SYMPTOMS

- Sneezing
- Watery nasal discharge
- Red, watery eyes
- Itchy ears, eyes, nose, and throat
- Nasal obstruction secondary to edema

DIAGNOSIS

Characteristic findings on physical exam, including:
- Boggy, bluish mucous membranes of the nose.
- Dark circles under the eyes.
- Allergic salute.
- Rabbit nose.
- A smear of nasal secretions will show a high number of eosinophils.

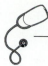

The most common location for epistaxis in children is from the anterior nasal septum, because Kiesselbach's plexus is located there.

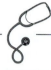

Blood in vomit may be present if a child has swallowed blood from an epistaxis; always ask about epistaxis if a patient presents with hematemesis.

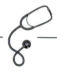

Allergic rhinitis is the most common atopic disease.

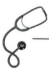

The "allergic salute," seen in allergic rhinitis— horizontal crease on the nose that occurs from constant rubbing.

Children with allergic rhinitis may exhibit rabbit-like nose wrinkling because of pruritus.

TREATMENT

- Avoid triggers.
- Antihistamines.
- Decongestants.
- Cromolyn nasal solution.
- Topical steroids.

Choanal Atresia

DEFINITION

A separation of the nose and pharynx by a membrane or bone (90%); may be unilateral or bilateral.

SIGNS AND SYMPTOMS

- Each child's presentation will differ depending on his or her ability to mouth breathe.
- Respiratory distress that improves as the child cries because the mouth is open.
- Cyanosis, especially when the child is feeding or sucking.

DIAGNOSIS

- Inability to pass a catheter through one or both nostrils.
- CT will show the extent of the atresia.

TREATMENT

- The ultimate treatment is surgical correction.
- Maintaining an open airway by an orogastric tube or large nipple.
- Tracheostomy or intubation may be required depending on the severity.

Nasopharyngeal Carcinoma

ETIOLOGY

Associated with the Epstein–Barr virus.

EPIDEMIOLOGY

- Male-to-female ratio is 2:1.
- Higher incidence in China.
- Children of Asian and North African ancestry are more commonly affected.

SIGNS AND SYMPTOMS

- Cervical adenopathy
- Epistaxis
- Associated with a paraneoplastic syndrome
- Mass placing pressure on surrounding tissues

DIAGNOSIS

- Biopsy
- CT or MRI

TREATMENT

- Surgical resection
- Radiation therapy
- Chemotherapy

Fifty percent of children with choanal atresia have other associated congenital anomalies:
Charge syndrome—
Coloboma
Heart disease
Atresia choanae
Retarded growth
Genital anomalies
Ear involvement

Restenosis of corrected choanal atresia is common.

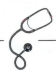

The paraneoplastic syndrome for nasopharyngeal carcinoma includes clubbing, fever, and the syndrome of inappropriate secretion of antiduretic hormone (SIADH).

Musculoskeletal Disease

NORMAL SKELETAL MATURATION

- The growth plate in the newborn is generally not constituted as an effective structure until 12 to 24 months.
- The metaphysis is the most metabolically active area.

PEDIATRIC SKELETON

- The anatomy, biomechanics, and physiology of the child's skeleton are very different when compared to adults, leading to differences in fracture pattern, diagnostic problems, and treatment regimens.
- Bone is more porous and elastic.
- The physis (growth plate) is the weakest site in a child's bone.
- A thick periosteal sleeve makes fractures more stable.
- Remodeling capabilities and rapid healing.

OSTEOMYELITIS

Definition

- Bone infection
- Can be acute (< 2 weeks) or chronic

Epidemiology

- Preschool-age children (50%)
- Male preponderance
- More common in African-American children

Etiology

- Most often bacterial.
- See Table 19-1 for causes of osteomyelitis by age group.
- Overall, *Staphylococcus aureus* is the most common bug.

Pathophysiology

- Primarily hematogenous
- Spread from contiguous infected structures
- Direct inoculation

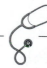

Children with sickle cell disease are prone to *Salmonella* osteomyeltis (but remember the most common cause even in these children is *S. aureus*).

The most common site for osteomyelitis is the rapidly growing end (metaphysis) of long bones.

TABLE 19-1. Causes of osteomyelitis by age.	
Age Group	**Organisms**
Infants < 1 year, especially under age 3 months	Group B streptococci *S. aureus* *E. coli*
1 year–15 years	*S. aureus* Group A streptococci *S. pneumoniae*

Consider osteomyelitis in any child with decreased use of a limb and fever.

A previously ambulatory 18-month-old girl refuses to walk. She has marked tenderness over the distal left femur. Her mother says she fell several times the previous day while playing. The child has a temperature of 101.6°F (38.7°C), erythrocyte sedimentation rate (ESR) of 72 mm/hr, and white blood cell count (WBC) of 18.5. Radiographs reveal no bony abnormalities. *Think:* Osteomyelitis.

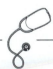

The ESR and CRP can be followed to assess response of osteomyelitis to therapy. They should decrease if treatment is working.

SIGNS AND SYMPTOMS

- Infants and young children:
  - Fever, irritability, and lethargy
  - Refusal to walk or bear weight
- Older children:
  - May localize pain
  - Limping
- Physical examination:
  - Painful local swelling
  - Point tenderness
  - Local warmth
  - Erythema

DIAGNOSIS

- Leukocytosis
- Elevated ESR: sensitive marker for osteomyelitis, mean ~70 mm/hr
- Elevated C-reactive protein (CRP)—peaks at 48 hours
- Growth on blood culture
- Radiographic findings (see Figure 19-1):
  - Lucent areas in bone represent cortical destruction.
  - Periosteal elevation.
  - Plain films may be normal for 7 to 10 days in up to two thirds of children.
- Radionuclide scintigraphy:
  - Common isotopes used include technetium and gallium.
  - Can detect osteomyelitis within 24 to 48 hours of onset with ~90% sensitivity.
  - False positives can occur with any condition that causes inflammation and new bone formation, including trauma, tumors, or soft tissue infections.

DIFFERENTIAL DIAGNOSIS

- Septic arthritis (can coexist)
- Fracture
- Cellulitis
- Toxic synovitis
- Ewing's sarcoma
- Slipped capital femoral epiphysis (SCFE)

TREATMENT

- Admit all children with osteomyelitis.
- Orthopedic consultation.

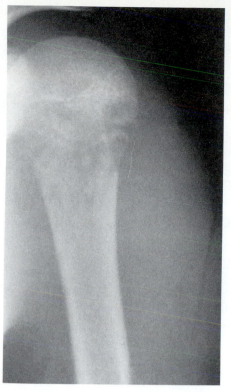

FIGURE 19-1. Acute hematogenous osteomyelitis of the proximal humerus. Mottling and patchy radiolucencies are present in the metaphyseal region. (Reproduced, with permission, from Wilson & Lin, *General Orthopedics.* New York: McGraw-Hill, 1997.)

- Parenteral antibiotics pending cultures (obtain blood, bone, and joint aspirate cultures before antibiotic administration).
- Infants and children: penicillinase-resistant penicillin (oxacillin) and cephalosporin (cefotaxime)
- Older children (> 5 years): nafcillin or vancomycin
- Consider surgical drainage if:
  - Pus is obtained from aspirate
  - No response to 24 to 48 hours of antibiotics

COMPLICATIONS

- Pathologic fractures
- Chronic osteomyelitis
- Leg length discrepancy

SEPTIC ARTHRITIS

DEFINITION

A microbial invasion of joint space.

ETIOLOGY

- Neonates:
  - Group B streptococci
  - *S. aureus*
  - Gram-negative enteric bacilli

Typical Scenario

A 14-year-old boy presents to the emergency department (ED) because of right knee pain for the past 2 days. Three days prior to the onset of the pain, he hit his knee on a pool table. Vitals: Temperature 100.6°F (38.1°C), pulse rate 100, respirations 24. On physical exam, the knee is slightly swollen and tender and is held in flexion. *Think:* The most important initial diagnostic procedure is aspiration of the knee for smear and culture.

Typical Scenario

A 5-year-old boy who has a definite history of penicillin allergy develops osteomyelitis. Smear of the aspirate shows gram-positive cocci in clusters. *Think:* Treat child with vancomycin.

- Older children (very similar to osteomyelitis):
  - *S. aureus*
  - *Streptococcus pyogenes*
  - *Streptococcus pneumoniae*

EPIDEMIOLOGY

Relatively common in infancy and childhood; can occur in all ages.

PATHOPHYSIOLOGY

Organisms may invade the joint by:
- Direct inoculation
- Contiguous spread
- Bacteremia (most common route)

SIGNS AND SYMPTOMS

- Pain
- Joint stiffness
- Erythema
- Edema
- Limp and unable to bear weight

LABORATORY

- Complete blood count (CBC)—a normal WBC does not rule out diagnosis
- Elevated ESR
- Blood culture
- Joint aspiration

MANAGEMENT

- Admit all children with septic arthritis.
- Orthopedic consultation.
- Joint aspiration.
- Parenteral antibiotics immediately after joint aspiration.

COMPLICATIONS

Potential for severe complications:
- Spread—results in osteomyelitis
- Avascular necrosis
- Angular deformities
- Leg length discrepancy

TOXIC SYNOVITIS

DEFINITION

Irritable hip.

ETIOLOGY

- Unclear
- Often follows an upper respiratory infection (URI)

SIGNS AND SYMPTOMS

- Unilateral hip or groin pain is the most common complaint.
- Painful limp.
- Usually afebrile.

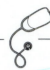

Most common cause of polyarticular septic arthritis is *Neisseria gonorrhoeae*.

Adolescent intravenous (IV) drug abusers are at risk for gram-negative septic arthritis.

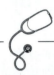

Candida albicans must also be considered in neonates and premature infants with septic arthritis.

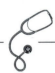

Most cases of septic arthritis occur in weight-bearing joints and involve a single joint (monoarticular).

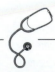

Fever is not necessary for diagnosis of septic arthritis.

Most common mimic of septic arthritis is transient synovitis. Examining the joint aspirate can differentiate.

Diagnosis

- Diagnosis of exclusion.
- Radiographs are usually normal.
- Plain films do not diagnose or exclude a hip effusion.
- The appearance of a septic arthritis of the hip may be identical.

Management

- First, rule out septic arthritis.
- Supportive therapy.
- Nonsteroidal anti-inflammatory drugs (NSAIDs).
- Complete recovery occurs within a few weeks.

OSGOOD-SCHLATTER DISEASE

Definition

Benign, self-limited extra-articular disease.

Etiology

- Traction apophysitis
- Chronic microtrauma to the tibial tuberosity secondary to overuse of the quadriceps muscle

Risk Factors

- Boys between 11 and 18 years of age
- Rapid skeletal growth
- Involvement in repetitive jumping sports

Signs and Symptoms

- Knee pain (tibial tuberosity pain).
- Reproduced by extending the knee against resistance.
- Knee joint examination is normal.
- Tibial tuberosity swelling.
- Absence of effusion or condylar tenderness.

Diagnosis

- Diagnosis is primarily clinical.
- X-ray of the knee may show evidence of fragmentation of the tibial tubercle (see Figure 19-2).

Treatment

- Relative rest
- Restriction of activities as tolerated (patients can still engage in activities even with pain; they will eventually grow out of it)
- Knee immobilizer only for severe cases
- Complete resolution through physeal closure

LEGG-CALVÉ-PERTHES DISEASE

Definition

Avascular necrosis of femoral head.

Etiology

- Idiopathic.
- Some precipitants include sickle cell disease, steroids, trauma, and infection.

Septic arthritis is an orthopedic emergency.

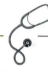

Septic arthritis may coexist with osteomyelitis at sites where the metaphysis lies *within* the joint capsule:

- Proximal femur—hip joint
- Proximal humerus—shoulder joint
- Distal lateral tibia—ankle joint
- Proximal radius—elbow joint

The major consequence of bacterial invasion of a joint is permanent damage to joint cartilage.

Toxic synovitis is the most common cause of limping and acute hip pain in children aged 3 to 10 years.

Osgood–Schlatter disease is a common cause of knee pain in the adolescent.

Typical Scenario

A 16-year-old boy complains of right knee pain. On examination, there is significant tenderness and swelling over the tibial tuberosity. He is otherwise healthy. *Think:* Osgood–Schlatter disease, and treat with activity restriction.

Classic presentation of Legg–Calvé–Perthes disease is a "painless limp."

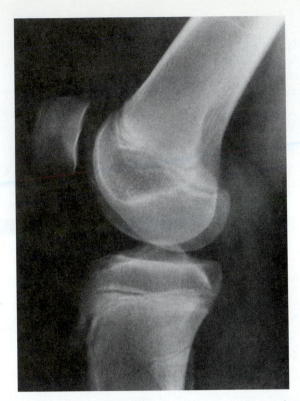

FIGURE 19-2. Osgood–Schlatter disease. Note the elevation and irregularity of the tibal tubercle. (Reproduced, with permission, from Wilson & Lin, *General Orthopedics.* New York: McGraw-Hill, 1997.)

EPIDEMIOLOGY

- Male-to-female ratio: 4:1.
- Highest incidence is during periods of rapid growth of the epiphyses (ages 4–8 years).

SIGNS AND SYMPTOMS

- Insidious onset. Symptoms generally begin with minor trauma.
- Limp.
- Pain (activity related and relieved by rest).
- Limited hip motion, particularly abduction and medial rotation.

RADIOLOGY

- Anteroposterior (AP) and frog-leg lateral position. X-ray findings correlate with the progression and extent of necrosis (see Figure 19-3).
    - Early: Effusion of the joint, widening of the joint space and periarticular swelling.
    - Few weeks: Decreased bone density around the joint, collapse of the femoral head (affected side appears smaller than the unaffected femoral head).
    - Late: New bone replaces necrotic bone.

MANAGEMENT

- Pediatric orthopedic consultation
- Protect joint

COMPLICATIONS

Limb length discrepancy.

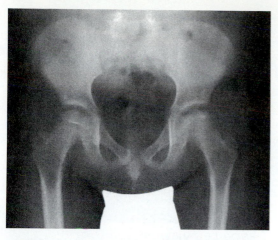
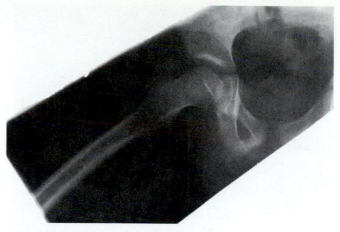

FIGURE 19-3. Radiograph of pelvis demonstrating changes of Legg–Calvé–Perthes disease. Note the sclerotic, flattened, and fragmented right femoral head.

SLIPPED CAPITAL FEMORAL EPIPHYSIS (SCFE)

DEFINITION

- Type of Salter I fracture of the proximal femoral growth plate.
- Displacement of the proximal femoral epiphysis through the physeal plate.
- Epiphysis is usually displaced medially and posteriorly.

ETIOLOGY

- Most cases are idiopathic.
- Weak growth plate (physis is weak prior to closure).
- Local trauma.

TYPES

- Acute (< 3 weeks)
- Chronic (> 3 weeks)

RISK FACTORS

- Obesity
- Hypothyroidism
- Hypogonadism
- Growth hormone administration
- Renal osteodystrophy
- Radiation therapy

SIGNS AND SYMPTOMS

- Pain can be located anywhere between the groin and medial knee.
- Limping.
- Internal rotation, flexion, and abduction are lost.

DIAGNOSIS

- AP and frog-leg lateral of both hips (Figure 19-4).
- Earliest sign is widening of epiphysis.
- Always examine and obtain x-ray of the contralateral hip.

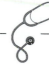

Knee pain in a child warrants a complete hip examination.

Typical Scenario

A 6-year-old boy presents with hip and knee pain. He has been limping. On exam, he is unable to abduct or internally rotate his hip. *Think:* Legg–Calvé–Perthes disease.

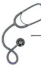

Magnetic resonance imaging (MRI) can reveal avascular necrosis whereas conventional radiographs may appear normal.

335

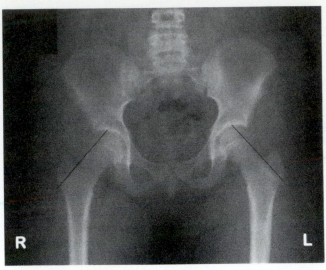

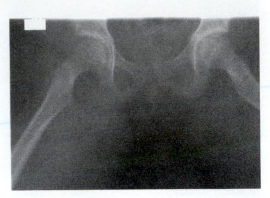

FROG LEG VIEW

ANTERO-POSTERIOR (AP) VIEW

FIGURE 19-4. Hip radiographs in a 13-year-old girl with mildly slipped capital femoral epiphysis (SCFE) on the right. Note on the AP view that a line drawn along the superior border of the femoral neck (Klein line) shows less femoral head superior to the line on the right than it does in the normal hip on the left.

SCFE is the most common orthopedic hip disorder occurring in adolescence.

Typical Scenario

An obese 14-year-old boy has pain in the left anterior thigh for 2 months. On physical exam, there is limited passive flexion and internal rotation of his hip. *Think:* The most likely diagnosis is SCFE.

COMPLICATIONS

- Avascular necrosis of capital femoral epiphysis
- Chondrolysis
- Nonunion
- Premature closure of the epiphyseal plate

TREATMENT

- Orthopedic consultation.
- Internal fixation using central percutaneous pin fixation with one or more cannulated screws is the treatment of choice (Figure 19-5)

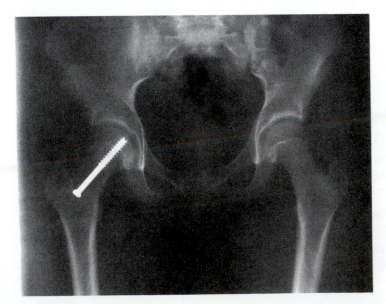

FIGURE 19-5. SCFE after screw fixation (same patient as Figure 18-4).

TENOSYNOVITIS

DEFINITION

Inflammation of the tendon and tendon sheath.

ETIOLOGY

- Trauma
- Overuse

TYPES

- de Quervain tenosynovitis of the wrist (i.e., abductor pollicis longus and extensor pollicis brevis tendons)
- Volar flexor tenosynovitis (i.e., trigger finger)

MANAGEMENT

- Rest
- NSAIDs
- Thumb spica wrist splint

Klein line: On the AP view of the hip, a line drawn along the superior border of the femoral neck should pass through a portion of the femoral head. If not, consider SCFE.

JUVENILE RHEUMATOID ARTHRITIS (JRA)

DEFINITION

Chronic disease characterized by inflammation of the joints.

ETIOLOGY

Unknown.

CLASSIFICATION

- **Polyarticular** (35%)
  - Five or more joints
  - Symmetric distribution
  - Both large and small joints
- **Pauciarticular** (50%)
  - Fewer than five joints
  - Asymmetric distribution
  - Often large weight-bearing joints
  - Iridocyclitis (50%)
- **Systemic** (20%)
  - Fever, rash, arthritis, and visceral involvement

Seek help from your radiology and orthopedic colleagues if clinical suspicion for SCFE is high but the films are negative.

DIAGNOSTIC CRITERIA

- Age of onset under 16 years.
- Arthritis in one or more joints.
- Duration ≥ 6 weeks.
- Exclusion of other causes.
- See Table 19-2 for diagnosis based on joint fluid analysis.

SIGNS AND SYMPTOMS

Polyarticular
- Symmetric, chronic pain and swelling of joints.
- Systemic features are less prominent.
- Long-term arthritis; symptoms wax and wane.

Pauciarticular Disease
- Asymmetric chronic arthritis of a few large joints.
- Systemic features are uncommon.

The most common cause of chest pain in children is costochondritis.

337

TABLE 19-2. Joint fluid analysis.

Disorder	Cells/μL	Glucose
Trauma	RBC > WBC < 2,000 WBC	Normal
Reactive arthritis	2,000–10,000 mononuclear WBC	Normal
Juvenile rheumatoid arthritis	5,000–60,000 WBC, mostly neutrophils	Low to normal
Septic arthritis	> 60,000 WBC > 90% neutrophils	Low to normal

Reproduced, with permission, from Hay et al. *Current Pediatric Diagnosis and Treatment,* 14th ed. New York: McGraw-Hill, 2002.

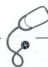
Systemic
- Salmon-pink macular rash.
- Systemic symptoms: arthritis, hepatosplenomegaly, leukocytosis, and polyserositis.
- Episodic, remission of systemic features within 1 year.

TREATMENT

The goal of treatment is to restore function, relieve pain, and maintain joint motion.
- NSAIDs
- Range-of-motion and muscle strengthening exercises
- Methotrexate, anti–tumor necrosis factor (TNF) antibodies, or antipyrimidine medication for patients who do not respond to NSAIDs

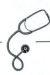
REITER'S SYNDROME

DEFINITION
Triad of asymmetric arthritis, urethritis, and uveitis.

ETIOLOGY
Thought to be a reactive arthritis after infection with gram-negative (*Salmonella, Shigella, Yersinia, Campylobacter, Chlamydia, Mycoplasma,* and *Ureaplasma*) in persons with human lymphocyte antigen (HLA)-B27.

DIAGNOSIS
- Bone density is preserved.
- Proliferative bone formation is present.

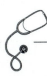
CHILDHOOD FRACTURES (NOT RELATED TO ABUSE)

Torus Fracture (Figure 19-6)
- Buckle fracture
- Impaction injury in children in which the bone cortex is buckled but not disrupted
- Stable fracture

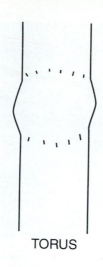

TORUS

FIGURE 19-6. Torus fracture.

Greenstick Fracture (Figure 19-7)

- Angulation beyond the limits of plastic deformation
- Incomplete fracture in which cortex is disrupted on only one side
- Represents bone failure on the tension side and a plastic or bend deformity on the compression side

Toddler Fracture (Figure 19-8)

- Nondisplaced spiral fracture of the tibia.
- Symptoms include pain, refusal to walk, and minor swelling.
- There is often no history of trauma.
- Differential diagnosis should include nonaccidental trauma.
- Treatment consists of immobilization for a few weeks to protect the limb and to relieve pain.

Reiter's Syndrome: Can't pee, can't see, can't climb a tree.

SALTER–HARRIS FRACTURE CLASSIFICATION

See Figure 19-9.

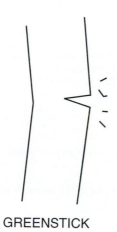

GREENSTICK

FIGURE 19-7. Greenstick fracture.

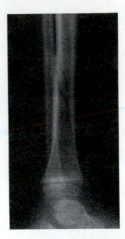

FIGURE 19-8. Toddler fracture. (Reproduced, with permission, from Schwartz & Reisdorff, *Emergency Radiology.* New York: McGraw-Hill, 2000.)

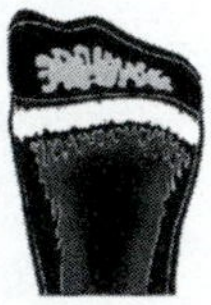

Salter–Harris Type I:
- Fracture through the physis (growth plate only)
- Often seen in children < 5 years
- Only visible radiographically if the physis is widened, distorted, or the epiphysis is distorted

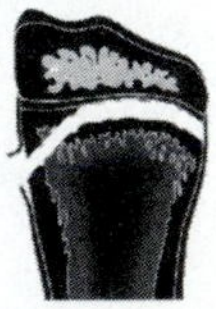

Salter–Harris Type II:
- Through the metaphysis and the physis
- Most common sites are distal radius & tibia

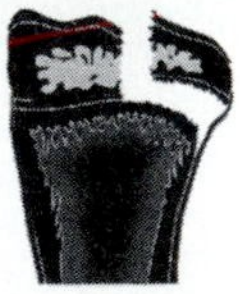

Salter–Harris Type III:
- Through the epiphysis and physis
- Most common sites are knee ankle

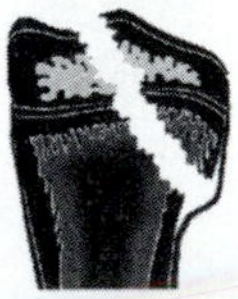

Salter–Harris Type IV:
- Through the epiphysis, physis, and metaphysis
- Most common site is lateral condyle of humerus
- Can produce joint deformity and chronic disability

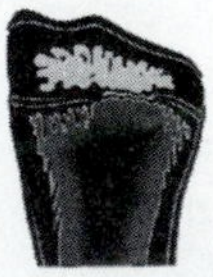

Salter–Harris Type V:
- Crush injury of the physis
- May appear as a narrowing of the growth plate lucency
- Often not radiographically visible
- May lead to premature fusion
- The proximal tibia is the most common site for growth disturbance
- Mechanism is axial compression

FIGURE 19-9. Salter–Harris fracture classification.

DEFINITION

- **Sprain:** Injury to ligament
- **Strain:** Injury to muscle–tendon unit

ANKLE SPRAIN

- **Inversion:** injury to lateral ligament (85%)
  - Anterior talofibular injures first
  - Posterior talofibular—severe pain
- **Eversion:** injury to medial ligament (15%)
  - Deltoid ligament injury most common
  - More severe than inversion

SIGNS AND SYMPTOMS

- Grade I—pain/tenderness without loss of motion
- Grade II—pain/tenderness, ecchymosis with some loss of range of motion
- Grade III—ligament is completely disrupted; pain/tenderness, swelling and ecchymosis, joint instability, and complete loss of range of motion

MANAGEMENT

- The goal of treatment is to decrease local edema and residual stiffness.
- RICE therapy—rest, ice, compression, elevation.
- Protection includes joint immobilization at a right angle, elastic (Ace) bandage wrap, and Jones's dressing for more severe injuries. Splinting the affected joint protects against injury and relieves swelling and pain.
- Crutches and crutch gait training.
- NSAIDs as needed for analgesia.

Sprain is a diagnosis of exclusion in children.

NURSEMAID'S ELBOW

DEFINITION

Subluxation of the radial head.

ETIOLOGY

- Slippage of the head of the radius under the annular ligament.
- Most common cause is axial traction.

EPIDEMIOLOGY

- Common age: 1 to 4 years
- More frequent under 2 years
- Left arm predominance
- Rare after the age of 6 years

SIGNS AND SYMPTOMS

- Suddenly refuses to use an arm
- Elbow fully pronated

DIAGNOSIS

- Diagnosis is made primarily by history.
- Imaging studies are often unnecessary.

MANAGEMENT

- Elbow is placed in full supination and slowly moved from full flexion to full extension.

Typical Scenario

A 2-year-old boy complains of left arm pain. He holds his arm in a flexed pronated position and refuses to supinate his forearm during examination. His mother remembers pulling him by the arm yesterday. *Think:* Subluxation of the radial head (nursemaid's elbow).

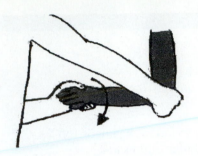

FIGURE 19-10. Reduction of nursemaid's elbow. (Artwork by Elizabeth N. Jacobson.)

- A click at the level of the radial head signifies reduction (see Figure 19-10).
- Relief of pain is remarkable.

OSTEOSARCOMA

DEFINITION

Malignant tumor arising from osteoblasts.

EPIDEMIOLOGY

- The most frequent sites of origin are the metaphyseal regions.
- Most osteosarcomas develop in patients 10 to 20 years of age.
- Osteosarcomas most frequently occur during periods of maximal growth.

SIGNS AND SYMPTOMS

- Bone pain
- Typically long bones (distal femur and proximal tibia) and flat bones (pelvis 10%)

RADIOLOGY

Radiographs show mixed sclerotic and lytic lesion arising in the metaphyseal region, often described as a *sunburst pattern* (Figure 19-11).

MANAGEMENT

Bone tumors generally are sensitive to radiation and chemotherapy. Amputation and limb salvage are effective in achieving local control.

PROGNOSIS

- Three- to ten-year survival is 55–85% (2001 statistics).
- Death is usually due to pulmonary metastasis.

EWING'S SARCOMA

DEFINITION

Malignant tumor of bone arising in medullary tissue.

EPIDEMIOLOGY

- Most common bone lesion in first decade
- Second to osteosarcoma in second decade
- However, still rare—only 200 new cases/year
- Very strong Caucasian and male predilection, hereditary

Osteosarcoma is the most common primary malignant neoplasm of bone (60%).

Osteosarcoma is the sixth most common malignancy in children and the third most common in adolescents.

Typical Scenario

A patient has had dull, aching pain for several months that has suddenly become more severe. *Think:* Osteosarcoma.

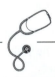

All patients with osteosarcoma should undergo computed tomographic (CT) scanning to detect metastatic pulmonary disease.

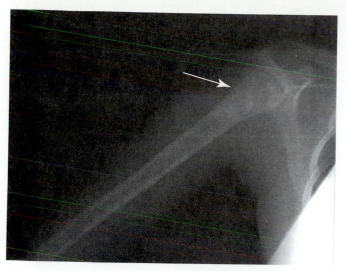

FIGURE 19-11. Osteosarcoma of proximal humerus. Note disorganized appearance of bony cortex (arrow).

SIGNS AND SYMPTOMS

- Bone pain
- Systemic signs: fever, weight loss, fatigue

RADIOLOGY

- Calcified periosteal elevation, termed *onion skin*.
- Radiolucent lytic bone lesions in the diaphyseal region.
- Evaluation of patients with Ewing's sarcoma should include a CT to define the extent of metastatic disease.

TREATMENT

- Radiotherapy
- Chemotherapy
- Surgical resection
- Autologous bone marrow transplant for high-risk patients

PROGNOSIS

Patients with a small localized tumor have a 50–70% long-term disease-free survival rate; patients with metastatic disease have a poor prognosis.

BENIGN BONE TUMORS

Osteoid Osteoma

DEFINITION

Reactive lesion of bone.

SIGNS AND SYMPTOMS

- Pain (evening or at night), relieved with aspirin
- Point tenderness
- Predominantly found in boys

RADIOLOGY

Osteosclerosis surrounds small radiolucent nidus.

Bone pain is a presenting symptom of Ewing's sarcoma in 80–90%.

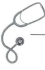

Primary site is split almost evenly between the extremities and central axis.

Typical Scenario

A 10-year-old boy complains of pain in his left leg. On examination, there is localized swelling and pain in the middle of his left femur. His temperature is 100.8°F (38.2°C), and ESR is elevated. Further questioning reveals a 2-month history of increasing fatigue and weight loss. *Think:* Ewing's sarcoma.

Metastasis is present in 25% of patients with Ewing's sarcoma at diagnosis. The most common sites of metastasis are the lungs, bone (spine), and bone marrow.

MANAGEMENT

- Salicylates relieve pain.
- Surgical incision of the nidus is curative.

PROGNOSIS

Prognosis is excellent. There have been no known cases of malignant transformation, although the lesion has been known to reoccur.

Enchondroma

DEFINITION

Cartilaginous lesions.

SIGNS AND SYMPTOMS

- Tubular bones of hands and feet
- Pathologic fractures
- Swollen bone
- Ollier's disease (if multiple lesions are present)

RADIOLOGY

- Radiolucent diaphyseal or metaphyseal lesion.
- Often described as "fingernail streaks in bones."

MANAGEMENT

Surgical curettage and bone grafting.

PROGNOSIS

Prognosis is excellent. Malignant transformation may occur, but is very rare in childhood.

Osteochondroma

DEFINITION

- Most common bone tumor in children
- Disturbance in enchondral growth
- Benign cartilage-capped protrusion of osseous tissue arising from the surface of bone

SIGNS AND SYMPTOMS

- Painless, hard, nontender mass
- Distal metaphysis of femur, proximal humerus, and proximal tibia

RADIOLOGY

Pedunculated or sessile mass in the metaphyseal region of long bones.

MANAGEMENT

Excision if symptomatic.

PROGNOSIS

Prognosis is excellent. Malignant transformation is very rare.

Baker Cysts

DEFINITION

- Herniation of the synovium in the knee joint into the popliteal region.
- A Baker cyst is lined by a true synovium, as it is an extension of the knee joint.

Osteoid osteomas are most common in the femur and tibia.

Enchondromas have a predilection for the phalanges.

Baker cysts are the most common mass in the popliteal fossa.

It is important to exclude deep vein thrombosis (DVT) in patients with a popliteal cyst and leg swelling.

SIGNS AND SYMPTOMS

- Popliteal mass
- Commonly transilluminates

DIAGNOSIS

Aspiration of mucinous fluid from popliteal fossa.

MANAGEMENT

- Baker's cysts are benign.
- Nearly always disappears with time in children.
- Avoid surgery (only for significant pain).

DEVELOPMENTAL DYSPLASIA OF THE HIP (DDH)

DEFINITION

Abnormal growth and development of the hip resulting in an abnormal relationship between the proximal femur and the acetabulum.

EPIDEMIOLOGY

- 1:1,000 live births
- 10-fold increased risk in sibling of child with DDH
- Female > male

PATHOPHYSIOLOGY

- At birth there is a lack of development of both acetabulum and femur
- Progressive with growth
- Reversible if corrected in first few days or weeks

SIGNS AND SYMPTOMS

Newborn
- Ortolani—reduction maneuver
- Barlow—provocative test
- Asymmetric skin folds (40%)

3 to 6 Months
- Limited abduction
- Allis or Galeazzi sign—knee is lower on affected side when hips flexed

12 Months (Unilateral Dislocation)
Trendelenburg sign—painless limp and lurch to the affected side with ambulation. When the child stands on the affected leg, there is a dip of the pelvis on the opposite side, due to a weakness of the gluteus medius muscle.

12 Months (Bilateral Dislocation)
- Waddling gait
- Lumbar lordosis due to flexion contractures

TREATMENT

- Newborn to 6 months: Pavlik harness (flexion and abduction of the hip)
- 6 months to 3 years: skin traction for 3 weeks to relax soft tissues around the hip prior to closed or open reduction
- > 3 years: operations to correct deformities of the acetabulum and femur

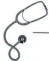

Associated anomalies with DDH:
- Torticollis
- Clubfeet
- Metatarsus adductus

Typical Scenario

While doing a physical exam on a 3-month-old female infant, the physician notices that her left knee is lower when her hips are flexed. The infant was born to a P1G1 mother via a breech vaginal delivery. *Think:* DDH.

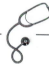

Ortolani test: Slowly abduct flexed hip. The femoral head will shift into the acetabulum producing a clunk.
Barlow test: Dislocate the hip by flexing and adducting the hip with axial pressure.

In DDH, after 3 to 6 months, muscle contractures develop, and the Barlow and Ortolani tests become negative.

X-ray is not helpful in the newborn. After 6 to 8 weeks, x-rays begin to show signs of dislocation (lateral displacement of the femoral head).

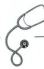

Signs of instability are more reliable than x-ray in DDH.

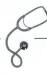

Double or triple diapers are not adequate to obtain a proper position and are no longer indicated treatment of DDH.

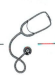

Forced abduction of the hips in DDH is contraindicated because of risk of avascular necrosis.

OI is the most common osteoporosis syndrome in children.

OSTEOGENESIS IMPERFECTA (OI)

DEFINITION

Rare, inherited disorder of connective tissue, characterized by multiple and recurrent fractures.

ETIOLOGY

- Molecular genetics have identified more than 150 mutations in the genes that encode for type 1 collagen.
- There are four types of OI. Types I and IV are mild and present with an increase risk of fractures. Type II is lethal in the newborn period, and Type III is a severe form causing significant bony deformity secondary to multiple fractures.

SIGNS AND SYMPTOMS

- Bone fragility
- Easy bruising
- Repeated fracture after mild trauma
- Deafness
- Blue sclera
- Hyperextensibility of ligaments
- Normal intelligence

DIAGNOSIS

- Radiographic findings:
  - Osteopenia
  - Thin cortices
  - Bowing
  - Normal callus formation
- Collagen synthesis analysis

TREATMENT

- Bisphosphonates
- Surgical correction of long-bone deformities
- Trauma prevention

PROGNOSIS

Prognosis is poor, and most patients are confined to wheelchairs by adulthood.

KLIPPEL–FEIL SYNDROME

DEFINITION

Congenital fusion of a variable number of cervical vertebrae.

ETIOLOGY

Failure of normal segmentation in the cervical spine.

SIGNS AND SYMPTOMS

- Classic clinical triad:
  - Short neck
  - Low hairline
  - Limitation of neck motion
- Associated with:
  - Renal anomalies
  - Scoliosis

- Spinal bifida
- Deafness

DIAGNOSIS

Children with Klippel–Feil syndrome should have the following tests performed:

- Renal ultrasound
- Hearing test
- Lateral flexion–extension radiographs of cervical spine

TREATMENT

- Annual evaluation.
- Avoid violent activities.
- Close evaluation of immediate family members.

TORTICOLLIS

DEFINITION

Twisted or wry neck.

ETIOLOGY

- **Congenital:** injury to the sternocleidomastoid muscle during delivery
- **Acquired:** rotatory subluxation of the upper cervical spine

MANAGEMENT

- **Congenital:** physical therapy
- **Acquired:**
  - Warm soaks
  - Analgesics
  - Mild anti-inflammatory agents
  - Soft cervical collar
  - Passive stretching

MUSCULAR DYSTROPHIES

Duchenne's Muscular Dystrophy (DMD)

DEFINITION

Degenerative disease of muscles. DMD is characterized by early childhood onset, typically within the first 5 years.

INHERITANCE

- X-linked recessive
- 1:3,000 male infants

SIGNS AND SYMPTOMS

- Clumsiness
- Easy fatigability
- Symmetric involvement
- Axial and proximal before distal
- Pelvic girdle, with shoulder girdle usually later
- Rapid progression
- Loss of ambulation by 8 to 12 years
- Pseudohypertrophy of calves

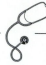

Type I collagen fibers are found in bones, organ capsules, fascia, cornea, sclera, tendons, meninges, and the dermis.

Typical Scenario

A 2-year-old child is brought in with a right radial fracture after lightly bumping his arm. An x-ray shows multiple healing fractures. On examination, the child has blue sclera, thin skin, and hypoplastic teeth. *Think:* OI.

Children with Klippel–Feil syndrome are at risk for:
- Atlantoaxial instability
- Neurologic impairment

Torqueo = to twist
Collum = neck

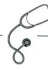

Torticollis is the most common cause of neck muscle strain.

DMD is the most common muscular dystrophy.

- Serum creatinine kinase (CK) is markedly elevated.
- Muscle biopsy is pathognomonic—degeneration and variation in fiber size and proliferation of connective tissue. No dystrophin present.

MANAGEMENT

- Encourage ambulation.
- Prevent contractures with passive stretching.

Typical Scenario

A 3-year-old boy must use his hands to push himself up when rising from a supine position. *Think:* Gower's maneuver.

Becker's Muscular Dystrophy (BMD)

DEFINITION

Milder form of muscular dystrophy.

INHERITANCE

X-linked recessive.

SIGNS AND SYMPTOMS

- Late childhood onset, typically between 5 and 15 years
- Slow progression
- Proximal muscle weakness
- Prominence of calf muscles
- Inability to walk occurs after 16 years

DMD is associated with:
- Mental retardation
- Cardiomyopathy

DIAGNOSIS

Muscle biopsy shows degeneration of muscle fibers. Dystrophin is reduced or abnormal.

Myotonic Muscular Dystrophy (MMD)

INHERITANCE

Autosomal dominant.

SIGNS AND SYMPTOMS

- Congenital MMD affects infants and is more severe than the adult form.
- Adult-onset MMD has a variable onset, typically in the teens to adulthood.
- Muscle weakness of voluntary muscles in the face, distal limbs, and diaphragm.
- Involuntary clenching of hands and jaw, ptosis, and respiratory difficulty.

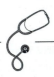

Death in patients with DMD occurs through cardiac or respiratory failure.

Limb Girdle Muscular Dystrophy

DEFINITION

Two types:
- Pelvifemoral (Leyden–Möbius)
- Scapulohumeral (Erb's juvenile)

INHERITANCE

Autosomal recessive, with high sporadic incidence.

SIGNS AND SYMPTOMS

- Variable age of onset; childhood to early adult (present in second or third decade)
- Pelvic girdle usually involved first and to greater extent
- Shoulder girdle often asymmetric

DIAGNOSIS

Muscle biopsy shows dystrophic muscle changes. Dystrophin is normal.

MANAGEMENT

- Promote ambulation.
- Physiotherapy.
- Mildy progressive, life expectancy mid to late adulthood.

Facioscapulohumeral Muscular Dystrophy

INHERITANCE

Autosomal dominant.

SIGNS AND SYMPTOMS

- Variable
- Slow progression
- Diminished facial movements: inability to close eyes, smile, or whistle
- Weakness of the shoulder girdle: difficulty raising arms over head
- Normal life span

DERMATOMYOSITIS/POLYMYOSITIS

DEFINITION

- **Polymyositis** primarily affects skeletal muscle.
- **Dermatomyositis** = skin eruption + myopathy.

EPIDEMIOLOGY

- Female > male
- 5 to 14 years old

SIGNS AND SYMPTOMS

- Symmetric proximal muscle weakness
- Violaceous rash—symmetric, erythematous rash on extensor surfaces, upper eyelids, and knuckles. Rash around eyes called "heliotrope rash."
- Worrisome triad (not common):
  - Dysphagia
  - Dysphonia
  - Dyspnea

DIAGNOSIS

- ESR, serum CK, and aldolase reflect the activity of the disease.
- Electromyography (EMG) is used to distinguish myopathic from neuropathic causes of muscle weakness.

TREATMENT

- Prednisone
- Intravenous immune globulin (IVIG), cyclosporine, or methotrexate in refractory cases

PROGNOSIS

Most children will recover in 1 to 3 years.

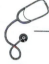

In adults, dermatomyositis and polymyositis are associated with malignancy and rheumatic disease. Myositis is not associated with cancer in children.

Dermatomyositis affects proximal muscles more than distal muscles, and weakness usually starts in the legs. An inability to climb stairs may be the first warning sign.

HIGH-YIELD FACTS

Musculoskeletal Disease

Marfan Syndrome

DEFINITION

Genetic defect of genes coding for the connective tissue protein fibrillin.

INHERITANCE

Autosomal dominant.

SIGNS AND SYMPTOMS

- Tall stature
- Long, thin digits (arachnodactyly)
- Hyperextensible joints
- High arched palate
- Dislocation of lenses of eye

The most worrisome complications of Marfan syndrome are aortic dilation, aortic regurgitation, and aortic aneurysms.

Ehlers–Danlos Syndrome (EDS)

DEFINITION

Connective tissue disorders.

ETIOLOGY

- Quantitative deficiency of collagen causing poor cross-linking of collagen
- Autosomal dominant

SIGNS AND SYMPTOMS

- Children with EDS are normal at birth.
- Skin hyperelasticity.
- Fragility of the skin and blood vessels.
- Joint hypermobility.
- Propensity for tissue rupture.

MANAGEMENT

- Symptomatic
- Preventive
- Prolonged wound fixation
- Genetic counseling

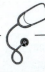

Type IV EDS is associated with a weakened uterus, blood vessels, or intestines. It is important to identify patients with EDS type IV because of the grave consequences of the disease. Women with EDS type IV should be counseled to avoid pregnancy.

Scoliosis

DEFINITION

More than 10-degree curvature of spine in the lateral plane due to the rotation of the involved vertebrae (see Figure 19-12).

ETIOLOGY

- Eighty percent of cases are idiopathic.
- Scoliosis is associated with:
    - Neurofibromatosis
    - Marfan syndrome
    - Cerebral palsy
    - Muscular dystrophy
    - Poliomyelitis
    - Myelodysplasia

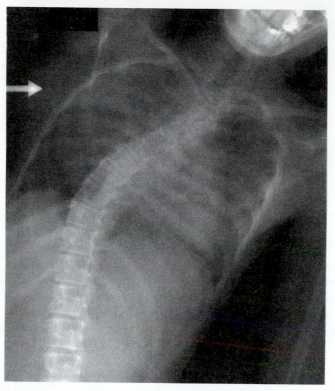

FIGURE 19-12. Radiograph of spine demonstrating marked scoliosis.

- Congenital vertebral anomalies (hemivertebrae, unilateral vertebral bridge)

EPIDEMIOLOGY

- Four to five times more common in girls
- Age of onset: 9 to 10 years for girls, 11 to 12 years for boys

SIGNS AND SYMPTOMS

- Usually asymptomatic.
- Severe curvature may lead to impairment of pulmonary function.

DIAGNOSIS

- X-ray of entire spine in both the AP and lateral planes.
- To examine children, have the patient bend forward 90 degrees with the hands joined in the midline. An abnormal finding consists of asymmetry of the height of the ribs or paravertebral muscles on one side.

MANAGEMENT

Treatment depends on the curve magnitude, skeletal maturity, and risk of progression:

- Curve < 20 degrees: Physical therapy and back exercises aimed at strengthening back muscles.
- Curve 20 to 40 degrees in a skeletally immature child: Orthopedic back brace. A back brace does not decrease the curve, but prevents further curve progression.
- Curve > 40 degrees: Spinal fusion to correct deformity.

Thirty percent of family members of patients with scoliosis are also affected. Siblings of affected children should be carefully examined.

Screening for scoliosis should begin at 6 to 7 years of age.

PROGNOSIS

- Curve > 60 degrees: Associated with poor pulmonary function. Large thoracic curves are associated with a shortened life span.
- Curve < 40 degrees: Usually do not progress. Small curves are well tolerated.

Kyphosis

DEFINITION

Posterior curvature of the spine due to some rotation of the involved vertebrae.

ETIOLOGY

Scheuermann thoracic kyphosis is a structural deformity of the thoracic spine.

SIGNS AND SYMPTOMS

- Pain
- Progressive deformity
- Neurologic compromise
- Cardiovascular complaints
- Cosmetic issues

RADIOLOGY

- Diagnosis is confirmed on lateral radiographs.
- X-ray shows anterior wedging of at least 5 degrees of three or more adjacent thoracic vertebral bodies.

Spondylolysis

DEFINITION

Fracture of the pars interarticularis due to repetitive stress to this area.

ETIOLOGY

Spondylosis occurs as a result of new bone formation in areas where the annular ligament is stressed.

TYPES

- **Congenital:** cervical
- **Acquired:** lumbar, most often at L5 (85% of cases)

SIGNS AND SYMPTOMS

- Cervical pain.
- Low back pain, worse during the adolescent growth spurt and with spine extension.
- Radicular symptoms are not common.

DIAGNOSIS

Oblique x-ray view of the spine will show the characteristic "Scottie dog sign."

TREATMENT

- NSAIDs
- Strength and stretching exercises
- Lumbosacral back brace

Spondylolysis is the most common cause of low back pain in adolescent athletes. This injury is most commonly seen in gymnasts, dancers, and football players.

Spondylolisthesis

DEFINITION

Anterior or posterior displacement of one vertebral body on the next due to bilateral pars interarticularis injury.

SIGNS AND SYMPTOMS

- A palpable "step-off" at the lumbosacral area
- Limited lumbar flexibility

DIAGNOSIS

Lateral x-ray views show displacement of one vertebral body from another.

MANAGEMENT

Treatment depends on grade of lesion:

- < 30% displacement: no restrictions on sports activities, but require routine follow-up
- > 50% displacement: in situ posterior spinal fusion or bracing

COMPLICATIONS

- Deformity
- Disability

Diskitis

DEFINITION

- Pyogenic infection of the intervertebral disk space
- An uncommon primary infection of the nucleus pulposus, with secondary involvement of the cartilaginous end plate and vertebral body

ETIOLOGY

- Most present prior to 10 years of age
- Spontaneous

SIGNS AND SYMPTOMS

- Moderate to severe pain.
- Pain is localized to the level of involvement and exacerbated by movement.
- Radicular symptoms.

LABS

- MRI is the radiographic study of choice.
- Elevated ESR.

MANAGEMENT

- Intravenous antibiotics.
- Surgery is often not necessary.

RENAL OSTEODYSTROPHY

DEFINITION

Bone diseases resulting from defective mineralization due to renal failure.

SIGNS AND SYMPTOMS

- Growth retardation
- Muscle weakness
- Bone pain

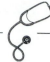

Grade 1: < 25% displacement
Grade 2: 25–50%
Grade 3: 50–75%
Grade 4: 75–100%
Grade 5: complete displacement

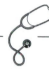

Children at highest risk for diskitis:
- Immunocompromised
- Systemic infections
- Postsurgery

The lumbar spine is the most common site of involvement for diskitis.

S. aureus is the most common organism causing diskitis.

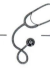

Plain radiographs are usually not helpful for early diagnosis of diskitis.

- Skeletal deformities
- Slipped epiphyses

In children, renal osteodystrophy resembles rickets.

DIAGNOSIS

- Normal to decreased serum calcium.
- Normal to increased phosphorus.
- Increased alkaline phosphatase.
- Normal parathyroid hormone (PTH) levels.
- Radiographs of the hands, wrists, and knees shows subperiosteal resorption of bone with widening of the metaphyses.

TREATMENT

- Low-phosphate formula.
- Enhance fecal phosphate excretion with oral calcium carbonate, an antacid that also binds phosphate in the intestinal tract.
- The goals of treatment include normalization of the serum calcium and phosphorus levels and maintenance of the intact PTH level in the range of 200 to 400 pg/mL.

Dermatologic Disease

CLASSIFICATION OF SKIN LESIONS

Primary Skin Lesions

Macule	Flat, nonpalpable, skin discoloration
Plaque	Elevated, > 2 cm diameter
Wheal	Elevated, round or flat-topped area of dermal edema, disappears within hours
Vesicle	Circumscribed, elevated, fluid-filled, < 0.5 cm diameter
Bullae	Circumscribed, elevated, fluid-filled, > 0.5 cm diameter
Pustule	Circumscribed, elevated, pus-filled
Papule	Elevated, palpable, solid, < 0.5 cm diameter
Nodule	Elevated, palpable, solid, > 0.5 cm
Petechiae	Red-purple, nonblanching macule, < 0.5 cm diameter, usually pinpoint
Purpura	Red-purple, nonblanching macule > 0.5 cm diameter
Telangiectasia	Blanchable, dilated blood vessels

Secondary Skin Lesions

Scale	Accumulation of dead, exfoliating epidermal cells
Crust (scab)	Dried serum, blood, or purulent exudate on skin surface
Erosion	Superficial loss of epidermis, leaving a denuded, moist surface; heals without scar
Ulcer	Loss of epidermis extending into dermis; heals with scar
Scar	Replacement of normal skin with fibrous tissue as a result of healing
Excoriation	Linear erosion produced by scratching
Atrophy	Thinning of skin
Lichenification markings	Thickening of epidermis with accentuation of normal skin

DIAGNOSTIC PROCEDURES USED IN DERMATOLOGY

Diascopy	Pressing glass slide firmly against red lesion—blanchable (capillary dilatation) or nonblanchable (extravasation of blood)
Gram stain	To identify some bacterial infections

Culture	To identify infectious agent and find antimicrobial susceptibilities
KOH prep	To identify fungi and yeast under microscope
Tzanck prep	To identify vesicular viral eruptions under microscope
Scabies prep	Scrape skin to identify mites, eggs, or feces under microscope
Wood's lamp	Tinea capitis will fluoresce green/yellow on hair shaft
Patch testing	Detects Type IV hypersensitivity reactions (allergic contact dermatitis)

PAPULOSQUAMOUS REACTIONS

Psoriasis (Figure 20-1)

DEFINITION

Chronic, noninfectious, hyperproliferative inflammatory disorder.

ETIOLOGY

Unknown, but has genetic predisposition.

PATHOPHYSIOLOGY

Increased epidermal cell proliferation due to a shortened epithelial cell cycle.

EPIDEMIOLOGY

- Rare under 10 years old
- Worse in winter

SIGNS AND SYMPTOMS

- Thick, adherent, well-demarcated, salmon-pink plaques with adherent silver-white scale
- On extensor surface of extremities, trunk, and scalp
- Nails commonly involved—pitting, "oil spots," onycholysis, subungual hyperkeratosis

DIAGNOSIS

- Clinical diagnosis
- Potassium hydroxide (KOH) test to rule out fungal infection

TREATMENT

- Topical coal tar, anthralin, corticosteroids, synthetic vitamin D analogue
- If extensive or resistant—ultraviolet B (UVB) phototherapy, PUVA (psoralen and ultraviolet A [UVA]), retinoids, methotrexate, cyclosporine

Salmon-pink plaques with silvery scale. *Think:* Psoriasis.

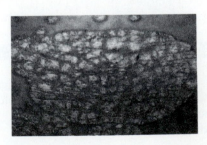

FIGURE 20-1. Silvery scale plaque of psoriasis.

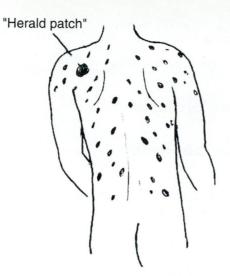

"Herald patch"

FIGURE 20-2. Pityriasis rosea. Note "Christmas tree" distribution of macules. Note "herald patch" that precedes other lesions.

Pityriasis Rosea (Figure 20-2)

DEFINITION

Common, self-limited eruption of single herald patch followed by a generalized secondary eruption.

ETIOLOGY

Suspected infectious agent.

EPIDEMIOLOGY

Affects children and young adults.

SIGNS AND SYMPTOMS

- Herald plaque—2- to 10-cm solitary, oval, erythematous, with collarette of scale
- Followed in 80% by generalized eruption of multiple smaller, pink, oval, scaly patches over trunk and upper extremities in Christmas tree distribution
- Pruritus

DIAGNOSIS

- Clinical
- Rapid plasma reagin (RPR) to rule out syphilis, KOH to rule out fungal infection

TREATMENT

- Self-limited, resolves in 6 to 12 weeks
- Symptomatic (no treatment shortens disease course)—baths, calamine, topical cortical steroids, oral antihistamines, UVB/sunlight

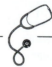

When there is a herald patch followed by a rash in a Christmas tree distribution (oriented parallel to the ribs), *think* pityriasis rosea.

ECZEMATOUS REACTIONS

Eczema: broad term used to describe several inflammatory skin reactions; used synonymously with dermatitis.

Atopic Dermatitis

DEFINITION
Hypersensitivity inflammatory reaction.

ETIOLOGY
Type I (IgE) immediate hypersensitivity response.

PATHOPHYSIOLOGY
Sensitized mast cells release vasoactive mediators.

EPIDEMIOLOGY
- Affects all ages, but onset is in first 6 months of life
- Two thirds outgrow by age 10
- Familial

SIGNS AND SYMPTOMS
- Pruritic.
- Lesions vary with patient's age.
- Infantile—red, exudative, crusty, and oozy lesions primarily affecting face and extensor surfaces.
- Juvenile/adult—dry, lichenified, pruritic plaques distributed over flexural areas (antecubital, popliteal, neck)
- Susceptible to secondary bacterial and viral infections

DIAGNOSIS
Clinical; supported by personal or family history of atopy.

TREATMENT
- Avoid scratching.
- Lubricate dry skin.
- Avoid wool, fragrances, and harsh cleansers.
- Oral antihistamines.
- Oral antibiotics *only* if clinical signs of secondary infection.
- Topical corticosteroids are the mainstay of therapy.
- Avoid oral corticosteroids because patients become steroid dependent or rebound when discontinued.

Contact Dermatitis

DEFINITION
Inflammatory skin reaction resulting from contact with an external agent.

ETIOLOGY
Irritant or allergic types.

SIGNS AND SYMPTOMS
- Sharply demarcated, erythematous vesicles and plaques at site of contact with agent.
- Chronic lesions may be lichenified.

DIAGNOSIS
- Clinical—consider location, relationship to external factors, particular configurations
- KOH to rule out fungal infection

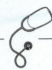

Atopic dermatitis is part of the atopic trilogy: allergic rhinitis, asthma, and eczema.

You can think of atopic dermatitis as "the itch that rashes."

Don't culture skin in atopic dermatitis—90% of atopic patients are carriers of *Staphylococcus aureus*.

Rhus dermatitis is an allergic dermatitis caused by contact with poison ivy or oak.

TREATMENT

- Remove offending agent
- Topical lubrication
- Wet dressings soaked in Burow's solution (aluminum acetate)
- Topical corticosteroids

Seborrheic Dermatitis

DEFINITION

Chronic and recurrent skin disease occurring at sites with sebaceous gland activity, characterized by erythema and scaling.

ETIOLOGY

Unknown.

PATHOPHYSIOLOGY

Unknown.

EPIDEMIOLOGY

- Affects children and adults
- Occurs more often in winter months

SIGNS AND SYMPTOMS

- Children age 0 to 3 months—"cradle cap": greasy scales covering scalp
- Adults—flaking, greasy scales on erythematous background over scalp (dandruff), ears, eyelids (blepharitis), nasolabial fold, and central chest

DIAGNOSIS

- Clinical
- KOH to rule out fungal infection

TREATMENT

Symptomatic—antiseborrheic shampoo, topical corticosteroids.

BULLOUS DISEASES

Pemphigus Vulgaris

DEFINITION

Potentially fatal, chronic, autoimmune, blistering disease of the skin and mucous membranes.

ETIOLOGY

Autoimmune.

PATHOPHYSIOLOGY

Circulating antibodies adhere to cell surface glycoproteins that hold epidermal cells together, causing intraepidermal blisters.

EPIDEMIOLOGY

Very rare in children, but occurs. Often follows a viral infection.

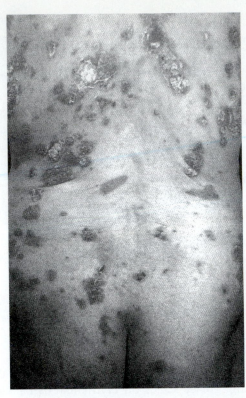

FIGURE 20-3. Pemphigus. (Reproduced, with permission, from Rycroft & Robertson, *A Color Handbook of Dermatology*. Stamford, CT: Appleton & Lange, 1999.)

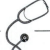

Nikolsky sign — direct pressure applied to surface of bulla causes it to extend laterally.

SIGNS AND SYMPTOMS

- Initially develop oral blisters that rupture easily (see Figure 20–3).
- Months later, flaccid bullae emerge and rupture, leaving eroded, denuded, and crusted surfaces.
- Localized to mouth or generalized on scalp, face, axillae, chest, and groin, sparing palms and soles.

DIAGNOSIS

- Clinical.
- Confirm by biopsy showing acantholysis (separation of keratinocytes).
- Intercellular immunoglobulin G (IgG) deposits on direct immunofluorescence.
- Circulating antibodies that correlate with disease activity.

TREATMENT

- Often fatal if not treated
- Systemic corticosteroids, immunosuppressive agents

Erythema Multiforme (Figure 20-4)

DEFINITION

General name used to describe an immune complex–mediated hypersensitivity reaction to different causative agents.

Herpes simplex viruses account for most cases of recurrent erythema multiforme that are not idiopathic.

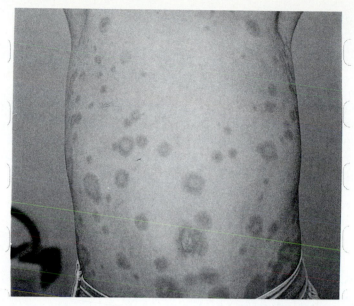

FIGURE 20-4. Erythema multiforme. Note the many different-sized lesions. (Reproduced, with permission, from Stead LG, Stead SM, Kaufman MS. *First Aid for the EM Clerkship.* New York: McGraw-Hill, 2001.)

ETIOLOGY

- Drugs (e.g., penicillin, sulfonamides, barbiturates, nonsteroidal anti-inflammatory drugs [NSAIDs], thiazides, phenytoin, vaccinations)
- Viruses (herpes simplex, hepatitis A and B)
- Bacteria (streptococcus)
- Fungi, mycoplasma, malignancy, radiotherapy, pregnancy
- 20–50% idiopathic

PATHOPHYSIOLOGY

Unknown, likely hypersensitivity reaction.

EPIDEMIOLOGY

Older children and adults.

SIGNS AND SYMPTOMS

Pruritus or pain.

Stevens–Johnson Syndrome (Erythema Multiforme Major)

DEFINITION

Severe variant of erythema multiforme with systemic illness.

ETIOLOGY

Often viruses (herpes) or drugs (see above).

SIGNS AND SYMPTOMS

- Systemic illness (fever, malaise)
- Mucous membrane involvement (oral, vaginal, conjunctival)
- Extensive target-like lesions and mucosal erosions covering < 10% of body surface area

- Ocular involvement (purulent uveitis/conjunctivitis) may result in scarring or corneal ulcers
- May evolve to toxic epidermal necrolysis

TREATMENT
- Symptomatic and supportive.
- Observe closely for strictures developing upon mucous membrane healing.
- Mouthwashes, topical anesthetics.

Toxic Epidermal Necrolysis

DEFINITION
Severe variant/progression of erythema multiforme with widespread involvement.

ETIOLOGY
Hypersensitivity, triggered by many of above list.

PATHOPHYSIOLOGY
Damage to basal cell layer of epidermis.

SIGNS AND SYMPTOMS
- Widespread, full-thickness necrosis of skin, covering > 30% body surface area
- Prodrome of fever and influenza-like symptoms
- Pruritus, pain, tenderness, and burning
- Complications—secondary skin infections, fluid and electrolyte abnormalities, prerenal azotemia
- 30% mortality rate

DIAGNOSIS
Clinical; confirm by biopsy.

TREATMENT
- Removal and/or treatment of causative agent
- Hospitalization for severe disease
- Fluid and electrolyte replacement
- Systemic corticosteroids

CUTANEOUS BACTERIAL INFECTIONS

Impetigo (Figure 20-5)

DEFINITION
Contagious, superficial, bacterial infection transmitted by direct contact.

ETIOLOGY
- *Staphylococcus aureus* (bullous lesions)
- Group A β-hemolytic *Streptococcus pyogenes* (GAS) (nonbullous lesions)

PATHOPHYSIOLOGY
Only epidermis is affected.

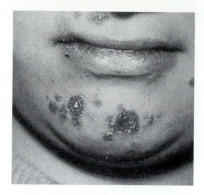

FIGURE 20-5. Impetigo. Note characteristic honey-colored crusted lesion, typically seen at corners of mouth and over face.

EPIDEMIOLOGY

- Common in children
- Warm and humid climates
- Crowded conditions

SIGNS AND SYMPTOMS

- Mild burning or pruritus.
- Initial lesion is a transient erythematous papule or thin-roofed vesicle that ruptures easily and forms a honey-colored crust.
- Lesions can progress for weeks if untreated.

DIAGNOSIS

Clinical; can confirm with Gram stain and culture showing gram-positive cocci in clusters (*S. aureus*) or chains (GAS).

TREATMENT

- Remove crusts by soaking in warm water.
- Antibacterial washes (benzoyl peroxide).
- Topical antibiotic if disease is limited (Bactroban).
- Oral antibiotics (pencillins or macrolide) if more severe.

Cellulitis

DEFINITION

Acute, deep infection of dermis and subcutaneous tissue.

ETIOLOGY

- *S. aureus*
- Group A β-hemolytic *Streptococcus pyogenes*
- *Haemophilus influenzae* (children)

PATHOPHYSIOLOGY

- Precipitating factors include injury, abrasions, burns, surgical wounds, mucosal infections, bites, underlying dermatosis, and preexisting lymphatic stress.
- Risk factors include drug and alcohol abuse, chronic lymphedema, cancer, chemotherapy, immunodeficiency, diabetes, cirrhosis, neutropenia, and malnutrition.

"Honey-colored crust" is classic for impetigo.

Dermatologic Disease

EPIDEMIOLOGY

Any age.

SIGNS AND SYMPTOMS

- Erythematous, edematous, shiny area of warm and tender skin with poorly demarcated, nonelevated borders.
- Fever, chills, and malaise can develop rapidly.

DIAGNOSIS

- Clinical; confirmed by Gram stain demonstrating gram-positive cocci in clusters or chains.
- Culture of lesion or blood will be positive only 25% of the time.

TREATMENT

- Penicillin
- If allergic to penicillin or methicillin-resistant *S. aureus* (MRSA) is involved, vancomycin or cephalosporins
- Cefotaxime or ceftriaxone for *H. influenzae*

Erysipelas

DEFINITION

- Variant of cellulitis
- Others include erysipeloid (hands from handling infected food) and necrotizing fasciitis (medical emergency)

ETIOLOGY

GAS.

EPIDEMIOLOGY

Increased incidence in young children and adults.

SIGNS AND SYMPTOMS

- Local pain and tenderness.
- Acute onset of fever, malaise, and shivering may precede lesion.
- Unlike cellulitis—well-demarcated, indurated, and elevated advancing border; less edematous.
- High morbidity rate if untreated.

DIAGNOSIS

Clinical; Gram stain reveals gram-positive cocci in chains.

TREATMENT

Oral antibiotics (penicillin, cephalosporin, macrolide, vancomycin).

TOXIN-MEDIATED DISEASES

Staphylococcal Scalded Skin Syndrome

DEFINITION

Toxin-mediated disease resulting in detachment of the epidermis.

ETIOLOGY

S. aureus.

PATHOPHYSIOLOGY

Pathogen colonizes nose or conjunctivae without causing clinical signs of infection, but produces exfoliatin and epidermolytic toxins that spread hematogenously to skin, resulting in blistering and sloughing of the epidermis.

EPIDEMIOLOGY

Newborns and infants (< 2 years old).

SIGNS AND SYMPTOMS

- Skin is initially red and tender with flaccid bullae.
- Epidermis sloughs off and appears wrinkled, usually beginning in the face, neck, axillae, and groin.
- Becomes widespread within 24 to 48 hours, resembling scalding.
- Direct pressure applied to surface of bulla causes it to extend laterally (Nikolsky sign).
- Self-limited in 5 to 7 days, though death can occur in neonates with extensive disease.

DIAGNOSIS

Clinical; confirmed by culture of colonized site (nose, eyes, throat) revealing gram-positive cocci.

TREATMENT

- Hospitalize newborns with extensive skin sloughing.
- Warm baths for debridement of necrotic epidermis.
- Systemic antibiotics (oxacillin, dicloxacillin).
- Intravenous (IV) fluids in severe cases.

Culture of epidermolytic skin in staphylococcal scalded skin syndrome will not demonstrate the pathogen.

Scarlet Fever

DEFINITION

Toxin-mediated disease characterized by sore throat, high fever, and mucous membrane erythema.

ETIOLOGY

GAS.

PATHOPHYSIOLOGY

Toxin mediated.

EPIDEMIOLOGY

- Children
- Untreated streptococcal infection of pharynx, tonsils, or wound

SIGNS AND SYMPTOMS

- Finely punctate pink-scarlet exanthem first appears on upper trunk 12 to 48 hours after onset of fever.
- As exanthem spreads to extremities, it becomes confluent and feels like sandpaper.
- Fades in 4 to 5 days, followed by desquamation.
- Linear petechiae evident in body folds (Pastia's sign).
- Pharynx is beefy red and tongue is initially white, but within 4 to 5 days the white coating sloughs off and tongue becomes bright red.

See "strawberry tongue," *think* scarlet fever.

DIAGNOSIS

- Clinical; confirmed by culture from throat or wound.
- Rapid direct antigen tests detect GAS antigens.
- Gram stain reveals gram-positive cocci in chains (GAS) or cocci (S. aureus).

TREATMENT

- Acetaminophen for fever and pain
- Antibiotics (penicillin, macrolide, or cephalosporin)
- Follow-up recommended if history of rheumatic fever present

CUTANEOUS VIRAL INFECTIONS

Verrucae (Warts)

DEFINITION

Viral infection of skin and mucous membranes spread by direct contact.

ETIOLOGY

Human papillomavirus (HPV).

EPIDEMIOLOGY

Increased incidence in atopic and immunocompromised patients.

SIGNS AND SYMPTOMS

- Tender if irritated
- Types:
  - Verrucae vulgaris—hands, fingers, knees; skin-colored papule
  - Verrucae plantaris—rough; over pressure points on plantar aspect of foot
  - Verrucae planar—flat; on face and dorsum of hands and fingers
  - Condyloma acuminata—anogenital warts

HPV subtypes 6, 11, 16, 18, 31, 33, 35, and 44 are associated with cervical dysplasia (precancerous).

DIAGNOSIS

Clinical—absence of normal skin lines and presence of black dots.

TREATMENT

Cryotherapy, topical keratolytic agents (e.g., salicylic acid), destructive agents (podophyllin), curettage and desiccation, topical imiquod.

Herpes Gingivostomatitis (Fever Blisters, Cold Sores)

DEFINITION

Highly contagious viral eruption characterized by painful vesicles, commonly occurring around the mouth (type I) and genitals (type II).

ETIOLOGY

Herpes simplex virus (HSV) types I and II.

PATHOPHYSIOLOGY

- Transmitted by direct contact with skin and mucous membranes.
- After primary infection, virus remains latent in a neural ganglion.
- Reactivation of latent virus results in recurrent disease commonly occurring in the same area.
- Recurrences become less frequent over time.

EPIDEMIOLOGY

- Primary infection affects children and young adults.
- Increased incidence of infection in immunocompromised patients.

SIGNS AND SYMPTOMS

- Grouped vesicles on an erythematous base, occurring primarily on lips, mouths, genitals, and eyes, but can occur at any site.

- Erosion and crusted lesions form after a couple of days.
- Fever, malaise, headache, and adenopathy may occur with primary infection.
- Prodrome of burning, tingling, or itching occurs with recurrent infection.
- Complications include ocular disease, secondary infection, and dissemination (especially in immunocompromised patients).

DIAGNOSIS

- Clinical
- Confirmed by Tzanck preparation, revealing multinucleated giant cells
- Viral culture of vesicle fluid

TREATMENT

- Oral acyclovir, valacyclovir, or famciclovir decrease viral shedding time and accelerate healing time.
- Suppressive therapy with acyclovir for more than six recurrences per year.

Molluscum Contagiosum (Figure 20-6)

DEFINITION

Self-limited, contagious, viral infection transmitted by direct contact.

ETIOLOGY

Molluscum contagiosum virus (poxvirus).

EPIDEMIOLOGY

- Affects children and sexually active adults
- Increased incidence in atopic and immunocompromised patients

SIGNS AND SYMPTOMS

- Single or multiple, 2- to 5-mm, firm, umbilicated, skin-colored or pearly-white papules.
- Commonly found on face, eyelids, axillae, and anogenital region.
- Multiple lesions on face suggest human immunodeficiency virus (HIV) infection.

DIAGNOSIS

Clinical; confirm with identification of inclusion bodies ("molluscum bodies") on smear of plug.

TREATMENT

Curettage, cryosurgery, electrodesiccation, or laser surgery.

Herpetic whitlow (herpes infected finger) — can occur in health care workers, but is less common now with the use of universal precautions.

Do not try to excise herpetic whitlow — opening the lesion will only serve to spill more virus onto surrounding skin and spread the infection.

See umbilicated, pearly papules, *think* molluscum contagiosum.

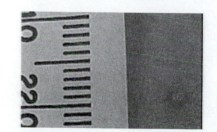

FIGURE 20-6. Molluscum contagiosum. (Photo courtesy of Danial Stuhlberg, MD, Utah Family Practice Residency, Provo, UT.)

Tinea (Dermatophytoses)

DEFINITION

- Group of noninvasive fungi that can infect keratinized tissue of epidermis, nails, and hair.
- Clinical presentation depends on anatomic site of infection and is named accordingly.

ETIOLOGY

Tricophyton, Microsporum, Epidermophyton.

EPIDEMIOLOGY

Exacerbated by warm, humid climates.

SIGNS AND SYMPTOMS

- Tinea pedis ("athlete's foot")
- Tinea cruris ("jock itch")—groin
- Tinea corporis ("ringworm")—body (see Figure 20-7)
- Tinea manuum—hand
- Tinea facialis—face
- Tinea capitis—scalp
- Tinea barbae—beard/mustache area
- Onychomycosis—nails
- Tinea versicolor—superficial, asymptomatic

DIAGNOSIS

- Clinical presentation and history.
- KOH preparation reveals multiple, septated hyphae.
- Wood's lamp reveals bright green fluorescence of hair shaft in tinea capitis.
- Fungal culture of affected area may demonstrate dermatophyte.

TREATMENT

- Prevention—wearing well-ventilated shoes and clothing
- Topical antifungal agents (imidazoles and terbinafine)
- Systemic antifungal agents if unresponsive to topical or have involvement of nails (griseofulvin, systemic azoles, terbinafine)
- Mild-potency topical corticosteroids if inflammation and pruritus are severe

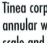

Tinea corporis lesions are annular with peripheral scale and central clearing.

Tinea versicolor has hyphae and yeast forms in a "spaghetti and meatball" distribution on KOH preparation.

Griseofulvin can cause elevation of liver enzymes.

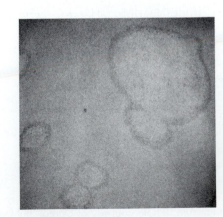

FIGURE 20-7. Tinea corporis (ringworm).

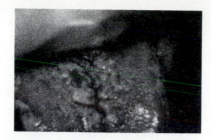

FIGURE 20-8. Oral candidiasis (thrush). (Reproduced, with permission, from Yong-Kwang T, Seow C. What syndrome is this? *Pediatric Dermatology* 2001;18(4):353.)

Candidal Skin Infections (Candida)

DEFINITION

Superficial infection occurring in moist cutaneous sites.

ETIOLOGY

Candida albicans.

PATHOPHYSIOLOGY

Predisposing factors—diabetes mellitus, obesity, immunosuppression, chronic debilitation, recent use of antibiotics.

SIGNS AND SYMPTOMS

- Pruritus and soreness
- Confluent, bright red papules and pustules forming a sharply demarcated eroded patch with pustular lesions at the periphery (satellite lesions)
- Distributed over intertriginous regions, including axillae; groin; web spaces; genital, anal, and inframammary areas
- Oral form is thrush: thick white plaque on tongue that can't be scraped off (Figure 20–8)

DIAGNOSIS

Clinical; confirmed by KOH preparation revealing pseudohyphae and budding spores and cultures of lesion.

TREATMENT

- Keep intertriginous areas dry.
- Topical antifungals (azoles).
- Topical corticosteroids for symptomatic relief.

Thrush is a candidal infection of mucosal surfaces, presenting as creamy white, easily removable papules on an erythematous mucosal surface (see Figure 20-8).

Diaper rash is often superinfected with *Candida*, which manifests as erythematous satellite lesions.

INFESTATIONS

Lice (Pediculosis)

DEFINITION

1. Pediculosis corporis—body
2. Pediculosis capitis—scalp hair
3. Pediculosis pubis—pubic hair

ETIOLOGY

1. *Pediculus humanus corporis*
2. *Pediculus humanus capitis*
3. *Pthirus pubis*

PATHOPHYSIOLOGY

These lice are obligate parasites, feeding on human blood.

1. Poor hygiene
2. Head-to-head contact, sharing hair items
3. Sexual contact

SIGNS AND SYMPTOMS

- Pruritus.
- Pyoderma may develop from scratching.
- Corporis—primary lesion is an intensely pruritic, small, red macule or papule with central hemorrhagic punctum on shoulders, trunk, or buttocks; secondary lesions include excoriations, wheals, and eczematous, secondarily infected plaques.

DIAGNOSIS

Nits detectable on hair/fibers.

TREATMENT

- Hot water laundering.
- Boil or dispose of implements.
- Comb hair.
- Permethrin rinse—once, then again at 1 week (alternatives—pyrethrin, lindane).

Cutaneous Larva Migrans (Figure 20-9)

DEFINITION

Eruption caused by several larval nematodes not usually parasitic to humans.

ETIOLOGY

Most often *Ancylostoma braziliense* (hookworm of dogs and cats).

PATHOPHYSIOLOGY

Parasite eggs are deposited in feces of animals, then hatch. Larvae penetrate human skin, then migrate along epidermal–dermal junction.

EPIDEMIOLOGY

Warm, moist areas.

SIGNS AND SYMPTOMS

- Raised, erythematous, serpiginous tracks, occasionally forming bullae
- Single or multiple
- Usually on an extremity or the buttocks, but can occur anywhere on the body

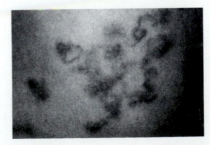

FIGURE 20-9. Cutaneous larva migrans. (Reproduced, with permission, from Berger MS. A serpiginous eruption on the buttocks. *American Family Physician* 2000;62:2493.)

DIAGNOSIS

Clinical.

TREATMENT

- Self-limited in weeks to months
- Thiabendazole if symptoms warrant treatment

Scabies

ETIOLOGY

Female mite *Sarcoptes scabiei hominis*.

PATHOPHYSIOLOGY

- Pregnant female mite exudes keratolytic substance and burrows into the stratum corneum, depositing eggs and feces daily.
- Eggs hatch; larvae molt into nymphs, mature in 2 to 3 weeks, and repeat the cycle.

EPIDEMIOLOGY

- Physical contact with infected individual
- Rarely transmitted by fomites, as isolated mites dies within 2 to 3 days

SIGNS AND SYMPTOMS

- Pruritus at initial infestation
- First sign—1- to 2-mm red papules, some of which are excoriated, crusted, or scaling
- Threadlike burrows
- Multiple types of lesions

DIAGNOSIS

Scraping for microscopic identification of mites, ova, and feces.

TREATMENT

- Lindane, neck down, scalp only if involved; leave on 8 to 12 hours; may be repeated after 1 week.
- Infants are particularly susceptible to the neurotoxicity of lindane.
- Alternatives include permethrin or sulfur ointment.

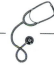

Threadlike burrows are classic for scabies, but may not be seen in infants.

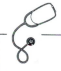

Transmission of scabies mites is unlikely 24 hours after treatment.

GROWTHS

Hemangioma

DEFINITION

Benign vascular proliferation that is usually present at birth or appears soon afterwards (e.g., capillary hemangioma, port-wine stain, cavernous hemangioma). (Figure 20–10)

ETIOLOGY/PATHOPHYSIOLOGY

Abnormal angiogenesis, perhaps incited by cytokines, such as basic fibroblast growth factor (bFGF) and vascular endothelial growth factor (VEGF).

EPIDEMIOLOGY

~0.5% of infants.

SIGNS AND SYMPTOMS

Capillary hemangioma—"strawberry"—red or purple papules or nodules that develop soon after birth and spontaneously involute by fifth year (see Figure 20-11).

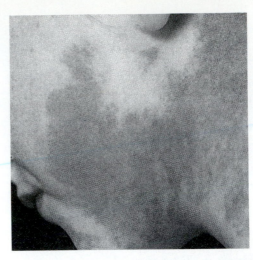

FIGURE 20-10. Port-wine stain seen in Sturge–Weber disease. (Reproduced with permission from Rycroft and Robertson,[D10] *A Color Handbook of Dermatology.* Stamford, CT: Appleton & Lange, 1999.)

TREATMENT

- Most resolve without treatment.
- Involvement of bone, soft tissue, or organ parenchyma may warrant excision of the hemangioma.

Melanocytic Nevus (Mole) (Figure 20-12)

DEFINITION

Benign proliferation of melanocytes, which are classified to location of clustering—dermal–epidermal junction (junctional), dermis (dermal), or both (compound).

EPIDEMIOLOGY

Nevi usually arise in childhood, peak during adolescence, and spontaneously regress during adulthood.

TREATMENT

- Serial observation
- Early excision of suspicious lesions

Malignant Melanoma

DEFINITION

Malignant proliferation of melanocytes.

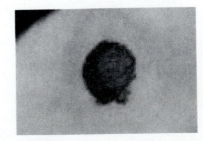

FIGURE 20-11. Capillary hemangioma.

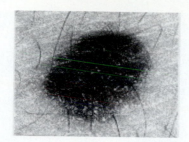

FIGURE 20-12. Melanocytic nevus. (Reproduced, with permission, from Wang SQ, Katz B, Rabinovitz H, Kopf AW, Oliviero M. Lessons on dermoscopy. *Dermatologic Surgery* 2000;26(4):397.)

ETIOLOGY

May arise from normal-appearing skin or from preexisting mole or skin lesion.

PATHOPHYSIOLOGY

- Horizontal growth phase—lateral extension within the epidermis and dermis
- Vertical phase—penetrates into dermis, greatly increasing risk of metastasis

EPIDEMIOLOGY

- Increased incidence in fair-skinned people and with sun exposure.
- Adolescents

SIGNS AND SYMPTOMS

Characteristics of a mole suspicious for melanoma:
- Asymmetric
- Border (irregular)
- Color (variegated and mottled)
- Diameter (> 0.6 cm)
- Elevated
- Enlarging

DIAGNOSIS

Prognosis based on thickness of the primary tumor.

TREATMENT

- Surgical excision with margins at least 1 cm, depending on depth of lesion
- Follow-up

Characteristics of mole suspicious for melanoma:
- Asymmetric
- Borders irregular
- Color uneven
- Diameter > 0.6 cm
- Elevated
- Enlarging

Xeroderma Pigmentosum

DEFINITION

Genetic defect in DNA repair mechanisms, predisposing to certain skin cancers.

ETIOLOGY

Autosomal recessive.

PATHOPHYSIOLOGY

Failure to repair ultraviolet-damaged DNA.

SIGNS AND SYMPTOMS

Predisposes patients to basal and squamous cell skin cancers.

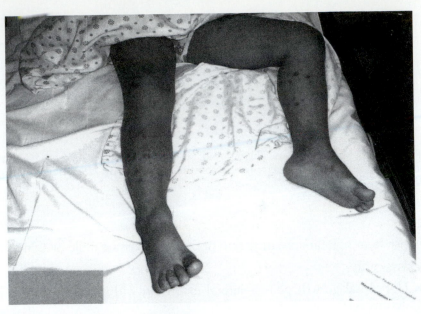

FIGURE 20-13. Henoch–Schönlein purpura.

OTHER SKIN CONDITIONS

Henoch–Schönlein Purpura (Figure 20-13)

DEFINITION
Classic example of vasculitis in children.

ETIOLOGY/PATHOPHYSIOLOGY
- Immunoglobulin A (IgA) mediated
- Occurs most commonly following streptococcal or viral infection

EPIDEMIOLOGY
Children.

SIGNS AND SYMPTOMS
- Palpable purpura
- Arthritis
- Abdominal pain

DIAGNOSIS
Clinical; may biopsy.

TREATMENT
Benign, self-limited.

Acne Vulgaris

DEFINITION
Disorder of pilosebaceous glands.

ETIOLOGY/PATHOPHYSIOLOGY
Results from a combination of hormonal (androgens), bacterial (*Propionibacterium acnes*), and genetic factors.

Palpable purpura is the classic sign of small-vessel damage.

374

EPIDEMIOLOGY

Adolescents.

SIGNS AND SYMPTOMS

- Comedone—plug of sebaceous and dead skin material stuck in the opening of a hair follicle; open follicle (blackhead) or almost closed (whitehead).
- Pustules, papules.
- Painful nodules and cysts if severe.
- Seborrhea of face and scalp (greasy skin).
- Depressed or hypertrophic scars may develop with healing.

DIAGNOSIS

Clinical; confirmed by presence of comedones.

TREATMENT

- Benzoyl peroxide wash
- Topical antibiotics (clindamycin or erythromycin)
- Intralesional corticosteroid injections (triamcinolone acetonide)
- Topical retinoid—increase cell turnover and prevent follicle occlusion
- Oral isotretinoin (Accutane) for severe, recalcitrant, nodular acne
- Dermabrasion for treatment of scars

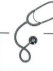

Accutane is teratogenic and should be prescribed with oral contraceptives; it also has many side effects.

Diaper Rash

DEFINITION

Rash occurring in the diaper area.

ETIOLOGY

- Irritant contact dermatitis—prolonged dampness, interaction of urine (ammonia) and feces with the skin, reactions to medications/creams, type of diaper.
- Candidal or bacterial secondary infection can occur.
- Atopic dermatitis.
- May be any other dermatologic condition in diaper distribution.

PATHOPHYSIOLOGY

Overhydration, friction, maceration, allergy, etc.

EPIDEMIOLOGY

Most children who wear diapers, to some degree.

SIGNS AND SYMPTOMS

- Red, scaly, fissured, eroded
- Patchy or confluent
- If secondarily infected: impetiginous or candidal

TREATMENT

- Keep infant dry, change diapers often.
- Avoid harsh detergents, wipes with alcohol, and plastic pants.
- Ointments can reduce friction and protect skin from irritation.
- Avoid powders, as they can injure infants' lungs.
- Nystatin or other antifungal cream for yeast infection.

Recurrent Minor Aphthous Ulcers/Stomatitis (Canker Sores)

DEFINITION

Chronic inflammatory disease causing recurrent oral ulcers of varying frequency.

ETIOLOGY

Local cell-mediated immunity, elevated inflammatory mediators, abnormal cell communication/epithelial integrity.

PATHOPHYSIOLOGY

Triggers may include toothpaste/mouthwash with sodium lauryl sulfate, mechanical trauma, stress, nutritional deficiencies, food sensitivities/allergies, hormones, infection, genetics, medical conditions, and medications.

EPIDEMIOLOGY

Twenty percent of the general population.

SIGNS AND SYMPTOMS

- Round/ovoid ulcer with grayish membrane and edges surrounded by reddish halo
- Occur on nonkeratinized skin—inside of the lips and cheeks, floor of the mouth, under the tongue, soft palate, and tonsillar areas
- High recurrence rate
- Usually heal uneventfully in 4 to 14 days

DIAGNOSIS

Clinical; rule out herpes stomatitis.

TREATMENT

- Avoid individual triggering factors.
- Symptomatic—oral numbing or coating medications.
- Antibacterial/cleansing rinses.
- Home remedies—Milk of Magnesia, warm salt water, alum rinses.
- Prescription anti-inflammatory or antibacterial collagenase inhibitors.

Vitiligo

DEFINITION

Pigmentary defect.

ETIOLOGY/PATHOPHYSIOLOGY

- Unknown, possibly autoimmune.
- Trauma may be associated with initiation of the lesions.

EPIDEMIOLOGY

Half of cases present before 20 years of age.

SIGNS AND SYMPTOMS

- Depigmented macules
- Predilection for hyperpigmented areas

DIAGNOSIS

Clinical, though melanocyte absence can be confirmed by electron microscopy of biopsy specimen.

- Many months of psoralen and UV therapy can partially or completely repigment areas.
- Potent topical steroids are used on areas such as lips not amenable to phototherapy.

Urticaria–Angioedema

DEFINITION

Allergic response leading to edema of the tissues.

ETIOLOGY/PATHOPHYSIOLOGY

Type I hypersensitivity reaction of immunoglobulin E (IgE) with mast cells causes the release of histamine, leading to vasodilation, increased vascular permeability, and axonal response.

EPIDEMIOLOGY

Can occur in response to a whole host of entities—ingestion, contact, infectious agents, environmental factors, or genetic conditions.

SIGNS AND SYMPTOMS

- **Urticaria**—well circumscribed, but can be coalescent, erythematous, raised lesions (wheals or welts) (see Figure 20-14)
- **Angioedema**—involves the deeper layers of skin, submucosa, and subcutaneous tissues

TREATMENT

- Usually self-limited.
- Antihistamines to relieve pruritus.
- Watch for signs of airway compromise (especially with angioedema).
- Epinephrine for severe cases.

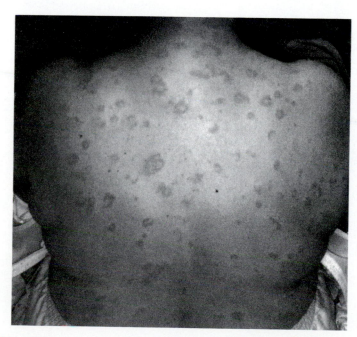

FIGURE 20-14. Urticaria.

See Table 20-2.

TABLE 20-2. Neonatal dermatologic conditions.

Condition	Etiology	Appearance	Resolution
Sebaceous hyperplasia	Maternal hormones	Shiny, yellow papules	A few weeks
Acne neonatorum	Maternal hormones	Similar to minor acne vulgaris	Peaks at 2 months
Milia	Retention of dead skin and oily material in hair follicles	White papules on face	Within first month
Erythema toxicum	Unknown, possible hypersensitivity	Blotchy red spots with overlying white or yellow papules or pustules	A few days
Mongolian spots	Melanocytes arrested in migration from neural crest to epidermis	Congenital, blue-gray macules, especially in nonwhite infants	First few years of life, though some never disappear

Note: All of these conditions are diagnosed clinically, are self-limited, and rarely require treatment.

See Table 20-3.

TABLE 20-3. Dermatologic manifestations of some infectious diseases.

Rubella (German measles)	■ Pink macules and papules, initially on face and spread inferiorly within 24 hours
Measles (rubeola) [a paramyxovirus]	■ Erythematous macules and papules initially along hairline, spreading inferiorly within 2–3 days, fade within 4–6 days with subsequent desquamation ■ Koplik's spots—bluish-white papules on erythematous base appear on day 1–2 of fever, over buccal mucosa, adjacent to second molars
Hand, foot, and mouth disease [coxsackie A virus]	■ Stomatitis—vesicles rapidly open to painful ulcers ■ Gray blisters on hands and feet on background erythema
Rocky Mountain spotted fever [Rickettsia rickettsii]	■ 2–6-mm blanchable macules that first appear peripherally on wrists, forearms, ankles, palms, and soles ■ Spreads to trunk, proximal extremities, and face within 6–18 hours ■ Evolve to deep red papules and petechiae over 1–3 days ■ Within 2–4 days, exanthem is no longer blanchable
Erythema infectiosum (fifth disease) [parvovirus B19]	■ "Slapped cheeks"—red papules coalesce on face ■ Reticulate rash on buttocks and upper arms that spreads ■ Palms and soles may be involved ■ Mucous membranes may have red spots
Meningococcemia [Neisseria meningitidis]	■ Discrete, pink macules, papules, and petechiae over trunk, extremities, and palate
Gonococcemia [Neisseria gonorrhea]	■ Erythematous macules over arms and legs evolve into hemorrhagic, painful pustules within 2–3 days
Syphilis [Treponema pallidum]	■ Primary—painless "button-like" chancre with indurated borders ■ Secondary—multiple, discrete, firm, "ham-colored" papules scattered symmetrically over trunk, palm, soles, and genitals; condyloma lata—soft, flat-topped, pink papules in anogenital region ■ Tertiary—some untreated develop brown, firm plaques on body
Lyme disease [Borrelia burgdorferi]	■ Erythema chronicum migrans—expanding, erythematous, annular plaque with central clearing
Kawasaki's disease [etiology unknown]	■ Erythematous macules and plaques appear in a stocking and glove distribution 1–3 days after onset of fever ■ Spreads to involve trunk and extremities within 2 days, lasts an average of 12 days

See Table 20-4.

TABLE 20-4. Dermatologic manifestations of systemic disease.

Tuberous sclerosis	■ *Ash leaf*—hypopigmented lesions anywhere on body ■ *Shagreen patches*—raised patches on lower back with orange-peel texture ■ *Adenoma sebaceum*—red, vascular nodules on face that may resemble aggravated acne ■ *Periungual fibromas*
Neurofibromatosis	■ *Café-au-lait spots*—flat, sharply demarcated, ovoid, light brown macules, with the long axis oriented along a cutaneous nerve track
Sturge–Weber syndrome	■ *Port-wine stain*—hemangioma variant; appears as a sharply marginated, red or purple macule, commonly distributed unilaterally on the face; present at birth and never disappears; lesion grows proportionally to the size of the individual and may develop papular and nodular areas (see Figure 20-13)
Bacterial endocarditis	■ *Osler's nodes*—tender, violaceous subcutaneous nodules on palms and soles ■ *Janeway lesions*—multiple, hemorrhagic, nontender macules on fingers and toes ■ Subungual splinter hemorrhages ■ Multiple, nonblanching red macules (petechiae) on upper chest and mucous membranes
Obesity, endocrinopathy, malignancy (GI)	■ *Acanthosis nigricans*—velvety, hyperpigmented plaques; occur in axillae and groin
Peutz–Jeghers syndrome	■ *Lentigines*—hyperpigmented macules on nose, mouth, oral cavity, hands, and feet

Psychiatric Disease

PSYCHIATRIC EXAMINATION OF CHILDREN

- Consult multiple sources:
  - Child—young children usually report information in concrete terms but give accurate details about their emotional states
  - Parents
  - Teachers
  - Child welfare/justice
- Methods of gathering information:
  - Play, stories, drawing
  - Kaufman Assessment Battery for Children (K-ABC)—intelligence test for ages 2½ to 12
  - Wechsler Intelligence Scale for Children–Revised (WISC-R)—intelligence quotient (IQ) for ages 6 to 16
  - Peabody Individual Achievement Test (PIAT)—tests academic achievement

MENTAL RETARDATION (MR)

See chapter on neurologic disease.

LEARNING DISORDERS

See chapter on neurologic disease.

BEHAVIORAL DISORDERS

DEFINITION
Behavioral disorders include oppositional defiant disorder and conduct disorder.

Oppositional Defiant Disorder (ODD)
DIAGNOSIS
- Recurrent pattern of negativistic, defiant, disobedient, and hostile behavior for 6 months, with four or more of the following:

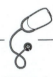

- Loses temper
- Argues with adults
- Refuses to comply with adult requests or rules
- Deliberately annoys
- Does not take responsibility for mistakes or behavior
- Sensitive, touchy, easily annoyed
- Angry, resentful
- Spiteful, vindictive
- Behavior causes impairment in social and academic functioning.
- Rule out other causes of clinical presentation.

PATHOPHYSIOLOGY

Low self-esteem, low frustration tolerance, precocious use of substances.

EPIDEMIOLOGY

- 2–16% prevalence
- May be a precursor of a conduct disorder
- Increased incidence of substance abuse, mood disorders, attention deficit–hyperactivity disorder (ADHD)

TREATMENT

- Behavioral therapy, problem-solving skills
- Family involvement, parenting skills training regarding limit setting and consistency

Conduct Disorder

DIAGNOSIS

A pattern of behavior that involves violation of the basic rights of others or of social norms and rules, with at least three of the following in 1 year:

- Aggression toward people and animals
- Destruction of property
- Deceitfulness
- Serious violation of rules

ETIOLOGY

Involves genetic and psychosocial factors.

EPIDEMIOLOGY

- 6–16% in boys, 2–9% in girls
- Up to 40% risk of developing antisocial personality disorder in adulthood
- Increased incidence of ADHD, learning disorders, mood disorders, substance abuse, and criminal behavior in adulthood

TREATMENT

Multimodal:

- Structured environment, firm rules, consistent enforcement
- Psychotherapy—behavior modification, problem-solving skills
- Adjunctive pharmacotherapy may help—antipsychotics, lithium, selective serotonin reuptake inhibitors (SSRIs)

DEFINITION

Three types predominantly:
- Inattentive
- Hyperactive–impulsive
- Combined

DIAGNOSIS

- Six or more of the following for 6 months:
  - Inattention—problems listening, concentrating, paying attention to details, organizing tasks, easily distracted, forgetful
  - Hyperactivity–impulsivity—unable to inhibit impulses in social behavior, leading to blurting out, interrupting, fidgeting, leaving seat, talking excessively
  - Onset before age 7 years
  - Behavior inconsistent with age and development
- Impairment in two or more social settings.
- Evidence of impairment in functioning.
- Rule out other causes of the clinical presentation.
- The above may lead to:
  - Difficulty getting along with peers and family
  - School underachievement secondary to poor organizational skills
  - Poor sequential memory, deficits in fine motor skills

ETIOLOGY

- Genetic predisposition
- Perinatal complications, maternal nutrition and substance abuse, obstetric complications, viral infections
- Neurochemical/neurophysiologic factors
- Psychosocial factors, including emotional deprivation and parental anxiety and inexperience

PATHOPHYSIOLOGY

- Catecholamine hypothesis, a decrease in norepinephrine metabolites
- Hypodopaminergic function, low levels of homovanillic acid

EPIDEMIOLOGY

- Three to ten percent prevalence among young and school-age children.
- Male-to-female ratio: 3:1.
- Increased incidence of mood disorders, personality disorders, conduct disorder, and ODD.
- Most cases remit in adolescence; 20% have symptoms into adulthood.

TREATMENT

- Pharmacotherapy:
  - Psychostimulants—methylphenidate (Ritalin), dextroamphetamine, pemoline
  - Tricyclic antidepressants (TCAs), SSRIs
- Psychotherapy—behavior modification
- Parental counseling—positive reinforcement, firm nonpunitive limit setting, reduce external stimulation
- Group therapy—social skills, self-esteem

Conduct disorder is the most common diagnosis in outpatient psychiatry clinics.

The three cardinal signs of ADHD:
- Inattention
- Hyperactivity
- Impulsivity

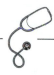

Symptoms must be present in two or more situations for a diagnosis of ADHD.

Typical Scenario

A 9-year-old boy's mother has been called to school because her son has not done his homework. He claims that he did not know about the assignments. He interrupts other kids and is always getting up during class. *Think:* ADHD.

Onset of ADHD occurs no later than age 7 years.

HIGH-YIELD FACTS

Psychiatric Disease

DEFINITION

- Group of conditions that involve problems with social skills, language, and behaviors
- Apparent early in life with developmental delay involving multiple areas of development
- Include autistic disorder, Asperger's syndrome, Rett syndrome, and childhood disintegrative disorder

TREATMENT

- There is no cure, but goal of treatment is to manage symptoms and improve social skills.
- Remedial education.
- Behavioral therapy.
- Neuroleptics such as haloperidol to control self-injurious and aggressive behavior and mood lability.
- SSRIs to help control stereotyped and repetitive behaviors.

Autistic Disorder

DIAGNOSIS

- Diagnosis made within the first 3 years and other causes of the clinical presentation ruled out
- At least six of the following (with at least two from qualitative impairment in social interaction, one from qualitative impairments in communication, and one from patterns of behavior):
  - Qualitative impairment in social interaction (at least two):
    - Marked impairment in the use of multiple nonverbal behaviors, including poor eye contact
    - Failure to develop peer relationships and attachments
    - Lack of spontaneous seeking to share enjoyment, interests, achievements
    - Lack of emotional or social reciprocity
  - Qualitative impairments in communication (at least one):
    - Delay or lack of spoken language (expressive language deficit)
    - Marked impairment in the ability to initiate or sustain a conversation with others
    - Stereotyped and repetitive use of language or idiosyncratic language
    - Lack of spontaneous make-believe play or social initiative
  - Repetitive and stereotyped patterns of behavior and activities (at least one)
    - Inflexible rituals
    - Preoccupations
  - Highly responsive to intimate environment, stimulus overselectivity, unable to cope with change in routine

ETIOLOGY

- Genetic predisposition (36% concordance rate in monozygotic twins, 0% in dizygotic twins)
- Prenatal neurologic insult
- Immunologic and biochemical factors

ADHD is the most common significant behavioral syndrome in childhood.

Two thirds of children with ADHD also have conduct disorder or ODD.

The most efficacious pharmacotherapeutic agents for ADHD are psychostimulants, though behavioral modification and firm limit setting should also be used. Seventy-five percent of patients have significant improvement on Ritalin.

Stimulants used appropriately for ADHD do not cause addiction.

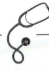

Two areas are particularly affected in autistic disorder:
- Communication
- Social interactions

PATHOPHYSIOLOGY

- Neuroanatomic structural abnormalities
- Abnormalities in dopamine and serotonin system—increase in serotonin

EPIDEMIOLOGY

- 10 to 15:10,000
- Male-to-female ratio: 4:1
- Onset—first year (25%), second year (50%), after 2 years (25%)
- Significant comorbidity with fragile X syndrome, tuberous sclerosis, mental retardation, and seizures

PROGNOSIS

Depends on presence or absence of underlying disorder and speech.

Asperger's Syndrome

DIAGNOSIS

- Impaired social interaction (at least two, similar to autistic disorder)
- Restricted or stereotyped behaviors, interests, or activities

EPIDEMIOLOGY

Male > female.

Rett Syndrome

DIAGNOSIS

- Normal pre- and perinatal development until between 5 and 48 months of age
- Normal head circumference at birth, but decreases rate of growth between the ages of 5 and 48 months
- Loss of previously learned purposeful hand skills between the ages of 5 and 30 months, followed by the development of stereotyped hand movements
- Early loss of social interaction, usually followed by subsequent improvement
- Problems with gait or trunk movements
- Severely impaired language and psychomotor development

EPIDEMIOLOGY

Classically restricted to females; males are beginning to be recognized due to genetic testing.

Childhood Disintegrative Disorder

DIAGNOSIS

- Normal development in the first 2 years of life
- Loss of previously acquired skills in at least two of the following:
  - Language
  - Social skills
  - Bowel or bladder control
  - Play
  - Motor skills

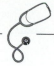

Half of children with autistic disorder never speak.

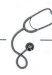

Those with autistic disorder who do speak exhibit echolalia, pronoun reversal, inappropriate cadence or intonation, impaired semantics, and failure to use language for social interaction.

Typical Scenario

A 3-year-old boy is brought in by his parents because they think he is deaf. He shows no interest in them or anyone around him and speaks only when spoken to directly. He often lines his toys up in a straight line. Hearing tests are normal. *Think:* Autism.

Computed tomography (CT) and magnetic resonance imaging (MRI) in autistic disorder show ventricular enlargement; polymicrogyria; and small, densely packed, immature cells in the limbic system and cerebellum.

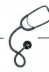

Unlike those with autistic disorder, children with Asperger's syndrome have normal language and cognitive development.

Typical Scenario

A 13-year-old boy has had uncontrollable blinking since he was 9 years old. Recently, he has noticed that he often involuntarily makes a barking noise that is embarrassing. *Think:* Tourette's disorder.

Tics in Tourette's disorder may be consciously repressed for short periods of time.

- At least two of the following:
  - Impaired social interaction
  - Impaired use of language
  - Restricted, repetitive, and stereotyped behaviors and interests

EPIDEMIOLOGY

- Onset ages 2 to 10 years
- Four to eight times higher incidence in boys
- Rare

TIC DISORDERS

Tics

- Involuntary movements or vocalizations.
- Most common motor tics involve the face and head (e.g., blinking of eyes).
- Examples of vocal tics include coprolalia (repetitive speaking of obscene words) and echolalia (exact repetition of words).

Tourette's Disorder

DIAGNOSIS

- Multiple motor and vocal tics occurring multiple times per day, almost daily for > 1 year (no tic-free period for > 3 months)
- Onset before age 18
- Distress or impairment in social functioning

EPIDEMIOLOGY

- Three times more common in boys
- Onset usually between the ages of 7 and 8 years
- High comorbidity with obsessive–compulsive disorder (OCD) and ADHD

ETIOLOGY

- Genetic—50% concordance rate in monozygotic twins, 8% in dizygotic
- Neurochemical—impaired regulation of dopamine in the caudate nucleus

TREATMENT

- Pharmacotherapy—haloperidol or pimozide
- Supportive psychotherapy

ELIMINATION DISORDERS

Enuresis

DIAGNOSIS

- Lack of involuntary urinary continence beyond age 4 for diurnal enuresis and age 6 for nocturnal enuresis
- Occurs at least twice per week for at least 3 consecutive months
- Types:
  - Primary—child never established continence
  - Secondary—most commonly occurs between ages 5 and 8 years
- Rule out the influence of a medical condition (e.g., urethritis, diabetes, seizures)

ETIOLOGY

- Genetic predisposition
- Physical factors—small bladder, low nocturnal levels of antidiuretic hormone (ADH)
- Delayed or stringent toilet training
- Psychosocial stressors

EPIDEMIOLOGY

- 7% male and 3% female prevalence at 5 years old
- 3% male and 2% female prevalence at 10 years old

SIGNS AND SYMPTOMS

Urination during the day, night, or both on the individual.

TREATMENT

- According to specific causative factors suggested by an adequate psychosocial evaluation.
- Enlist child in cure, offer positive reinforcement, do not punish; older children participate in cleaning up.
- No liquids after dinner; urinate before going to bed.
- Behavior modification therapy (e.g., buzzer to wake up child when wetness is detected).
- Pharmacotherapy—antidiuretics (DDAVP) or TCAs (imipramine).

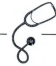

Most cases of enuresis spontaneously remit by age 7.

Encopresis

DIAGNOSIS

- Repeated passage of feces into inappropriate places (e.g., clothing or floor) whether involuntary or intentional.
- At least one such event a month for at least 3 months.
- Individual must be at least 4 years old.
- Rule out the influence of a medication or a general medical condition (e.g., hypothyroidism, lower gastrointestinal [GI] problems, dietary factors).

ETIOLOGY

- Anxiety about defecating in a particular place
- A more generalized anxiety in response to stressful environmental factors
- Oppositional behavior
- Physiologic conditions—lack of sphincter control, constipation with overflow incontinence

EPIDEMIOLOGY

- One percent prevalence in 5-year-old children.
- Incidence decreases with age.
- More common in males than females.
- Associated with other conditions such as conduct disorder and ADHD.

TREATMENT

- According to the specific causative factors suggested by an adequate psychosocial evaluation.
- Enlist child in cure, positive reinforcement; do not punish.
- Older children participate in cleaning up.
- Choose a specific time every day to attempt bowel movement.
- Stool softeners, if related to constipation.
- Psychotherapy, family therapy, and behavioral therapy.

Encopresis in a 7-year-old child likely indicates a more serious disturbance than thumb-sucking in a 4-year-old, which is more serious than a nightmare in a 5-year-old, breath-holding spells in a 2-year-old, and nocturnal enuresis in a 6-year-old.

Major Depressive Disorder (MDD)

DEFINITION

- Pathologic sadness or despondency not explained as a normal response to stress and causing an impairment in function
- Recurrent condition that generally continues into adulthood

ETIOLOGY/PATHOPHYSIOLOGY

- Genetic predisposition.
- Catecholamine hypothesis: Depression is caused by a deficit of norepinephrine at nerve terminals throughtout the brain.
- Cortisol hypothesis: Larger quantities of cortisol metabolites in blood and urine, abnormal diurnal variation.

EPIDEMIOLOGY

- Seven percent of general pediatric patients.
- Twenty-eight percent of child psychiatry clinic patients.
- Fifteen to twenty percent incidence in adolescents.
- Two to three times higher in postpubertal girls than boys.
- Other mental disorders frequently co-occur with major depressive episode including anxiety/panic disorders, OCD, eating disorders, substance abuse, borderline personality disorder, ADHD, and ODD.

DIAGNOSIS

- At least five of the following for a 2-week period:
  - Depressed mood
  - Loss of interest in activities
  - Sleep disturbance
  - Weight change or appetite disturbance
  - Decreased concentration
  - Suicidal ideation
  - Psychomotor agitation or retardation
  - Fatigue or loss of energy
  - Feelings of worthlessness or inappropriate guilt
- Always rule out other causes of the clinical presentation (e.g., hypothyroidism, nutritional deficiency, chronic infection/systemic disease, substance abuse).

COMPLICATIONS

- Can persist into adulthood.
- Up to 15% of patients with depression commit suicide each year.

TREATMENT

- If suicidal or homicidal, admit to the hospital
- Biopsychosocial approach
- Individual and/or group therapy
- Family intervention
- TCAs, monoamine oxidase inhibitors (MAOIs), SSRIs
- Electric shock therapy for catatonic syndrome or intractable depression

Suicide

DEFINITION

- Suicide is a complex human behavior with biologic, sociologic, and psychological roots that results in a self-inflicted death that is intentional rather than accidental.

Fifty to sixty percent of individuals with a single depressive episode can be expected to have a second episode.

Electroencephalography (EEG) in depression shows decreased slow-wave (delta) sleep, shortened time before onset of rapid eye movement (REM), and longer duration of REM.

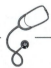

In suspected cases of depression, be sure to look for other signs or risk factors such as school failure or family history of mental health disorders.

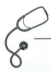

A combination of treatments for depression may be necessary. Childhood depression should be treated with behavior modification before medication.

- Suicide ideation, with or without a plan.
- Suicide gesture—for attention, without intent for death.
- Suicide attempt.

ETIOLOGY

- Genetic predisposition
- Psychiatric disorders—correlations of suicidal behavior and mood or disruptive disorders, substance abuse
- Environmental factors—stressful life events; family disruption due to death or separation, illness, birth, or siblings; peer pressure; physical or sexual abuse
- Parental influence—psychiatric illness, substance abuse, violence, physical or sexual abuse

PATHOPHYSIOLOGY

Multiple abnormalities, which may indicate risk for depression, not directly for suicide:

- Low levels of cerebrospinal fluid (CSF) 5-hydroxyindoleacetic acid (5-HIAA), a serotonin metabolite
- Decreased imipramine binding in the frontal cortex
- Abnormal dexamethasone suppression tests suggesting presence of hypothalamic–pituitary–adrenal axis hyperactivity
- High levels of cortisol urinary metabolites
- Enlarged adrenal glands

EPIDEMIOLOGY

- Attempted suicides:
  - 0.7% 5 to 14 years old
  - 13% 15 to 24 years old
- Third leading cause of death for young adults aged 15 to 24 years old.
- In the United States, there are about 50 to 200 attempts for each complete suicide.
- Males more frequently complete suicide, but females attempt more often.
- The rate of suicide is higher in Alaskan, Asian-American, and Native American youth.
- Of the 1–2% of those who attempt suicide, 10% will eventually complete the act.
- Risk factors: Look for psychiatric disorders, family clustering of suicides, substance use/abuse, history of sexual abuse, or serotonin abnormalities.

DIAGNOSIS

- Even though risk factors for suicide are known, it is not possible to predict who will commit suicide.
- Assess signs and symptoms, correlate with other clinical variables such as psychiatric and substance abuse history, gender, age, race, prior history of suicide attempts, and recent traumatic life events.
- Key questions: Are you having any thoughts about harming yourself? taking your life? Have you developed a plan? What is your plan?

TREATMENT

- Immediate hospitalization; remove all potentially lethal items.
- Psychotherapeutic intervention, trustful atmosphere, coping strategies; remove motivation for suicide; involve parents and relatives, guidance counselor.
- Pharmacotherapy depends on the accompanying diagnosis.

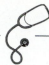

One percent of suicide gestures are lethal.

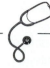

Seventy-five percent of those who go on to attempt suicide convey their suicidal intentions directly or indirectly.

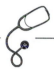

Thirty to seventy percent of suicides occur with significant alcohol or drug abuse. Substance abuse disinhibits the individual to complete the act.

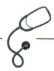

Suicide completers: male, older, history of depression, alcoholism, schizophrenia, careful planning, high lethality, firearms. Suicide attempters: female, younger, history of depression, alcoholism, personality disorder, impulsive, no planning, low lethality, drug overdose.

Suicidal ideation, when accompanied by a specific plan, must be taken seriously, and these patients need to be hospitalized for assistance and suicide precautions.

VIOLENT BEHAVIOR

EPIDEMIOLOGY

- From 1983 to 1993 the firearm homicide rate more than tripled from 5 to 18 in 100,000.
- Rates of homicide are higher in males than in females.
- Death by firearm homicide is highest in the 15- to 24-year-old age group.

RISK FACTORS

Look for clinical entities associated with violent behavior such as mental retardation, moderate to severe language disorder, learning disorder, ADHD, mood disorders, anxiety disorders, personality disorders, conduct disorders, and ODD.

SCREENING

Ask about recent involvement in physical fights, carrying a weapon, firearms in household, concerns that an adolescent has about his/her safety, past episodes of trauma, and social problems in school or neighborhood.

SUBSTANCE ABUSE

EPIDEMIOLOGY

- Alcohol and cigarettes are the most prevalent drugs among school-age young adults.
- Marijuana is the most commonly reported illicit drug used.
- The prevalence of substance abuse varies according to age, gender, geographic region, race, and other demographic factors.

SIGNS AND SYMPTOMS

See Table 21-1 for signs and symptoms of intoxication and withdrawal due to substances of abuse.

ANXIETY DISORDERS

Separation Anxiety

DEFINITION

- Excessive anxiety beyond that expected for the child's developmental level related to separation or impending separation from the attachment figure.
- Separation anxiety is normal until age 3 to 4 years.

EPIDEMIOLOGY

- 4% of school-age children.
- Males and females are affected equally.

ETIOLOGY

Contribution by parental anxiety/excessive concern expressed.

SIGNS AND SYMPTOMS

- May refuse to sleep alone or go to school
- May complain of physical symptoms in order to avoid anxiety-provoking activities

TABLE 21-1 Substances of abuse—intoxication and withdrawal.

Substance	Intoxication/Overdose	Withdrawal
Alcohol	Decreased fine motor control Impaired judgment and coordination Ataxic gait and poor balance Lethargy, difficulty sitting upright Respiratory depression	Irritability, insomnia, disorientation, tremor, diaphoresis (6–24 hours) Alcoholic hallucinosis (1–2 days) Delirium tremens (2–5 days)—grand mal seizures Rx: benzodiazepines
Sedative–hypnotics (benzodiazepines, barbiturates)	Drowsiness, slurred speech Incoordination, ataxia Mood lability, impaired judgment Nystagmus Respiratory depression, coma, death Rx: benzodiazepines—Flumazenil (careful, may precipitate seizures); barbiturates—alkalinize urine; both—activated charcoal	Autonomic hyperactivity Insomnia, anxiety, tremor Nausea, vomiting Delirium, hallucinations Seizures—may be life threatening
Stimulants (cocaine, amphetamines)	Euphoria, sweating, chills, nausea Autonomic instability, cardiac arrhythmias Psychomotor agitation, dilated pupils Vasoconstriction—MI, CVA Rx: benzodiazepines (haloperidol if severe)	Not life threatening Dysphoric "crash," depression, anxiety Hunger, craving Constricted pupils
Opioids (heroin, codeine, morphine, methadone, meperidine)	Drowsiness, slurred speech Nausea, vomiting, constipation Constricted pupils Seizures Respiratory depression Rx: nalaxone/naltrexone, methadone taper	Not life threatening Dysphoria, insomnia Lacrimation, rhinorrhea Yawning, weakness, muscle ache Sweating, piloerection, dilated pupils Nausea, vomiting Rx: Clonidine, methadone taper
Hallucinogens (mushrooms, mescaline, LSD)	Perceptual changes, papillary dilation Tachycardia, palpitations Tremors, incoordination Rx: "talk down"	May have flashbacks later due to reabsorption of lipid stores
PCP (hallucinogen)	Violence, recklessness, impulsivity Impaired judgment, nystagmus, ataxia Hypertension, tachycardia Muscle rigidity, high pain tolerance Seizures, coma Rx: benzodiazepines, acidify urine	As with other hallucinogens, flashbacks may occur
Marijuana (THC)	Euphoria, impaired concentration Mild tachycardia Conjunctival injection Dry mouth, increased appetite	No withdrawal syndrome, but mild irritability, insomnia, nausea, and decreased appetite may occur in heavy users
Inhalants	Impaired judgment, belligerence, impulsivity Perceptual disturbances, slurred speech Ataxia, dizziness Nystagmus, tremor, hyporeflexia Lethargy, euphoria, stupor, coma Respiratory depression, cardiac arrhythmias	Does not usually occur, but can Irritability, nausea, vomiting, tachycardia Occasional hallucinations

(continues)

HIGH-YIELD FACTS

Psychiatric Disease

Substance	Intoxication/Overdose	Withdrawal
Caffeine	Anxiety, insomnia, twitching Flushed face, rambling speech GI disturbance, diuresis	Headache, nausea, vomiting, drowsiness Anxiety, depression
Nicotine	Restlessness, insomnia, anxiety Increased GI motility	Dysphoria, anxiety, irritability, insomnia Increased appetite, craving

Rx, treatment; MI, myocardial infarction; CVA, cerebrovascular accident; LSD, lysergic acid diethylamide; PCP, phencyclidine; THC, tetrahydrocannabinol; GI, gastrointestinal.

- Become extremely distressed when forced to separate, and may worry excessively about losing their parents forever

TREATMENT

- Family therapy
- Supportive psychotherapy
- Low-dose antidepressants

School Phobia

DEFINITION

- A child who develops emotional upset at the prospect of going to school in the absence of severe antisocial behavior
- Related to separation anxiety

ETIOLOGY

- Environmental, hostile, or dependent relationship between a parent and child; stressful events at home or school
- Concurrent psychiatric disorders, depression, separation anxiety, generalized anxiety, posttraumatic stress, somatoform disorder, avoidant personality disorder

PATHOPHYSIOLOGY

Neurotransmitter systems implicated, noradrenergic, gamma-aminobutyric acid (GABA), serotonergic in frontal lobe and limbic system.

EPIDEMIOLOGY

- More common in lower socioeconomic classes, younger children in the family, early teenage years, lack of parental interest or education
- Equal in both males and females
- Most frequent among younger children
- 5% of elementary school children
- 2% of junior high school children

SIGNS AND SYMPTOMS

- Avoidance behavior in relation to school; seek situations that provide comfort and security; once in school, comfortable and productive, fear of school recurs the next day despite positive experience the day before
- Physical complaints secondary to anxiety—anorexia, headache, abdominal pain

DIAGNOSIS

- Marked and persistent fear that is excessive and unreasonable, instigated by the anticipation of the school situation.
- Exposure to school provokes an immediate anxiety response.
- School is avoided.
- School phobia interferes with academic and social functioning.
- Duration of at least 6 months.
- Other mental disorders ruled out.

TREATMENT

- Mainstay of treatment is returning the child to regular school attendance.
- Behavioral therapy, recognize and control anxiety symptoms.
- Anxiolytics or antidepressants for a short period of time when the symptoms are most severe.

EEG in school phobia — decreased α activity, stage I, and REM; increased β activity.
Findings secondary to inhibition of the autonomic nervous system.

Obsessive–Compulsive Disorder (OCD)

DEFINITIONS

- **Obsessions**—self-aware; senseless, unnecessary, unwanted thoughts, images, impulses involuntarily intruding into consciousness causing distress and functional impairment
- **Compulsions**—actions that are responses to a perceived internal obligation to follow certain rituals and rules, which may be motivated directly by obsessions or efforts to ward off certain thoughts or fears

DIAGNOSIS

- Impaired social, academic, or vocational functioning with four or more of the following:
  - Preoccupied with details, rules, lists, order, organization, or schedules resulting in loss of the goal of activity
  - Perfectionism that prohibits task completion
  - Social impairment secondary to preoccupation with work and level of productivity
  - Overconscientious, scrupulous, and inflexible about matters of morality, ethics, or values
  - Unable to discard objects of no worth or sentimental value
  - Preference to work as an individual and not in a group
  - Miserly spending in order to save for future catastrophes
  - Unflexible, rigid, stubborn
- Characteristics must be ego-dystonic and functionally disruptive versus ego-syntonic and functionally adaptive in OCD.

ETIOLOGY

Genetic predisposition, higher concordance among monozygotic versus dizygotic twins.

PATHOPHYSIOLOGY

- CT/MRI show increased ventricle size and abnormal frontal cortex, cingulate gyrus, and lenticular nuclei.
- Decreased CSF 5-HIAA, a metabolite of serotonin.

EPIDEMIOLOGY

High comorbidity with ADHD and tic disorders.

- Unproductive because of preoccupation with details, rules, lists, schedules, organization, order.
- Uncompleted tasks secondary to perfectionist tendencies.
- Work habits interfere with social interactions.
- Impossible standards of morals, ethics, or values.
- Inflexible, stubborn, cheap; prefers to work as an individual and not in a group.

TREATMENT

- Long-term therapy is required.
- Maintain a professional distance from the patient.
- Establish ground rules for therapy.
- Behavioral therapy such as self-observation, extinction, operant conditioning, and modeling.
- Pharmacotherapy:
  - First-line agents are SSRIs (i.e., fluoxetine, fluvoxamine, paroxetine, sertraline).
  - Clomipramine is a second-line agent.
  - Also lithium, L-tryptophan.

Habit

DEFINITION

Repetitive patterns of movement used to discharge tension.

ETIOLOGY

- A stressful environment at home or school
- Concurrent psychiatric disorders including anxiety or depression

PATHOPHYSIOLOGY

- Exacerbated following exposure to agents that increase dopaminergic activity, due to altered receptor function in the midbrain.
- Purposeful movement loses original meaning and becomes repetitive and a means to discharge anxiety or provide comfort.

EPIDEMIOLOGY

- Highest prevalence among 7- to 11-year-olds
- 1 to 13% males
- 1 to 11% females

SIGNS AND SYMPTOMS

- Bruxism (teeth grinding or clenching)
- Tics, repetitive movement, gesture or utterance that mimics some aspect of normal behavior
- Stuttering, impairment in speech fluency characterized by frequent repetitions or prolongations of sounds or syllables
- Thumb-sucking, self-nurturing and comforting behavior

Individual is often unaware of habitual behavior.

Habit reversal: substituting another more benign behavior for the previous habit.

TREATMENT

Behavior therapy: identify habit, under what circumstances it most often occurs, work on habit reversal.

Selective Mutism

DEFINITION

Not speaking in certain situations (e.g., school).

- Onset usually around age 5 or 6
- Girls > boys
- May be preceded by a stressful life event

TREATMENT

Supportive psychotherapy, behavior therapy, family therapy.

GENDER IDENTITY DISORDER

DEFINITION

- Intense, persistent, and pervasive preoccupation with becoming a member of the opposite sex.
- Patients exhibit a strong and persistent cross-gender identification and a sense of inappropriateness about their assigned sex.

EPIDEMIOLOGY

- 1:30,000 males, 1:100,000 females.
- Coexisting separation and/or generalized anxiety disorder or depression is common.
- Increases risk of suicide.

SIGNS AND SYMPTOMS

For genetic men—overidentification with the mother, overtly feminine behavior, little interest in usual male pursuits, peer relationships primarily with girls.

DIAGNOSIS

- Persistent discomfort with his or her sex
- Four or more of the following:
  - Stated desire to be or that he or she is the other sex
  - Wearing clothes appropriate to the opposite sex
  - Persistent role playing or fantasies of being the opposite sex
  - Interest in the habits of the opposite sex
  - Preference for playmates of the opposite sex

TREATMENT

- Sexual reassignment surgery
- Hormonal therapy
- Electrolysis to remove hair
- Psychotherapy aimed at helping individual to accept his or her anatomic sex, adjustment in social and occupational areas
- Psychotherapy after surgery—the emotionally unstable person before surgery is the same person after surgery

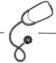

Social and occupational adjustment is usually no better after surgery for gender identity disorder.

EATING DISORDERS (EDs)

Anorexia Nervosa

DIAGNOSIS

- Refusal to maintain body weight at or above 85% of ideal weight for age and height
- Even though underweight, an intense fear of gaining weight
- Disturbance in self-perception of body weight and lack of insight into the seriousness of physical condition
- The absence of at least three consecutive menstrual cycles in women

HIGH-YIELD FACTS

Psychiatric Disease

ETIOLOGY

- Genetic predisposition (6–10% of female relatives of anorexic patients have the condition, twin studies confirm)
- Psychological need to control, perfectionism
- Conforming to society's ideal of beauty
- Stressful life events such as leaving home for college or death in the family

PATHOPHYSIOLOGY

- A primary hypothalamic disturbance secondary to increased corticotropin-releasing factor
- Central neurotransmitter dysregulation affecting dopamine, serotonin, and norepinephrine
- Reduced norepinephrine activity and turnover
- Endocrine abnormalities, increased growth hormone levels, loss of cortisol diurnal variation, reduced luteinizing hormone (LH), follicle-stimulating hormone (FSH), impaired response to luteinizing hormone–releasing hormone (LHRH), abnormal glucose tolerance test

EPIDEMIOLOGY

- Predominance in females (female-to-male ratio 10:1).
- One percent prevalence among women.
- Bimodal onset at 14 and 18 years.
- More common in industrialized countries.
- Incidence has increased over the last two decades.
- More common in activities such as ballet, gymnastics, and modeling.

SIGNS AND SYMPTOMS

- Extreme dieting, special diets such as vegetarianism
- Refusal to eat meals with family members or in public
- Rituals surrounding meals
- Preoccupation with food and its preparation
- Intense fear of becoming obese, which does not diminish as weight loss progresses
- Disturbance in the way in which one's body, weight, size, and/or shape is experienced such as "feeling fat" although one may be emaciated
- Denial of hunger
- Obsessive interest in physical exercise
- Abuse laxatives, diuretics, or stimulants in an effort to enhance weight loss
- Studiousness and academic success
- Affects all organ systems:
  - Amenorrhea
  - Hypothermia
  - Constipation
  - Low blood pressure, bradycardia
  - Lanugo, hair loss
  - Petechiae
  - Pedal edema, dry skin
  - Osteopenia
  - Electrolyte abnormalities—alkalosis, hypokalemia
- Lab abnormalities—leukopenia, elevated liver function tests (LFTs), elevated triglycerides, carotenemia

Typical Scenario

A 16-year-old girl has a 6-month history of amenorrhea and a 25-lb. weight loss. She is thin, with Tanner stage 4 development of breasts and pubic hair. Thyroid cascade is normal. *Think:* Anorexia nervosa.

The most common cause of death in anorexia nervosa is cardiac arrhythmias due to electrolyte disturbances, particularly hypokalemia.

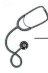

Electrocargiography (ECG) in anorexia nervosa may show low-voltage T-wave inversion and flattening, ST depression, supraventricular or ventricular arrhythmias, and/or prolonged QT intervals.

TREATMENT

- Individual and family psychotherapy—target abnormal and destructive thought processes
- Behavior modification techniques to restore normal eating behavior, set specific weight goals
- Nutritional rehabilitation—restore nutritional state and weight
- Pharmacologic therapy, especially antidepressants or anxiolytics

Bulimia Nervosa

DIAGNOSIS

- Recurrent episodes of eating within a 2-hour period of larger-than-normal proportions accompanied by a sense of lack of control over actions (binge eating).
- Recurrent compensatory behavior in order to prevent weight gain—self-induced vomiting, laxatives, diuretics, enemas, excessive exercise.
- Episodes occur at least twice a week for 3 months.
- Body shape and weight is the basis of self-evaluation.
- Does not occur exclusively during episodes of anorexia nervosa.

ETIOLOGY

Biopsychosocial.

PATHOPHYSIOLOGY

- A primary hypothalamic disturbance secondary to increased corticotropin-releasing factor
- Central neurotransmitter dysregulation affecting dopamine, serotonin, and norepinephrine
- Reduced norepinephrine activity and turnover
- Endocrine abnormalities, low triiodothyronine (T_3), high T_3 receptor uptake (T_3RU), impaired thyrotropin-releasing hormone (TRH) responsiveness, abnormal dexamethasone suppression test

EPIDEMIOLOGY

- Predominantly found in women (4% prevalence)
- Predominant in whites
- More common in industrialized countries
- Culturally dependent

SIGNS AND SYMPTOMS

- Secretive binge-eating and purging behaviors
- Often of normal weight
- Abuse laxatives, diuretics, or stimulants in an effort to enhance weight loss
- Obsessive interest in physical activity
- Physical manifestations include parotid gland enlargement, dental caries, scars on dorsum of fingers (due to teeth scraping during self-induced vomiting)
- Laboratory abnormalities include dehydration, hypokalemia, hypochloremia, hypomagenesemia, elevated blood urea nitrogen (BUN), and amylase

TREATMENT

Similar to anorexia nervosa.

The long-term mortality of anorexia nervosa is 10%.

Beware of complications occurring during rehabilitation for anorexia nervosa, including congestive heart failure (CHF), cardiac arrhythmias, and overcorrection of electrolyte abnormalities.

Typical Scenario

A 15-year-old girl has bilateral parotid gland swelling and erosion of the posterior aspect of the dental enamel of her upper incisors. *Think:* Bulimia nervosa.

Eating Disorder Not Otherwise Specified (NOS)

DEFINITION

Abnormal eating behaviors or exhibits characteristics of other eating disorders without meeting all criteria. Examples include:

- Meets all criteria for anorexia nervosa except weight falls within normal range or does not have amenorrhea
- Meets all criteria for bulimia nervosa but binge eating does not meet duration/frequency criteria
- Binge eating in the absence of purging activities

Rumination

DIAGNOSIS

- Repeated regurgitation and rechewing of food for a period of at least 1 month following a period of normal functioning.
- Onset is between 3 and 12 months in normal infant; later in the mentally retarded.
- Other medical and psychiatric conditions have been ruled out.

ETIOLOGY

- Adverse psychosocial environment
- Mental retardation

PATHOPHYSIOLOGY

- Unsatisfactory mother–infant relationship that causes the infant to seek an internal source of gratification
- Positive reinforcement when attention follows rumination
- Negative reinforcement when rumination reduces anxiety

EPIDEMIOLOGY

Highest prevalence in normal infants and mentally retarded adults.

SIGNS AND SYMPTOMS

- Presents with "spitting up" or frequent vomiting.
- Effortless regurgitation, does not involve retching.
- Infants are irritable and hungry between episodes of regurgitation.
- Malnutrition, weight loss, failure to thrive.
- 25% mortality rate.

TREATMENT

- Behavioral intervention.
- Aversive techniques, noxious stimulus is paired with rumination.
- Nonaversive techniques, differential reinforcement or other incompatible responses.
- In infants, the disorder frequently remits spontaneously.

Pica

DIAGNOSIS

- Persistent eating of nonnutritive substances for a period of at least 1 month (e.g., clay, dirt, etc.).
- The eating of nonnutritive substances is inappropriate to the level of development.
- Behavior is not culturally sanctioned.
- Rule out other psychiatric disorders.

Rumination comes from the Greek root, *ruminare*, meaning "to chew the cud."

ETIOLOGY

- Mental retardation
- Vitamin or mineral deficiencies (e.g., iron deficiency anemia, particularly in pregnancy)
- Poverty, neglect, lack of parental supervision, developmental delays
- Cultural belief

EPIDEMIOLOGY

- In children aged 18 months to 2 years, the ingestion and mouthing of nonnutritive substances is normal behavior.
- Most common during the second and third years.
- The prevalence increases with the severity of mental retardation.

SIGNS AND SYMPTOMS

- Presenting complaint—"puts everything in his or her mouth"
- Direct observation of pica
- Complications:
  - Ingestion of paint chips can lead to lead poisoning.
  - Hair or large objects can cause bowel obstruction.
  - Sharp objects such as pins or nails can cause intestinal perforation.
  - Ingestion of feces or dirt can cause toxoplasmosis and toxocariasis.

TREATMENT

- Often remits spontaneously.
- Treat underlying vitamin deficiency, if present.
- Psychotherapy—assess why pica is occurring.
- Behavior modification.
- Direct observation and removal of potential pica.

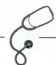

Pica is found commonly in pervasive developmental disorder and schizophrenia.

SOMATOFORM DISORDERS

See Table 21-2 comparing somatoform disorders, factitious disorders, and malingering.

DEFINITION

- Symptoms without physical cause.
- Symptoms must cause clinically significant distress or impairment in social, occupational, or other areas of functioning.
- Includes somatization disorder, undifferentiated somatoform disorder, conversion disorder, pain disorder, hypochondriasis, body dysmorphic disorder, and somatoform disorder NOS.

TREATMENT

- Psychodynamic therapy—gain insight into unconscious conflicts and understand how psychological factors have influenced maintenance of the symptoms.
- Identify and eliminate sources of secondary gain in order to avoid reinforcing the symptoms.
- Improve self-esteem, promoting assertiveness, and teaching nonsomatic ways to express distress.
- Group therapy—learn better coping strategies and improved social skills.

Somatization Disorder

- History of many physical complaints, including at least:
  - Four pain sites

Disorder	Development of Symptoms	Reason for Symptoms
Somatoform disorders	Unconscious	Unconscious
Factitious disorder	Conscious	Unconscious (primary gain)
Malingering	Conscious	Conscious (secondary gain)

- Two nonpain GI symptoms
- One sexual or reproductive complaint
- One pseudoneurologic complaint
- Age of onset < 30 years old

Conversion Disorder

DIAGNOSIS

- One or more symptoms affecting motor or sensory function that suggest a neurologic or general medical condition.
- Initiation of the symptom or deficit preceded by a psychological stressor.
- Unintentional and involuntary.
- Appropriate investigation leaves no medical explanation of symptoms.
- Symptoms cause impairment in social functioning.
- Other etiologies for the clinical presentation are ruled out.

ETIOLOGY

- Psychodynamic theory—certain developmental predispositions respond to particular types of stress with conversion symptoms
- Behaviorists—a learned excess or deficit that follows a particular event or psychological state and is reinforced by a particular event or set of conditions
- Sociocultural—predisposition of various ethnic and social groups to respond to stress with conversion symptoms

EPIDEMIOLOGY

- More common in women, rural areas, and lower socioeconomic classes
- Rare in children < 10 years
- Incidence increased in children who have experienced physical or sexual abuse and in those whose parents are seriously ill or have chronic pain

SIGNS AND SYMPTOMS

- Paralysis, abnormal movements, inability to speak, blindness, deafness, pseudoseizures.
- Usually occurs within the context of a primary illness such as major depression, schizophrenia, or somatization disorder.
- La belle indifference, the lack of interest in potentially life-altering symptoms, is common in adults, but rarely occurs in children.

Hypochondriasis

DIAGNOSIS

- Preoccupation with fear of having a disease based on the individual's misinterpretation of normal bodily sensations.

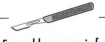

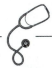

Favorable prognosis for conversion disorder is associated with acute onset, definite precipitation by a stressful event, good premorbid health, and the absence of previous psychiatric illness.

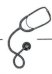

Conversion disorder may be associated in some cases with history of a traumatic brain injury.

A proportion of patients diagnosed with conversion disorder go on to develop demonstrable organic pathology (e.g., multiple sclerosis or seizure nidus)

- Persistent preoccupation despite adequate medical evaluation and assurance.
- Preoccupation causes impairment in social functioning.
- Duration of at least 6 months.
- Other psychiatric diseases ruled out.

ETIOLOGY

- Associated with anxiety, depression, and narcissistic traits
- Past experience with serious illness as a child or of a family member

EPIDEMIOLOGY

- There is a 1–9% prevalence in young adults.
- Affects males and females equally.
- The most common age of onset is early adulthood.

SIGNS AND SYMPTOMS

- Complaints involving most organ systems.
- Multiple visits to different doctors and deterioration of doctor–patient relationships.
- Individuals often believe that they are not receiving proper care so they pursue more opinions.
- Receive many evaluations and unnecessary surgeries.
- May become addicted to drugs as a result of their chronic ongoing physical complaints.

TREATMENT

- The primary aim of therapy is to help the patient identify and manage the fear of serious illness.
- In addition to techniques helpful for somatoform disorders:
  - Behavior modification techniques—earn points to participate in daily routine despite feeling sick.
  - Educate about physiologic mechanisms.

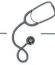

Hypochondriasis can lead to strained social relationships because of preoccupation with perceived condition and the patient's expectation of receiving special treatment.

Body Dysmorphic Disorder

Preoccupation with imagined defect in appearance or excessive concern about a slight physical anomaly (e.g., large nose, small muscles).

Pain Disorder

DIAGNOSIS

- Pain in one or more anatomic sites of sufficient severity to warrant medical attention but with no physical findings to account for the pain or its intensity.
- Pain causes impairment in social functioning.
- Psychological factors are directly related to the onset, severity, exacerbation, or maintenance of the pain.
- Pain is not intentionally produced or feigned.
- Rule out other causes of the clinical presentation.

ETIOLOGY

Psychiatric—common in conditions such as schizophrenia, somatization disorder, anxiety, dissociation, conversion, and depression.

PATHOPHYSIOLOGY
- A defect in ego function underlying the experience and expression of feelings.
- Psychologically stressful events are converted into somatic symptoms rather than the development and appropriate expression of emotions.

EPIDEMIOLOGY
Affects males and females equally.

> Alexithymia is the inability to express emotion.

FACTITIOUS DISORDERS

Munchausen Syndrome

DEFINITION
Intentional production or feigning of symptoms (e.g., thermometer manipulation, self-injury, ingestion, injection) for primary gain (e.g., relief of anxiety, being in the sick role).

ETIOLOGY
- Children or adults who make themselves sick may have been victims of Munchausen by proxy.
- Experience of misuse of illness to get attention and reinforcement of these actions.

TREATMENT
- Younger children are more likely than older children/adolescents to admit to deception if approached in a direct and concerned (not accusatory) way.
- Family therapy—recognize how family communicates through illness and identify more effective ways of communication and getting what they need from family members.
- Involvement of primary care doctor/pediatrician in confrontation.

Munchausen by Proxy (MBP)

DEFINITION
- Intentional fabrication or actual production of symptoms in a child by a caregiver (usually the mother) in order to gain attention for themselves
- A form of child abuse

EPIDEMIOLOGY
- Adults who commit MBP may have a history of factitious disorders themselves.
- Ninety-eight percent of perpetrators are women.
- Mortality rate is 9%.
- Up to 75% of the morbidity involved relates to physicians trying to treat the unknown conditions.

SIGNS AND SYMPTOMS
- Conditions that do not respond to treatment or whose courses are puzzling and persistent, often:
  - Vomiting/diarrhea (ingestion, syrup of ipecac)
  - Rashes (due to scrubbing with solvents)
  - Failure to thrive
  - Seizures

- Infections
- Adding blood or other substances to urine specimens
- Physical or laboratory findings that are unusual, discrepant, or clinically impossible or do not occur in the absence of the parent
- Medically knowledgeable/fascinated mother who appears to enjoy the hospital setting, who is reluctant to leave child, and herself is dramatic and desires attention
- Family history of similar problems or unexplained death in sibling
- Signs or history of factitious disorder in mother

TREATMENT

- Appropriate physician suspicion, good medical records, and reporting of abuse (often multiple doctors have been visited, with little continuity)
- Caregiver requires psychiatric therapy, such as for other factitious disorders

Malingering

DEFINITION

Intentional creation of symptoms for secondary gain (e.g., getting out of going to school or doing chores).

PSYCHOLOGICAL IMPACT OF ADOPTION AND FOSTER CARE

DEFINITION

- **Adoption**—acquiring legal guardianship of an individual
- **Foster care**—temporary placement of an individual who has been removed from an unsafe environment
- **Kinship**—placement with relatives

ETIOLOGY

- Questions of who the other parents are and why they left him or her and the subsequent impact of the perceived abandonment.
- Parental assumptions of the behavior and personalities of the people whose union produced the child causes them to be hypervigilant.

PATHOPHYSIOLOGY

- A narcissistic injury resulting in the assumption that they were unlovable, dirty, bad, or unrewarding to the biological parents.
- Some blame the biological parents, assuming they were bad, alcoholic, or mentally ill.
- Assume abandonment could happen again.
- Unconscious rage at having been abandoned.

EPIDEMIOLOGY

- Adoption is common among individuals who are unable to have children and want a family.
- Two percent of population is adopted.
- Foster care is common among children who have been abandoned by their parents or were removed from a dysfunctional environment.
- There are 430,000 children in foster care.

SIGNS AND SYMPTOMS

- Adolescent curious about his or her origins and early life creates conflict within the individual.

- Continually search strangers' faces for resemblances.
- Expression of feelings of abandonment and the desire to find biological parents.
- Foster child relationships may have been disrupted several times before, so the child is ambivalent toward the parents.
- Rage, stemming from initial abandonment, causes aggressive and antagonist behavior.

TREATMENT

- Individual and family therapy.
- Address disruptive behavior and the etiology.
- Location of birth parents with the agreement of biological parents.
- Address issues of abandonment.
- Enhance communication between child and parents.
- When to tell the child he or she is adopted?
    - Controversial
    - Sooner is better (age 3–4 or earlier)
- How to tell the child he or she is adopted?
    - According to development level

Pediatric Life Support

PEDIATRIC BASIC LIFE SUPPORT (BLS)

The great majority of pediatric cardiopulmonary arrests outside the hospital setting occur with parents or their surrogates (i.e., teachers, coaches, day care workers, baby-sitters) nearby. BLS courses should be particularly targeted toward these individuals.

EPIDEMIOLOGY

- Primary cardiac arrest is rather uncommon in children.
- The incidence of pediatric arrests is highest during infancy (age < 1) and during adolescence.
- During **infancy,** the leading causes of arrest are *injuries* (intentional and unintentional), *respiratory diseases, airway obstruction* (e.g., foreign body aspiration), *sepsis, drowning,* and *sudden infant death syndrome* (SIDS).
- During **childhood** and **adolescence,** the leading cause of arrest is *injury* (intentional and unintentional).
- **Injuries** should be viewed as *preventable* (not accidents), and education about injury prevention is an important aspect of pediatric BLS.

Most cardiac arrests in children are caused by *progressive respiratory failure* and *circulatory collapse.*

Injury is the leading cause of pediatric arrest in children over age 1 year.

FATAL PEDIATRIC INJURIES

Most common causes of fatal pediatric injuries:
1. **Motor vehicle injuries.**
   - Nearly 50% of all pediatric injuries or deaths.
   - Risk factors include misuse of child seat restraints, seat belts, and airbags; adolescent drivers; and intoxicated drivers.
2. **Pedestrian injuries**—leading cause of injury in ages 5 through 9.
3. **Bicycle injuries**—helmets reduce morbidity of head and brain injuries by 85–90%.
4. **Drownings.**
   - Twenty percent of drowning victims who survive suffer permanent brain injury secondary to prolonged hypoxia.
   - Children younger than age 4 are at especially high risk.
   - Alcohol is often associated with adolescent drownings.
5. **Burns.**
   - Eighty percent of all fatalities occur from house fires (mostly from smoke inhalation).
   - Smoke detectors can reduce morbidity and mortality of house fires by 90%.

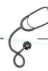

Remember, injury in children is not always an accident.

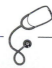

Motor vehicles are the number 1 cause of pediatric injuries.

Parent and child education is vital to preventing injuries:
- Look both ways before crossing streets.
- Wear bike helmets.
- Learn to swim.
- Watch young children at all times.
- Use smoke detectors.
- Keep pot handles turned in.

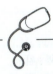

Be on the lookout for abuse in burn patients.

- Contact burns, electrical burns, and scaldings most often affect children below the age of 4.

6. **Firearms.**
   - Second leading cause of death in all adolescent males and the leading cause of death in African-American adolescents.
   - Two thirds of American households have firearms; one third have a handgun.

BURNS

Upper extremities most frequent, followed by face and neck.

PATHOPHYSIOLOGY

Disruption of three functions of skin:
- Regulation of heat loss
- Preservation of body fluids
- Barrier to infection

EPIDEMIOLOGY

Occur commonly in toddlers.

CLASSIFICATION

Four criteria:
- *Depth:*
  - First degree: superficial. Wound is painful, red, dry, and hypersensitive (sunburn).
  - Second degree: partial thickness.
    - Superficial second-degree burns are red and may blister.
    - Deep second-degree burns are white, dry, blanch with pressure, and have decreased sensitivity to pain.
  - Third degree: full thickness. Wound is dry, depressed, leathery, and without sensation.
- *Percent body surface area*
- *Location:*
  - Assess risk for disability.
  - Worse on face, eyes, ears, feet, perineum, or hands.
- *Association with other injuries*

TREATMENT

Superficial and Partial Thickness
- Rapid and effective analgesia.
- Cold compresses.
- Antiseptic cleansing.
- Debride open blisters.
- Topical antibiotic (silver sulfadiazine).
- Protect with bulky dressing.
- Reexamine in 24 hours and serially after for healing and infection.

Full Thickness or Extensive Partial Thickness
- ABCs (airway, breathing, circulation) of trauma, especially airway.
- Fluid and electrolyte replacement (4 mL/kg per percentage of body surface area affected for first 24 hours with half in first 8 hours).
- Sedation and analgesia is usually necessary.
- Clean and manage as above.

1. Determine unresponsiveness: stimulate and check for responsiveness.
2. If unresponsive, shout for help and provide 1 minute of BLS to the child.
3. Activate emergency medical services (EMS) system.
4. Airway (open and assess)—head tilt–chin lift maneuver or jaw thrust maneuver (if cervical spine injury is suspected).
5. Breathing—look for a rise and fall of the chest, listen for exhaled air, and feel for exhaled air; provide rescue breaths if no spontaneous breathing is present.
   - **Infants** (< 1 year old)—place mouth over infant's mouth and nose, creating a seal.
   - **Children** (> 1 year old)—pinch nose and create mouth-to-mouth seal.
   - Give two slow breaths (the correct volume is different depending on the size and age of the child—use the rise and fall of the chest wall as a gauge).
   - If the chest does not rise, or the breath does not go in easily, reposition the head and try again.
6. Circulation—pulse check in brachial artery for infants and the carotid artery for children > 1 year (*Note:* pulse check should be taught to health care providers but is not expected of laypersons).
   - *If pulses are present,* provide rescue breathing at a rate of 20 per minute; activate EMS system (if not done already) after one cycle of 20 rescue breaths.
   - If pulses are absent, or heart rate is less than 60 beats per minute, begin chest compressions and coordinate with ventilations; activate EMS after 1 minute (if not done already).

Infant Compressions

For < 1 year of age:
- Place one hand on the head to maintain open airway for ventilation.
- Place the two middle fingers of the other hand on the sternum one fingerbreadth below the nipple line to be used for chest compressions.
- Chest compressions of 0.5"–1" in depth at a rate of *at least* 100 per minute
- Coordinate compressions with pauses for ventilation at a ratio of 5:1.

Child Compressions

For child age 1 to 8 years:
- Place one hand on the head to maintain open airway for ventilation.
- Place the heel of the other hand on the lower half of the sternum (take care to avoid the xiphoid).
- Chest compressions of 1" to 1 1/2" in depth at a rate of 100 per minute.
- Coordinate compressions with pauses for ventilation at a ratio of 5:1.

Foreign Body Airway Obstruction

- Foreign body airway obstruction should be considered in any child who suddenly demonstrates signs of respiratory distress, gagging, coughing, wheezing, or stridor.
- Please note that these symptoms of airway obstruction can also be caused by infection. Infectious etiologies of airway obstruction are pediatric emergencies and should be suspected if fever, congestion, hoarseness, drooling, lethargy, or atony are present.

BLS
Determine unresponsiveness, call for help, and remember your **ABC**s:
Airway
Breathing
Circulation

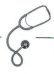

One minute of BLS is provided to children before activating the EMS system, because most cardiopulmonary arrest in children is caused by the development of hypoxemia, and 1 minute of ventilatory and circulatory support may delay or prevent the development of cardiac arrest.

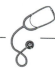

Improper opening of the airway is the most common cause of ineffective rescue breaths.

Infant Compressions
Two fingers
0.5"–1" depth
Rate > 100 per min
5:1 ratio

HIGH-YIELD FACTS

Pediatric Life Support

Child Compressions
Heel of palm
1″ to 1.5″ depth
Rate 100 per min
5:1 ratio

Ninety percent of foreign body deaths are children under age five; two thirds of these are infants.

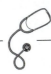

Airway obstruction caused by infection requires immediate transport to the hospital.

Infant airway obstruction = back blows + chest thrusts

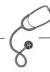

Child (> 1 year of age) airway obstruction = Heimlich maneuver

- If an infectious cause of airway obstruction is being entertained, the child must be transported immediately to the nearest hospital capable of emergent pediatric intubation.

Infant Airway Obstruction (< 1 Year of Age)

Back blows and chest thrusts:
1. Activate EMS.
2. Hold the choking infant in one arm, with the infant face down, firmly holding the jaw and allowing the body to rest on your forearm.
3. Deliver five **back blows** using the heel of your free hand directly between the infant's shoulder blades.
4. If no improvement, turn the infant over to the face-up position, maintaining support of the head and neck.
5. Deliver five quick **chest thrusts** using the same technique as for infant chest compressions.
6. Repeat above steps, alternating back blows and chest thrusts, until object is removed or the child loses consciousness.

Child Airway Obstruction (> 1 Year of Age)

- Heimlich maneuver—if **conscious:**
  1. Ask patient if she is choking and if she can speak.
  2. If not, tell patient you are going to help her and activate EMS.
  3. Stand behind the conscious victim, and wrap your arms around the abdomen.
  4. Place the thumb of one fist in the midline of the abdomen just above the umbilicus (well below the xiphoid).
  5. Grasp the fist with the other hand and deliver quick thrusts inward and upward.
  6. Continue until object is expelled or victim becomes unconscious.
- If the victim becomes **unconscious** (witnessed):
  1. Place victim supine.
  2. Open the airway with head-tilt chin-lift; *if you see the object*, attempt a finger sweep to remove it.
  3. Attempt rescue breathing.
  4. If unsuccessful, reposition head and attempt rescue breathing.
  5. If still unsuccessful, straddle the victim, placing the heel of one hand on the child's abdomen in the midline just above the umbilicus (avoiding the xiphoid).
  6. Place the other hand on top of the first and deliver five quick inward and upward thrusts.
  7. Repeat steps 2 through 6 until ventilation is successful or EMS arrives and takes over.

PEDIATRIC ADVANCED LIFE SUPPORT (PALS)

- Goals: To provide rapid assessment and definitive management of the pediatric arrest situation using advanced airway management techniques, cardiac monitoring equipment, and pharmacologic therapy.
- Respiratory problems are rather common among children, and respiratory arrest is the major cause of cardiac arrest in the pediatric population.
- If respiratory arrest is treated before it progresses to cardiac arrest, survival is likely.

- If respiratory arrest progresses to pulseless cardiac arrest, the chances of survival are poor.
- Early recognition of respiratory failure and effective management of respiratory problems are key elements taught in PALS.

Anatomic Differences in the Pediatric Airway

- Smaller airway.
- Tongue occupies a greater percentage of the oropharynx.
- Vocal cords are more superior and anterior.
- The tonsils and adenoids are more prominent.
- The epiglottis is shorter, stiffer, and more narrow.
- The tracheal rings are less rigid.
- The narrowest part of the airway is just below the vocal cords at the nondistensible cricoid cartilage; endotracheal tube (ETT) size is thus determined by the size of this opening.
- Smaller amounts of vocal cord edema can drastically reduce the diameter of the airway (resistance is inversely proportional to the fourth power of the radius).
- The angle between the base on the tongue and the glottis is more acute.

Pediatric Respiratory Distress

- Recognize signs and symptoms of respiratory distress (tachypnea, nasal flaring, grunting, retractions).
- Provide oxygen in the highest concentration available to any child experiencing respiratory difficulty (face tent, blow-by stream, mask, partial nonrebreather).
- Suction secretions as needed.
- Continually reassess for signs of decompensation; if a trend of worsening respiratory status is noted, assisted ventilation is required to prevent respiratory failure.

Management of Respiratory Failure and Pediatric Intubation

- Airway—Open the airway.
- Breathing—Support breathing using bag–valve–mask ventilation until definitive airway is established (i.e., endotracheal intubation).
- Circulation—Assess circulation, establish intravenous (IV) access, chest compressions if necessary.

Endotracheal Intubation

1. Select and prepare all equipment prior to attempting intubation (make sure all are *functioning* well).
   - Laryngoscope blade:
     Infant—Miller (straight) 0
     Age < 1—Miller (straight) 1
     Age 1–5—Miller (straight) 2
     Age > 5—Mac (curved) 2
   - ETT size: (Age [years]/4) + 4.
   - Uncuffed tubes are used for pediatric intubation in children < 8 years of age.
   - Suction catheter.
   - Magill forceps.
   - Cardiac monitor and pulse oximetry.
2. Position the patient.

Do not do blind finger sweeps in choking children; do so only if you see the offending object.

The narrowest part of pediatric airway is the **cricoid cartilage.**

Poiseuille's equation: Resistance (airway) $\propto 1/r^4$

Straight laryngoscope blades are more effective to visualize the pediatric airway.

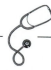

Signs of respiratory distress:
- Tachypnea
- Nasal flaring
- Retractions
- Grunting

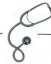

Give oxygen to any child in respiratory distress or with altered mental status.

3. Preoxygenate with bag–valve–mask.
4. Open airway, visualize epiglottis, insert straight blade beyond epiglottis and lift.
5. Directly visualize larynx and pass uncuffed tube through cords.
6. Secure tube.
7. Observe for symmetrical chest rise.
8. Confirm placement with end-tidal CO_2 indicator.
9. Listen in both lung fields for equal breath sounds and confirm absent gastric insufflation:
   - If bradycardia or hypoxia develop, suspend intubation attempt, oxygenate with bag–valve–mask, and reattempt when patient is more stable.
   - Uncuffed ETTs are used to avoid injury to the cricoid cartilage.

Vascular Access

CANNULATION OF PERIPHERAL VEINS

Upper Extremity
- Median cubital vein
- Cephalic vein (and tributaries in the dorsum of the hand)
- Basilic vein

Lower Extremity
- Saphenous veins (especially great saphenous at the ankle)
- Veins of the dorsal arch
- Median marginal veins

INTRAOSSEOUS CANNULATION
- Previously recommended only in children < 6 years; now permitted in older children as well
- During cardiopulmonary resuscitation (CPR), should be employed after three failed attempts to cannulate peripheral veins (or 90 seconds)
- Should be inserted into the anteromedial aspect of the tibia, 1 to 3 cm distal to the tibial tuberosity
- Can safely administer fluids, blood products, and drugs

CANNULATION OF CENTRAL VEINS
- Complications (bleeding, infection, pneumothorax, etc.) are more common in the pediatric age group.
- Central catheters should be used only when the benefit outweighs the risks (i.e., when central venous pressures need to be monitored).
- Catheters are inserted using the Seldinger (guidewire) technique.
- Common sites include:
  - Femoral vein
  - Internal jugular vein
  - Subclavian vein

Shock and Fluid Resuscitation
- All forms of shock require consideration of fluid administration during initial therapy.
- **Hypovolemia** is the worldwide leading cause of shock (inadequate fluid intake plus diarrhea and vomiting can lead to hypovolemic shock).
- **Septic shock, neurogenic shock,** and **anaphylactic shock** are all characterized by vasodilation, increased capillary permeability, and third-space fluid loss that results in an intravascular hypovolemia.

Pulse oximetry is considered a vital sign and should be obtained whenever respiratory distress or altered mental status is considered.

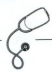

Laryngoscope Blade Sizes
Infant — Miller 0
Age < 1 — Miller 1
Age 1–5 — Miller 2
Age > 5 — Mac 2

ETT Size
(Age/4) + 4

ETT diameter is approximately equal to that of a child's little finger.

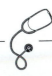

Place **intraosseous line** in anteromedial tibia *1 to 3 cm distal to tibial tuberosity.*

- **Cardiogenic shock** may even require initial fluid administration before the initiation of inotropic and chronotropic agents ("you must fill the tank before starting the engine").

Administration of Fluid Bolus

- Initial bolus should be a rapid infusion of 20 mL/kg (in < 20 minutes).
- Reassess after initial bolus and consider administering repeat bolus of 20 mL/kg.
- Remember that only about 25% of crystalloid will remain in the intravascular space; thus, you may need to administer three times the estimated fluid loss (3:1 rule).
- **Blood** is the preferred fluid replacement for trauma victims demonstrating persistent hypovolemic shock *after* two to three boluses of crystalloid (i.e., 40–60 mL/kg).

Classification of Shock

Hemorrhagic/Hypovolemic Shock

Class I
- 0–15% volume loss
- Normal pulse
- Normal blood pressure
- Normal capillary refill
- Normal respiratory rate
- Urine output 1–2 mL/kg/hr

Class II
- 15–30% volume loss
- Mild tachycardia
- Mildly decreased blood pressure
- Mildly prolonged capillary refill
- Mild tachypnea
- Urine output 0.5–1.0 mL/kg/hr

Class III
- 30–40% volume loss
- Tachycardia
- Decreased blood pressure
- Prolonged capillary refill
- Tachypnea
- Urine output 0.25–0.5 mL/kg/hr

Class IV
- > 40% volume loss
- Severely tachycardic, bradycardic, or absent pulse
- Very low blood pressure
- Greatly prolonged capillary refill
- Severe tachypnea
- Urine output 0 mL/kg/hr

Pressor Support in Pediatric Shock

- First attempt multiple fluid boluses.
- Try to identify and treat the underlying cause.
- Choose pressor agent according to the type of shock present.

The number 1 worldwide cause of shock is hypovolemia.

Initial fluid resuscitation: Normal saline or lactated Ringer's (isotonic)

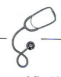

Initial fluid bolus: 20 mL/kg

3:1 Rule
May need to administer three times estimated fluid loss

Class I Shock
0–15% loss
Normal vitals

Class II Shock
15–30% loss
Mildly increased heart rate
Prolonged capillary refill
Mild anxiety

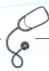

Class III Shock
30–40% loss
Increased heart rate
Decreased blood pressure
Decreased urine output
Poor capillary refill
Confused

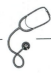

Class IV Shock
> 40% loss
Very low blood pressure
Negligible urine output
Lethargic
Pale or cyanotic

Shock Management
- Hypovolemic — *fluids!*
- Septic — multiple boluses, dopamine, epinephrine
- Cardiogenic — initial bolus, dobutamine or epinephrine

Hypovolemic Shock
Multiple crystalloid boluses will be necessary (up to 60–80 mL/kg).

Septic Shock
- Multiple crystalloid boluses will be necessary (up to 60–80 mL/kg).
- Consider dopamine 5 to 20 µg/kg/min if patient is *normotensive*.
- Consider epinephrine 0.1 to 1.0 µg/kg/min if patient is *hypotensive*.

Cardiogenic Shock
- Initial fluid bolus is usually necessary.
- Consider dobutamine 5 to 20 µg/kg/min if patient is *normotensive*. (*Note:* Dobutamine may not be effective in infants and young children due to lack of stroke volume response.)
- Consider epinephrine 0.1 to 1.0 µg/kg/min if the patient is *hypotensive*.

Cardiac Arrhythmias

- Tachycardias
- Bradycardias
- No pulse—asystole, pulseless electrical activity (PEA), ventricular fibrillation (VF)

Tachyarrhythmias

SINUS TACHYCARDIA

- Defined as a rate of sinus node discharge faster than normal for age.
- Age-specific heart rates:
  - 0–3 months (85–205 bpm)
  - 3 months–2 years (100–190 bpm)
  - 2–10 years (60–140 bpm)
  - > 10 years (60–100 bpm)
- Typically a response to a *need for increased cardiac output.*
- Common causes include fever, pain, anxiety, blood loss, sepsis, and shock.
- Always assess—*and reassess*—ABCs.
- Therapy entails treating the underlying cause.

SUPRAVENTRICULAR TACHYCARDIA (SVT)

- SVT is *rapid, regular,* often *paroxysmal.*
- Often exceeds 240 bpm in infants, exceeds 180 bpm in children.
- P waves are absent or indistinguishable.
- QRS complex is narrow (< 0.08 s).
- SVT is most commonly caused by reentry mechanism.

SVT Algorithm

1. Assess ABCs, support as needed.
2. Administer 100% oxygen, ventilate as needed.
3. Document electrocardiogram (ECG)/rhythm tracing.
4. IV access.
5. Adenosine 0.1 mg/kg rapid intravenous push (IVP), immediate 5 mL saline flush (max first dose: 6 mg).
6. If above unsuccessful, repeat adenosine at 0.2 mg/kg rapid IVP, immediate 5 mL saline flush (max second dose: 12 mg).
7. Synchronized cardioversion 0.5 to 1.0 J/kg (consider sedation).
8. Obtain cardiology consult as needed.

9. If patient becomes unstable at any time, proceed directly with synchronized cardioversion.

Ventricular Tachycardia (VT) (with pulse)

- Wide QRS complex (> 0.08 s)
- P waves not present
- Very uncommon in children
- Risk factors include: prolonged QT syndrome, cardiac anomalies, drug ingestions, electrolyte abnormalities, underlying cardiac disease

VT Algorithm

1. Assess ABCs, support.
2. Administer 100% oxygen, ventilate, prepare to intubate.
3. IV/IO access.
4. Consider medication alternatives: lidocaine 1 mg/kg IV bolus and start lidocaine 20 to 50 μg/kg/min infusion *or* amiodarone 5 mg/kg IV over 20 to 60 minutes *or* procainamide 15 mg/kg IV over 30 to 60 minutes. (Do not administer amiodarone and procainamide together.)
5. Identify and treat possible causes:
   4Hs:
   - Hypovolemia
   - Hypoxemia
   - Hypothermia
   - Hyper/hypokalemia
   4Ts:
   - Tamponade
   - Tension pneumothorax
   - Toxins
   - Thromboembolism
6. Synchronized cardioversion 0.5 to 1.0 J/kg (consider sedation).
7. Obtain cardiology consult, 12-lead ECG.
8. If patient becomes unstable at any time, proceed directly with synchronized cardioversion.

Bradyarrhythmias

Bradycardia Algorithm

1. Assess ABCs, support.
2. Administer 100% oxygen, ventilate, prepare to intubate.
3. Establish IV/IO access.
4. Cardiac monitor, pulse oximetry, blood pressure cuff.
5. Reassess ABCs:
   - If stable, continue to support ABCs, admit for observation.
   - If unstable (poor perfusion, hypotension, heart rate < 60, continued hypoxia despite 100% oxygen administration):
     1. Begin chest compressions.
     2. Identify and treat possible causes: hypoxemia, hypothermia, head injury, heart block, heart transplant, drugs/toxins/poisons.
     3. Epinephrine.
        IV/IO 0.01 mg/kg (1:10,000, 0.1 mL/kg), *or*
        ETT 0.1 mg/kg (1:1,000, 0.1 mL/kg)
        Repeat every 3 to 5 minutes.

Sinus tachycardia is usually a metabolic response to a need for increased cardiac output.

SVT is *rapid* and *regular* with a narrow QRS:
Infants > 240 bpm
Children > 180 bpm

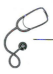

Management of SVT:
Stable — vagal maneuvers and/or adenosine
Unstable — synchronized cardioversion

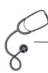

IV access is necessary in SVT because intraosseous (IO) administration of adenosine is *not* effective.

Ventricular tachycardia:
QRS wide
No P waves
Rare in children

4. Atropine 0.02 mg/kg IVP.
   Min dose: 0.1 mg
   Max dose: 0.02 mg/kg to maximum of 1.0 mg
   ETT dose: Two to three times dose in 5 mL normal saline
5. Consider external pacing.

Pulseless Arrhythmias

Ventricular Fibrillation (VF)/Pulseless VT

1. Assess ABCs.
2. Continue CPR.
3. Confirm rhythm in more than one lead.
4. Intubate and hyperventilate with 100% oxygen.
5. IV/IO access (do not delay defibrillation for access).
6. Defibrillate × 3 (2 J/kg, 4 J/kg, 4 J/kg).
7. Epinephrine, first dose; then defibrillate 4 J/kg 30 to 60 seconds after dose; then repeat dose every 3 to 5 minutes
   - IV/IO 0.01 mg/kg (0.1 mL/kg of 1:10,000)
   - ETT 0.1 mg/kg (0.1 mL/kg of 1:1,000)
8. Lidocaine 1 mg IV/IO/ETT; then defibrillate 4 J/kg 30 to 60 seconds after dose
   or
   Amiodarone 5 mg/kg bolus IV/IO, then defibrillate 4 J/kg 30 to 60 seconds after dose
9. Epinephrine 0.1 mg/kg (0.1 mL/kg of 1:1,000) given IV/IO/ETT every 3 to 5 minutes; then defibrillate 4 J/kg 30 to 60 seconds after each administration.
10. Consider magnesium 25 to 50 mg/kg IV/IO for torsades de pointes (max dose: 2 g).
11. Identify and treat possible causes (4Hs and 4Ts).

Pulseless Electrical Activity (PEA)

- PEA in children, while rare, usually occurs as a result of **progressive respiratory and/or circulatory failure.**
- As with adult PEA, the *differential diagnosis* for pediatric PEA is essential to successful resuscitation.

PEA Algorithm

1. Assess ABCs.
2. Continue CPR.
3. Confirm rhythm in more than one lead.
4. Intubate and hyperventilate with 100% oxygen.
5. IV/IO access.
6. Consider possible causes of PEA (and specific treatments)
   - Hypovolemia (volume—normal saline infusion)
   - Hypoxia (oxygen, intubation, ventilation)
   - Hypothermia (warmed normal saline infusion)
   - Massive pulmonary embolism
   - Acidosis (sodium bicarbonate)
   - Tension pneumothorax (needle decompression)
   - Cardiac tamponade (pericardiocentesis)
   - Hyperkalemia (sodium bicarbonate)
   - Massive acute myocardial infarction
   - Drug overdose from TCAs, digoxin, β blockers, calcium channel blockers

7. Epinephrine (first dose):
   IV/IO 0.01 mg/kg (0.1 mL/kg of 1:10,000)
   ETT 0.1 mg/kg (0.1 mL/kg of 1:1,000)
8. Epinephrine (subsequent doses):
   IV/IO/ETT 0.1 mg/kg (0.1 mL/kg of 1:1,000)

ASYSTOLE

- Most common pulseless rhythm in children.
- Airway management and hyperventilation are the most important interventions.

Asystole Algorithm

1. ABCs.
2. CPR.
3. *Confirm rhythm in more than one lead.*
4. Intubate and hyperventilate with 100% oxygen.
5. IV/IO access.
6. Epinephrine (first dose):
   IV/IO 0.01 mg/kg (0.1 mL/kg of 1:10,000)
   ETT 0.1 mg/kg (0.1 mL/kg of 1:1,000)
7. Epinephrine (subsequent doses—repeat every 5 minutes):
   IV/IO/ETT 0.1 mg/kg (0.1 mL/kg of 1:1,000)
8. Consider external pacing.

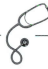

Always confirm asystole in more than one lead and ensure that leads are properly connected.

Note that atropine and bicarbonate are *not* part of the algorithm for asystole.

NEONATAL ADVANCED LIFE SUPPORT (NALS)

- Newborn resuscitation ideally should be performed in the delivery room, neonatal intensive care unit (NICU), or other unit with personnel experienced with treating newborns and equipment appropriate for the task.
- NALS establishes guidelines and procedures to assist health care practitioners for newborn resuscitations outside the delivery room.

Preassessment and Triage

Always ask the following questions when presented with an expectant mother in active labor:

1. How many weeks gestation is the pregnancy (i.e., will you be treating a full-term infant or a premature infant)?
2. What number pregnancy is this? How many minutes apart are the contractions (gives you an indication of how much time you have before delivery)?
3. Do you have any medical problems? Were there any complications during this pregnancy?
4. Was the amniotic fluid clear or was it thick and green (i.e., will you need to be concerned about meconium aspiration precautions during delivery)?
5. How many children are you expecting (allows preparation for enough equipment and personnel)?

Neonatal hypothermia is associated with respiratory depression.

Newborn Assessment

- **Temperature:** Neonatal hypothermia can be associated with neonatal respiratory depression. Upon delivery, warming and drying with a towel or blanket is often adequate to stimulate breathing in a newborn.

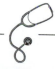

Suction newborn airway aggressively.

Start CPR on neonate if pulse < 60.

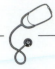

Newborn ABCs
- Position
- Suction
- Stimulate cry
- Warm and dry

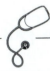

If meconium is present during a delivery, aggressively suction hypopharynx as soon as head is delivered.

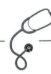

Have low threshold for intubation and direct tracheal suctioning if any signs of distress of a neonate delivered in the presence of meconium.

- **Airway:** Position the airway and suction any secretions. (*Note:* If meconium is present, aggressive suctioning of the hypopharynx should be performed immediately upon delivering the head.)
- **Breathing:** Observe chest rise and fall, give 100% oxygen if necessary, initiate adequate bag–valve–mask ventilation if necessary (i.e., heart rate < 100 bpm and unresponsiveness; absent or depressed respirations).
- **Circulation:** Assess heart rate and color, provide chest compressions as necessary (if heart rate absent, if heart rate < 60 despite 30 seconds of assisted ventilation).

Newborn Resuscitation

Assess every newborn (and give the appropriate support).
1. Delivery outside the delivery room
2. ABCs—assess and support
   - Airway (*position* and *suction*)
   - Breathing (*stimulate* to cry)
   - Circulation (*heart rate* and *color*)
   - Temperature (*warm* and *dry*)
3. Oxygen (100%)
4. Establish effective ventilation:
   - Bag–valve–mask
   - Laryngeal mask airway (LMA) can be an effective alternative for establishing an airway when bag–valve–mask fails
   - Endotracheal intubation (only by trained rescuer competent in neonatal intubations)
5. Chest compressions if pulse < 60
6. Medications as dictated by the situation

Neonatal Resuscitation

- **Ventilation rate:** 40 to 60/min (always use 100% oxygen).
- **Compression rate:** 120 events/min (90 compressions/30 ventilations/min).
- **Compression/ventilation ratio:** 3:1.
- **Compression technique:** The two thumb-encircling hands is now the preferred method of neonatal chest compressions; the two-finger compression technique is also acceptable.

Meconium Deliveries

1. Deliver head.
2. Aggressively suction hypopharynx while infant is still in birth canal.
3. Complete delivery of infant.
4. Assess temperature and ABCs. If the infant is active and vigorous, continue supportive measures. If any signs of distress (absent or depressed respirations, heart rate < 100, poor muscle tone) proceed with algorithm.
5. Direct tracheal suctioning either following endotracheal intubation or by using ETT as suction catheter.

APGAR

See chapter on gestation and birth.

Awards

AWARDS WITH A PEDIATRIC FOCUS

American Academy of Pediatrics (AAP) Resident Section Annie Dyson Child Advocacy Award

This award celebrates the outstanding efforts of pediatricians-in-training as they work in their communities to improve the health of children. Any resident-sponsored and/or resident-led project that seeks to advocate on behalf of children is eligible for this award. Medical student members of the AAP working with pediatric residents also qualify for this opportunity. This award seeks to showcase projects that are designed and implemented by residents, which aim to improve the lives of children. Please contact Jackie Burke at the AAP, at (800) 433-9016, extension 4759, or e-mail her at jburke@aap.org for further details. Deadline: August 1.

Society for Pediatric Research (SPR)/American Pediatric Society (APS) Award

The SPR and APS offer a medical student research training program to encourage gifted medical students to consider careers in research related to pediatrics. This program is specifically designed for students seeking a research opportunity at an institution other than their own medical school. Students selected for the program are able to choose or are assigned to leading research laboratories. Currently, our Directory of Laboratories lists research opportunities at more than 500 laboratories in the United States and Canada. Each research experience allows the student to spend eight to ten weeks at 30 to 40 hours per week in a research environment. The program provides students with a stipend of $50.43/day (as of August 8, 2002) for a maximum stipend of $3,732.

Further information can be obtained from the Student Research Program Coordinator at student-research@aps-spr.org. Deadline: January 28, 2004.

The Elizabeth Glaser Pediatric AIDS Foundation Student Intern Award

The goal of this program is to encourage students to choose a career in pediatric HIV/AIDS research and care. The program provides $2,000 for 320 hours of work (a minimum of 4 hours per week) as a stipend to the student. Students must apply through a sponsor (MD, PhD, CCSW) who has expertise in pediatric HIV/AIDS clinical care or research. Contact Chris Hudnall, Programs Coordinator, at chris@pedaids.org for further information.

St. Jude Children's Research Hospital—Professional Oncology Education Program

This program is designed to allow students to participate in oncology research for 8 to 16 weeks and to encourage them to enter into the field of oncology. The program provides a stipend of $1,200 per month to the student. Trainees are responsible for travel, housing, and living expenses. Contact Suzanne Gronemeyer, PhD, Director, Professional Oncology Education Program, Diagnostic Imaging Department, Room C-1150C, 332 North Lauderdale Street, Memphis, TN 38105; (901) 495-2488; Fax: (901) 527-0054; E-mail: suzanne.gronemeyer@stjude.org; Web site: *www.stjude.org*. Deadline: March 1.

American Academy of Child & Adolescent Psychiatry (AACAP)—James Comer Minority Research Fellowship

This fellowship encourages outstanding minority medical students to pursue careers in child and adolescent psychiatry research and provides early exposure to state-of-the-art research on child and adolescent mental disorders. Students participate in the program for an entire summer and attend the 5-day AACAP Annual Meeting. The receive a stipend of $2,500. Contact James Comer Minority Research Fellowship, Marilyn Benoit, MD, Program Director, AACAP Office of Research and Training, 3615 Wisconsin Avenue, NW, Washington, DC 20016; (202) 966-7300; E-mail: smahone@aacap.org; Web site: *www.aacap.org*. Deadline: April 1. AACAP—Jeanne Spurlock Minority Medical Student Clinical Fellowship in (1) Child and Adolescent Psychiatry or (2) Research Fellowship in Drug Abuse and Addiction for Minority Medical Students.

Funded through the Center for Mental Health Services, the first award offers outstanding minority medical students early exposure to child and adolescent psychiatry. The research fellowship offers early exposure to state-of-the-art research in child and adolescent psychiatry and drug abuse and addiction, as well as a personal mentorship opportunity with an active researcher. Students receive a $2,500 stipend. Selected students will work with a child and adolescent psychiatrist/mentor plus attend the 5-day AACAP Annual Meeting. Contact Jeanne Spurlock Minority Clinical Fellowship, Marilyn Benoit, MD, Program Director, AACAP Office of Research and Training, 3615 Wisconsin Avenue, NW, Washington, DC 20016, (202) 966-7300; E-mail: smahone@aacap.org; Web site: *www.aacap.org*. Deadline: April 1.

Epilepsy Foundation Health Sciences Student Fellowship

This program stimulates individuals to pursue careers in epilepsy/pediatric epilepsy in either research or practice settings. Predoctoral training students in the health sciences may be accepted at any point in their schooling—following acceptance but before beginning the first year, or in the period immediately following their final year. Contact the Epilepsy Foundation at 4351 Garden City Drive, Landover, MD 20785-7223; (800) 332-1000, for further information.

AWARDS WITH A FAMILY PRACTICE FOCUS

First-Time Student Attendee Award

Grants of $600 each are awarded to 20 students to attend their first National Conference of Family Practice Residents and Medical Students. Students are to write a 500-word essay on why they are interested in attending the National Conference and becoming a family physician. Winners will be notified by mail the first week of June. Contact the American Academy of Family Physicians, 1140 Tomahawk Creek Parkway, Leawood, KS 66211-2672; (800) 274-2237, ext. 6726 or 6720. Deadline: May.

Family Practice Research Presentations Awards

Awards of $1,000 each are presented for first-place presentations by family practice residents and medical students. Runners-up receive awards of $250. On-site oral paper presentations at the Assembly include Category I: Original Research, and Category II: Case Study or Literature Review. Winners will be announced at AAFP Assembly. Contact the American Academy of Family Physicians, 1140 Tomahawk Creek Parkway, Leawood, KS 66211-2672; (800) 374-2237, ext. 6568. Deadline: early April.

Family Medicine Interest Group (FMIG) Leadership Award

Up to 20 students will receive a $600 grant to attend the National Conference of Family Practice Residents and Medical Students. Student members will be actively involved in FMIG activities. An application is required. Recipients are asked to write a short essay to appear in the Exchange newsletter. Winners will be notified by mail the first week of June. Contact the American Academy of Family Physicians, 1140 Tomahawk Creek Parkway, Leawood, KS 66211-2672; (800) 374-2237, ext. 6722 or 6724. Deadline: May.

Minority Scholarship Program for Students

Twenty-five students and 15 residents will receive a $600 grant to attend the National Conference of Family Practice Residents and Medical Students. Student applications must be signed by the Dean or Program Director and include a 500-word essay on the impact of family practice on underserved populations. Winners will be notified by mail the first week of June. Contact the American Academy of Family Physicians, 1140 Tomahawk Creek Parkway, Leawood, KS 66211-2672; (800) 374-2237, ext. 6726 or 6720. Deadline: May.

Student Community Outreach Award

Two winners receive a plaque of recognition and a $600 grant to attend the National Conference of Family Practice Residents and Medical Students. Student members must be actively involved in a community service project including clinical work and patient education, not part of an offered or required rotation in the curriculum. Winners notified by mail the first week of June. Contact the American Academy of Family Physicians, 1140 Tomahawk Creek Parkway, Leawood, KS 66211-2672; (800) 374-2237, ext. 6722. Deadline: May.

Student Liaison Membership Award

Three medical school student membership liaisons will be selected to receive paid attendance to the National Conference (including coach airfare, hotel accommodations for up to 4 nights, $50 daily per diem, and registration). One student liaison is selected from each medical school for each academic year. A student must be a student member of the AAFP. Student liaisons promote student membership in the AAFP to students at medical schools. They are responsible for distributing applications, buttons, and posters. Contact the American Academy of Family Physicians, 1140 Tomahawk Creek Parkway, Leawood, KS 66211-2672; (800) 374-2237, ext. 6827.

James G. Jones, MD, Student Health Policy Scholarship (Administered by the AAFP Foundation)

This scholarship will provide funds for a medical student to attend the Political Leadership Institute (PLI) sponsored by the American Medical Student Association. The scholarship will support travel expenses and cover miscellaneous expenses of attending the PLI. Constituent chapter foundations and constituent chapters are asked to nominate medical students who have demonstrated leadership ability, a commitment to public health, and an interest in politics. One nomination will be accepted from each state. Interested medical students should contact their state chapter to apply. Nominations from chapters due by mid-January. The winner will be notified in early February. Contact the American Academy of Family Physicians, 1140 Tomahawk Creek Parkway, Leawood, KS 66211-2672.

Pisacano Leadership Foundation, Inc. (The Pisacano Scholars Program)

This program provides funding for outstanding third- or fourth-year medical students for a 4- or 5-year period. Students must make a commitment to the specialty of family practice. The funding program is designed to reimburse medical school debt incurred by the student at the conclusion of the student's residency. Students are evaluated each year to ensure eligibility for continuation. There is no service commitment for students upon completion of the scholarship. For additional information, contact Robert Cattoi, Pisacano Leadership Foundation, Inc., 2228 Young Drive, Lexington, KY 40505-4294; toll free: (888) 995-5700. www.njpmf.org/appfrm.html. Deadline: March.

Philip Huffman Summer Preceptorship in Family Medicine

Sponsored by the UCSF-Fresno Department of Family and Community Medicine, this is an 8-week preceptorship introducing students to the research, teaching, and patient care activities of the Selma Community Health Clinic, which primarily serves low-income Hispanic medicine farm workers. Students receive a stipend of $1,200. Deadline: March 15.

New York State Academy of Family Physicians Summer Fellowship

The New York State Academy of Family Physicians offers 4- to 6-week summer fellowships for student members of the Academy. Students receive a stipend of $1,000 and must find their own placements. Call Nancy McGowan, Institute for Urban Family Health, (212) 633-0800, for placements. Call NYS Academy of Family Physicians, (800) 822-0700, by January 15 for application.

Delaware Academy of Family Physicians Research & Education Foundation Platt Family Physician Preceptorship

The Delaware Academy of Family Physicians Research & Education Foundation offers 6-week preceptorships in which students will spend time with various family doctors in Delaware. Stipend is $1,500. Deadline: February 7. Contact: P.O. Box 8158, Wilington, DE 19803; (302) 479-5515.

Samuel H. Trichter Preceptorship in Family Practice

Sponsored by the St. Joseph's Medical Center Family Practice Department, this is a 4-week program in which first-year students will spend time at a family health center accompanying faculty and residents during patient sessions in order to familiarize them with the specialty and the special qualities that family practitioners bring to their patients. The student will also participate in an educational project that will be of medical benefit to patients. Stipend is $1,000. Contact Dr. Paul Gross, Dept. of Family Practice, St. Joseph's Medical Center, 127 South Broadway, Yonkers, NY 10701-4080; (914) 378-7586.

Joseph Collins Foundation Award

This award is based on both financial need and scholastic record and standing (upper half of class), a demonstrated interest in arts and letters or other cultural pursuits outside the field of medicine, indication of intention to consider specializing in neurology or psychiatry or becoming a general practitioner, and evidence of good moral character. Other preferences and procedures in file. Average grant is now $2,500. Deadline: March 1. Contact: Joseph Collins Foundation. Attn: Secretary–Treasurer, 153 East 53rd Street, New York, NY 10022.

GENERAL AWARDS

American Society of Hematology (ASH) Medical Student Awards Program

This program is intended to encourage medical students to take time to work with a hematologist on a project that will give them an exciting and rigorous introduction to the field of hematology.

ASH provides each participating institution one award per calendar year in the form of $4,500 in research support and $500 for travel to the Society's annual meeting. Institutions may select more than one medical student to participate in the program if the award amount can accommodate more than one research project. Please note that the Society prefers to work with the institution's hematology or hematology-related (hematology/oncology, pediatric hematology/oncology, hematopathology, etc.) program director to identify the participating students.

Either laboratory research or clinical investigation is appropriate. ASH encourages applicants to be creative in developing opportunities for medical students that will favorably introduce them to the discipline of hematology.

If you have any questions or require any additional information regarding the ASH Medical Student Awards Program, please contact Greg Volkar, Director of Training & Professional Development, by phone at (202) 776-0544.

Roswell Park Cancer Institute Summer Oncology Research Program

The Roswell Park program provides competitive stipend support ($280 per week) for students in the health professions (medicine, dentistry, osteopathy) to engage in clinical and/or basic scientific research for an 8-week period. Some funding is available to defray costs of room and board. Approximately 25 Fellowships will be awarded. Roswell Park Cancer Institute is one of the nation's largest and oldest comprehensive cancer centers. All Institute programs revolve around the cancer problem. The Institute is situated on a 25-acre site located in downtown Buffalo, New York. The strength of the Institute's research program is attested to by the fact that in excess of $25 million in grants and contracts are awarded to the Institute each year.

For further information, call or write Arthur M. Michalek, PhD, Dean, Department of Educational Affairs, Roswell Park Cancer Institute, Carlton and Elm Streets, Buffalo, NY 14263; (716) 845-2339; E-mail: arthur.michalek@roswellpark.org. Applications due: February 14.

The Pharmaceutical Research and Manufacturers of America Foundation Medical Student Research Fellowship

This fellowship is offered to medical or dental students who have substantial interests in research and teaching careers in pharmacology/clinical pharmacology and who are willing to spend full time in a specific research effort within a pharmacology or clinical pharmacology unit. Fellowships are available for a minimum period of 3 months or any period of time up to 24 months with a maximum stipend of $18,000. The commitment must be full time. The principal aim of this program is to generate interest in research careers in pharmacology, including clinical pharmacology, among medical and dental students. Both students who are not already in a training sequence leading to a research career and students already in an MD/PhD program for whom additional financial support is appropriate are both eligible to apply. Contact Pharmaceutical Research and Manufacturers of America Foundation, 1100 Fifteenth Street NW, Washington, DC 20005.

Radiologic Society of North America Medical Student/Scholar Assistant Grant Program

The purpose of this award is to make radiology research opportunities available for medical students early in their training and encourage them to consider academic radiology as a career option. A 1-year grant of $5,000, payable to the RSNA Scholar's Department in two equal installments, is available. Applicants must be nominated by a current RSNA Scholar grant recipient and work with the scholar on his/her designated research project. Nominees must be full-time medical students at an accredited North American medical school, and be a citizen of a North American country or hold permanent resident status.

For questions about the application form itself or submission procedures, please contact Scott A. Walter, Manager–Grant Review Process, RSNA Research and Education Foundation, 820 Jorie Boulevard, Oak Brook, IL 60523; (630) 571-7816; E-mail: walter@rsna.org.

Crohn's & Colitis Foundation of America Student Research Fellowship Awards

Up to 16 Student Research Fellowship Awards per year at $2,500 each are available for medical students or students not yet engaged in thesis research in accredited North American institutions to conduct full-time research with a mentor investigating a subject relevant to inflammatory bowel disease (IBD). The duration of the project is a minimum of 10 weeks. Submission deadline is March 15 of each year; awards begin on or about June 15.

Please contact the Research and Scientific Programs Department for an electronic version of the guidelines and forms. You can contact the following staff: Carol Cox (ccox@ccfa.org) or Natasha Rampersaud (nrampersaud@ccfa.org), Crohn's & Colitis Foundation of America, 386 Park Avenue South, 17th Floor, New York, NY 10016; (800) 932-2423.

American Dermatological Association Medical Student Fellowship Program

This award offers a $700 monthly stipend for a maximum of 3 months. Preference will be given to applicants seeking to work in a department or division of dermatology. The work undertaken must be done at a university or college in the United States or Canada. Work done and research experience gained by recipients cannot be used as a credit for a degree. Awards will be made to U.S. citizens or Canadian citizens or candidates lawfully admitted to the United States or Canada for permanent residence.

Applications relating to proposed research involving human subjects must be accompanied by institutional approval of the type required by the U.S. Public Health Service. Applications, inquiries, and correspondence should be sent to the American Dermatological Association, Inc., P.O. Box 554, Millwood, NY 10546, Attn: Michelle Gratz; Phone/Fax: (914) 923-8540. Deadline: April 15, 2003

Society of Nuclear Medicine Student Fellowship Award

The Student Fellowship Award sponsored by the Education and Research Foundation of the Society of Nuclear Medicine provides financial support for students to spend time assisting in clinical and basic research activities in Nuclear Medicine, with the expectation that this exposure will serve as an incentive to consider a career in some aspect of nuclear medicine. Awards will be limited to a maximum of $3,000 to provide support for at least 3 months of full-time effort in research. Shorter durations of fellowships will be considered at a stipend rate of $1,000 a month. The minimum fellowship period is 2 months.

For more information, contact the Education and Research Foundation, Society of Nuclear Medicine, c/o Sue Weiss, CNMT, Executive Director, 1060 Arbor Lane, Northfield, IL 60093. Deadline: November 15th.

AMERICAN ACADEMY OF PEDIATRICS—BENEFITS FOR MEDICAL STUDENT MEMBERSHIP

- Membership in the AAP Resident Section as an Affiliate Member.
- Free admission to the AAP National Conference and Exhibition.
- Resource list for obtaining lists of residency training programs (categorical), combined training programs, and fellowship training programs.
- Connection to local AAP Chapter.
- Medical Student Reception at the National Conference and Exhibition.
- Discounts on AAP products and publications.
- Online Access to the Members Only Channel through the AAP Web site.
- *AAP News*, the official news magazine of the American Academy of Pediatrics
- AAP Grand Rounds, timely synopses and critiques of important new studies relevant to pediatric practice, reviewing methodology, significance, and practical impact.
- AAP BookStore, your source for the best in pediatrics.
- CME Courses, cover a wide range of cutting-edge topics and feature a high faculty/participant ratio.
- *NeoReviews*, the Academy's new online-only journal devoted to neonatal and perinatal topics.
- *PediaLink*, designed to help you direct, focus, and manage your continuing professional development.
- *Pediatrics*, the official journal of the American Academy of Pediatrics.
- *Pediatrics in Review*, a monthly online continuing education journal.
- *Pediatrics Review and Education Program (PREP)*, our self-study course designed to prepare pediatricians for their initial certification or recerti-

fication exam. Course content is coordinated with the American Board of Pediatrics (ABP) and consists of a self-assessment exercise.

- PedJobs, an Internet-based, interactive, secure job search Web site.
- Policy statements.
- ResAssist, Internet booking engine for members to book their own air reservations
- Complimentary publications.
- Resident Section newsletter.
- Pediatric career information.

ALL THIS FOR $15/year!

For more information on becoming a medical student affiliate member of the Resident Section of the American Academy of Pediatrics, please contact the Division of Member Services at (800) 433-9016. American Academy of Pediatrics, Division of Member Services, 141 Northwest Point Blvd., Elk Grove Village, IL 60007; (800) 433-9016 or (847) 434-4000; Fax: (847) 228-7035; E-mail: membership@aap.org.

Index

Pages followed by f indicate figure; those followed by t indicate table.

lead poisoning, 242
Reye's syndrome, 151
Tourette's syndrome, 299
types
  adrenoleukodystrophy, 299
  hepatic, 298
  HIV/AIDS, 298
  lead, 298
  mitochondrial, 297–298
  Sydenham's chorea, 299
Wilson's disease, 152
Enchondroma
  definition/signs and symptoms/radiology, 344
  management/prognosis, 344
Encopresis
  diagnosis/etiology/epidemiology/treatment, 387
Endocarditis
  aneurysms, 306
  etiology/pathophysiology/signs and symptoms, 193
  predisposing conditions/diagnosis/treatment, 194
  prophylaxis recommendations, 194–195
Endocrine disease
  acute adrenal insufficiency, 272
  anorexia nervosa, 396
  bulimia nervosa, 397
  chronic mucocutaneous candidiasis, 101
  congenital adrenal hyperplasia, 270–271
  Cushing's syndrome, 271–272
  diabetes, 265–266, 265t
  diabetes insipidus, 276–277
  diabetic ketoacidosis, 266
  failure to thrive, 37
  gestation and birth, 19
  gigantism/acromegaly, 276
  hemochromatosis, 267
  hyperinsulinism, 266–267
  hyperparathyroidism, 269–270
  hyperpituitarism, 273
  hyperthyroidism, 267–268
  hypoglycemia, 267
  hypoparathyroidism, 270
  hypopituitarism, 274
  hypothyroidism, 268–269
  menstruation, 281–282
  pheochromocytoma, 273
  pituitary tumor, 274
  pseudohermaphroditism, 283
  sexual development, 278–280, 278f, 279f
  short stature, 274–275
  syndrome of inappropriate antidiuretic hormone secretion, 277
  tall stature, 276
  testicular feminization, 282
  thyroid neoplasm, 269
  true hermaphroditism, 282–283
Endoderm, 16t
Endogenous hypertriglyceridemia
  lipids/clinical manifestations/treatment/genetics, 93t
Endometritis, 282
Endoscopy, 161
Endotracheal intubation, 409–410
End-stage renal disease (ESRD)
  definition/treatment, 221
  hypoplasia, renal, 223
  polycystic kidney disease, 222
  vesicoureteral reflux, 230

Entamoeba, 138
Enterochromaffin cells, 142
Enteropathogens, 43
Enterotomy, 133
Enteroviruses, 294
Enuresis. See Incontinence
Enzyme-linked immunosorbent assay (ELISA), 27, 111, 113
Enzymopathies, hemolytic
  glucose-6-phosphate dehydrogenase deficiency, 248
  hexokinase deficiency, 249
  pyruvate kinase deficiency, 248–249
Eosinopenia, 271
Eosinophilia, 123
Eosinophils, 226, 327
Epicanthal folds, 76
Epidermolysis bullosa, 128
Epidermophyton, 368
Epididymitis, 117
Epidural hematoma
  epidemiology/etiology/signs and symptoms/diagnosis, 308–309, 308t
Epidural hematomas, 24
Epiglottitis
  definition/etiology/pathophysiology, 159
  laryngotracheobronchitis and, differentiating between acute, 158, 159
  signs and symptoms/diagnosis/treatment, 160, 160f
Epilepsy
  Angelman's syndrome, 74
  definition/epidemiology/signs and symptoms, 287–288
  myoclonus epilepsy with ragged-red fibers, 297
  treatment/common syndromes, 288–290, 288t–289t
Epinephrine
  anaphylaxis, 96
  asthma, 175
  laryngotracheobronchitis, acute, 158, 159
  pulseless arrhythmias, 415
  urticaria, 96, 377
  Von Gierke's disease, 89
Epiphyseal–metaphyseal injury, 67
Epiphysis, 276, 335–336, 336f, 354
Episcleritis
  definition/etiology/signs and symptoms/treatment, 319
Epistaxis, 254
  definition/etiology/signs and symptoms/treatment, 327
Epstein–Barr virus (EBV), 105, 328
Erb's palsy, 24, 24f
Erysipelas
  definition/etiology/epidemiology, 364
  signs and symptoms/diagnosis/treatment, 364
Erythema. See also Rash; Stevens–Johnson syndrome
  blepharitis, 319
  chronicum migrans, 118, 118f
  dacryostenosis, 320
  episcleritis/scleritis, 319
  hordeolum, 320
  Kawasaki's disease, 197, 198
  Lyme disease, 118
  multiforme
    definition/etiology/pathophysiology, 361
    epidemiology/signs and symptoms, 361
  orbital cellulitis, 321

osteomyelitis, 330
periorbital cellulitis, 321
rheumatic fever, 192
scarlet fever, 365
septic arthritis, 332
toxicum, 22
vaccines
  diphtheria/tetanus/pertussis, 58
  Haemophilus influenzae, 58
  influenza, 60
  pneumococcus, 60
  varicella, 59
Erythrocyte sedimentation rate (ESR)
  amebic abscess, 154
  chronic granulomatous disease, 104
  dermatomyositis/polymyositis, 349
  diskitis, 353
  endocarditis, 194
  intracranial pressure, 305
  Kawasaki's disease, 197
  lymphoma, 263
  osteomyelitis, 330
  septic arthritis, 332
  Wegener's granulomatosis, 199
Erythroderma, 106
Erythromycin
  acne, 374
  chlamydia, 26
  diphtheria, 168
  pertussis, 167
  pharyngitis, 164
  pneumonia, 165, 166
  pyloric stenosis, 128
Erythropoietin, 221, 251
Escherichia coli, 25, 104, 107, 229, 252
Esophageal atresia, 129, 178
  definition/signs and symptoms, 125, 126f
  diagnosis/treatment, 125
Esophagoscopy, 126
Estrogen, 22, 231, 232, 279
Ethambutol, 112, 169
Ethylenediaminetetraacetic acid (EDTA), 242
Ethylene glycol, 63t
Eustachian tube anatomy, 322
Euvolemic hypernatremia, 50
Euvolemic hyponatremia, 49
Ewing's sarcoma
  definition/epidemiology/signs and symptoms, 342–343
  radiology/treatment/prognosis, 343
Exercise
  amenorrhea, 281
  anorexia nervosa, 397
  asthma, 173
  cystic fibrosis, 170, 171
  diabetes mellitus, 266
  juvenile rheumatoid arthritis, 338
  obesity, 53
  proteinuria, 225
  spondylolysis, 352
  tetralogy of Fallot, 202
Exophthalmos, 100, 268
Extracellular fluid (ECF), 47, 47t
Extrahepatic biliary atresia
  definition/signs and symptoms/diagnosis/treatment, 146–147
Eyes. See also Conjunctivitis; Vision
  abuse, child, 68
  amblyopia, 317
  ataxia–telangiectasia, 101

435

436